| 10,000 人の症例 | ten thousand cases |
| --- | --- |
| 人口 100,000 人 | a [one] hundred thousand population,<br>a population of one hundred thousand |

★¹ 0 を読まない．または zero point eight ともいう．
★² 0 を読まない．または zero point-two-five milligrams ともいう．

## 単位の換算表（概算）

| 体重 | | 身長 | | | 体温 | |
| --- | --- | --- | --- | --- | --- | --- |
| キログラム | ポンド | センチメートル | インチ | フィート／インチ | 摂氏 | 華氏 |
| kg | lb | cm | in | ft/in ★¹ | ℃ | °F |
| 80 | 176 | 180 | 71 | 5'11" ★² | 40 | 104.0 |
| 70 | 154 | 170 | 67 | 5'7" | 39 | 102.2 |
| 60 | 132 | 160 | 63 | 5'3" | 38 | 100.4 |
| 50 | 110 | 150 | 59 | 4'11" | 37 | 98.6 |
| 40 | 88 | 140 | 55 | 4'7" | 36 | 96.8 |

◎重さ　ポンド　　　　lb＝(kg)×2.2
　　　　キログラム　　kg＝(lb)×0.45
◎長さ　インチ　　　　in＝(cm)×0.4
　　　　センチメートル　cm＝(in)×2.54
◎温度　華氏　　　　°F＝(℃×1.8)＋32
　　　　摂氏　　　　℃＝(°F−32)×5/9

★¹ フィート　1 foot＝12 inches
★² 5'11" は 5 ft 11 in (five feet eleven inches) と読む．

# そのまま使える
# 病院英語表現
# 5000

### 第2版

**森島祐子**
筑波大学医学医療系准教授

**仁木久恵**
聖路加国際大学名誉教授

**Nancy Sharts-Hopko**
ヴィラノヴァ大学看護学部教授

医学書院

**著者略歴**

**森島 祐子**(もりしま ゆうこ)
　米国生まれ．筑波大学医学専門学群在学中，カナダのマギル大学，マックマスター大学にて Clinical Clerkship を行う．医学博士．米国内科学会フェロー (FACP)．現在，筑波大学医学医療系呼吸器内科准教授．

**仁木 久恵**(にき ひさえ)
　津田塾大学卒業後，テキサス大学大学院にて MA 取得．津田塾大学大学院博士課程修了．聖路加国際大学教授，明海大学教授を経て，現在，聖路加国際大学名誉教授．

**Nancy Sharts-Hopko**(ナンシー・シャーツ・ホプコ)
　米国インディアナ大学卒業後，ニューヨーク大学大学院にて PhD 取得．聖路加国際大学客員講師を経て，現在，ヴィラノヴァ大学看護学部教授．

執筆協力者：F. Miyamasu　仁木 淳

## そのまま使える病院英語表現 5000

| | | |
|---|---|---|
| 発　行 | 2006年10月 1日 | 第1版第1刷 |
| | 2012年 2月15日 | 第1版第7刷 |
| | 2013年10月 1日 | 第2版第1刷© |
| | 2023年 1月15日 | 第2版第9刷 |
| 著　者 | 森島祐子　仁木久恵　ナンシー・シャーツ・ホプコ | |
| 発行者 | 株式会社　医学書院 | |
| | 代表取締役　金原　俊 | |
| | 〒113-8719　東京都文京区本郷 1-28-23 | |
| | 電話 03-3817-5600（社内案内） | |
| 印刷・製本 | 三美印刷 | |

本書の複製権・翻訳権・上映権・譲渡権・貸与権・公衆送信権（送信可能化権を含む）は株式会社医学書院が保有します．

ISBN978-4-260-01830-2

本書を無断で複製する行為（複写，スキャン，デジタルデータ化など）は，「私的使用のための複製」など著作権法上の限られた例外を除き禁じられています．大学，病院，診療所，企業などにおいて，業務上使用する目的（診療，研究活動を含む）で上記の行為を行うことは，その使用範囲が内部的であっても，私的使用には該当せず，違法です．また私的使用に該当する場合であっても，代行業者等の第三者に依頼して上記の行為を行うことは違法となります．

**JCOPY**〈出版者著作権管理機構　委託出版物〉
本書の無断複製は著作権法上での例外を除き禁じられています．複製される場合は，そのつど事前に，出版者著作権管理機構（電話 03-5244-5088，FAX 03-5244-5089，info@jcopy.or.jp）の許諾を得てください．

# 第 2 版　はじめに

　病気になると誰しも不安や迷いに揺れますが，そんな時，外国人の患者さんは言葉の壁にはばまれて心細い思いをします．一方，医療サイドからみると，十分なコミュニケーションがとれないため治療やケアに支障をきたす事態が起こるでしょう．

　本書は，医師やナースをはじめ病院スタッフの方々が，問診・診察・検査を行い，そしてよりよい治療やケアを目指すために編まれた実用的な英会話マニュアルです．病院内で起こりうる様々な状況を想定して，臨床の現場ですぐに使える基本的な英語表現を収録しました．

　改訂するにあたり，最新情報を取り入れるとともに，病院英会話のヒントとなるコラムの充実をはかりました．特に，医療コミュニケーションの中でもとりわけ慎重さを要するデリケートな話題，例えば，「悪い知らせの伝え方」，「臨終の場面での言葉かけ」，あるいは「訊きにくい性生活についての質問」などの英語表現例を提示しました．外国人の患者さんは文化背景・個性・知識レベルが一人ひとり異なることから，あくまでも参考として，個別の状況に対応してご活用下されば幸いです．また，新たに「リハビリテーション」と「医療福祉相談」の2章を追加し，巻末には患者満足度のアンケートを入れました．インフォームド・コンセントや紹介状のサンプルなどと合わせて資料として使うことができます．本書を活用して，外国人の患者さんと積極的にコミュニケーションをとっていただくことを期待します．

　最後に，出版に際してお世話になった阪本稔・志澤真理子両氏ほか医学書院の皆さんにお礼申し上げます．

　2013 年 9 月

著者

## 初版　はじめに

　病気になると誰しも不安や迷いに揺れますが，そんな時，外国人の患者さんはことばの壁にはばまれて心細い思いをします．一方，医療サイドからみると，十分なコミュニケーションがとれないため治療やケアに支障をきたす事態が起こるでしょう．

　本書は，医師やナースが，問診により正確な病歴をとり，診察や検査を行い，そしてよりよい治療やケアを目指すために編まれた実用的な英会話マニュアルです．病院内で起こりうる様々な状況を想定して，臨床の現場ですぐに使える基本的な英語表現を収録しました．また，病院英会話のヒントなども入れてあります．巻末には，インフォームド・コンセントの例文，紹介状のサンプル，駐日大使館リストが収録してあり，資料としても使うことができます．

　医学生，看護学生，医療通訳を目指す方々は，病院英会話の学習用テキストとして本書を役立てることができるでしょう．また，医師やナースばかりでなく，薬剤師，検査技師，その他の病院スタッフの方々も，本書を活用して，英語を話す患者さんと積極的にコミュニケーションをとっていただくことを期待します．

　なお，本書の作成にあたっては，内容全般にわたってお世話くださいました医学書院の方々にこの紙面を借りて心よりお礼申し上げます．

　2006年7月

著者

## 本書の特色と使い方

1. **基本的かつ平易な英語**
   病院内でコミュニケーションをとる上で必要と思われる基本的な表現を，状況ごとに収録してある．患者さんにはわかりにくい専門医学用語や特殊な表現は避け，できるだけ日常会話で用いられる平易なものとした．

2. **Yes/No で答えてもらえる，具体的な表現**
   患者さんから正確なデータを得るためには，自由形式の質問（open-ended questions）をすることが望ましいが，返答がまちまちになって，英語の聞き取りに慣れない医療従事者には，ポイントがつかみにくかったり，患者さんとの間に誤解が生じたりする恐れがある．そのため本書では，一般的な質問のあとに，Yes/No で答えられる具体的な質問をして，正確な情報を引き出せるように工夫した．

3. **1つ1つチェックしやすい**
   質問および説明は活用しやすいように，同じページの左側に日本語，右側に英語を並べて対訳形式にしてある．また，自分が使う頻度の多い項目には，英文の前にある四角のマス目（□）に印をつけておいて復習ができる．時には，その質問および説明箇所を見せて，患者さん自身に（□）に印をつけてもらうこともできる．

4. **コラムの充実**
   「病院会話のヒント」「痛みの表現」「頻度の表現」「悪い知らせの伝え方」などの囲み項目をもうけて，臨床の現場で役立つようにした．

5. **標準的なアメリカ英語**
   用例は，原則として標準的なアメリカ英語を収録してある．

6. **それぞれの活用を！**
   医学の世界は日進月歩なので，新しい表現が次々に生まれて医療現場に入り込んでくる．個々の医療従事者はそれぞれの状況に応じ，本書の内容及び表現を取捨選択しながらお使いいただきたい．

なお医療の現場で使われる英語表現を繰り返し練習し，身につけるにあたっては，実践編となる『そのまま使える医療英会話【CD付】』(医学書院)を本書と合わせてご活用いただければ幸いである。

## 記号

1. 〔　〕に入っている語（句）は，その直前の語（句）と入れ替えて用いることが可能であることを示す．

    例：アメリカ人〔カナダ人〕ですか．　□ Are you American〔Canadian〕?
    →語を入れ替えることで，色々な表現にすることができる．

2. ［　］に入っている語（句）は，その直前の語（句）と置き換え可能であることを示す．

    例：お名前をお聞かせ下さい．　　　□ May I have [ask] your name?
    →May I have your name? あるいは May I ask your name? と言ってよい．

3. (　)に入っている語（句）は，省略可能であることを示す．

    例：住所はどちらですか．　　　　□ What's your (home) address?
    →What's your home address? あるいは What's your address? と言ってよい．

## 外国人の患者さんとの効果的なコミュニケーション10か条

1. 初診時には自己紹介し，患者さんの名前を言って確かめる．
2. 患者さんと目を合わせながら話す．コンピュータ画面やカルテからできるだけ目を離す．
3. 自分のほうから声をかけて笑顔で接する．患者さんの気持ちを和らげるように努力する．
4. ゆっくり，そしてはっきり話す．患者さんの母語が英語であるとはかぎらない．
5. 平易な英語で話し，専門用語はなるべく使わない．
6. 必要に応じてジェスチャーを使う．イラストや資料を用いて説明する．また病名などの単語は文字で示すとわかりやすい．
7. 重要な情報は再確認する．患者さんが話す内容を正確に把握する．
8. 診察や検査を行う前にはきちんと説明する．
9. 自分が話した内容を患者さんに繰り返し言ってもらう．情報が正確に伝わったかを確認する．
10. 患者さんが退出するときには目を合わせて挨拶する．

最後に，患者さんとの信頼関係を築くために医療従事者も忍耐強い姿勢が大切である．Be patient！

# 目次

## Chapter 1　患者さんのプロフィール　　1

■個人に関する一般情報 …………2
● 名前・年齢 ……………………2
● 出生地・国籍 …………………2
● 住所・電話番号・E メールアドレス
　…………………………………3
● 日本語能力 ……………………4

■婚姻歴・家族 ……………………5
● 同居人 …………………………5
● 婚姻歴 …………………………5
● 子供・両親 ……………………6

■学歴・職歴 ………………………7
● 最終学歴 ………………………7
● 職業 ……………………………7
● 仕事の環境 ……………………8
● 家族の仕事 ……………………9

■宗教 ………………………………10

■健康保険・支払い………………11
● 保険 ……………………………11
● 支払い …………………………11

## Chapter 2　診察室に患者さんを迎える　　13

■受付で……………………………14
■診察室でのあいさつ……………16
● 初診のあいさつ………………16

● 再診のあいさつ………………17
■主訴を訊く………………………18

## Chapter 3　病歴を訊く　　21

■現病歴……………………………24
● 主要症状………………………24
　発熱…24　痛み（頭痛，胸痛，腹痛，腰背部痛）…27　全身倦怠感…42　めまい…43　浮腫…46　腫瘤・腫脹・リンパ節腫大…48　外傷…50
● 系統別レビュー………………54
1．眼………………………………54
　一般的な質問…54　視力・視野　54

　目の痛み…56　目のかゆみ・目やに・涙…56　目の中の異物…57　その他の症状…57　既往歴・家族歴…58
2．耳鼻咽喉・頸部…………………60
　一般的な質問…60　耳…60　鼻…63　咽喉頭…66　頸部…68
3．歯・口腔………………………70
　一般的な質問…70　歯痛・炎症…70　顎の痛み…71　口腔…72　その他…75

4．呼吸器 ……………………76
　一般的な質問…76　咳・痰…76　息切れ…79　いびき・睡眠時無呼吸…81　既往歴・生活習慣・家族歴…81

5．心・血管 …………………84
　一般的な質問…84　動悸…84　四肢の冷感・疼痛・腫脹…86　既往歴・家族歴…87

6．消化器 ……………………92
　一般的な質問…92　嚥下障害…92　消化不良…93　吐き気・嘔吐…93　便通異常(血便・便秘・下痢)…96　食欲…99　体重変化…100　黄疸…100　既往歴・家族歴…101

7．腎・泌尿器 ………………103
　一般的な質問…103　尿の性状…103　排尿回数・尿量…104　尿失禁…105　排尿困難…106　排尿痛…106　既往歴・生活習慣・家族歴…108

8．男性生殖器 ………………110
　一般的な質問…110　痛み…110　分泌物・精液…111　随伴症状…112　性機能…112　性生活…114　既往歴…114

9．乳房・女性生殖器 …………117
　一般的な質問…117　乳房変化…117　月経…118　不正出血…121　帯下(おりもの)…122　更年期症状…122　性生活…123　既往歴・家族歴…125

10．代謝・内分泌 ……………127
　一般的な質問…127　体重変化…127　口渇・多飲・多尿…129　前頸部腫瘤…130　その他…131　既往歴・家族歴…132

11．血液 ……………………134
　一般的な質問…134　貧血…134　出血傾向…136

12．筋・骨格 …………………139
　一般的な質問…139　痛み…139　運動制限…142　こわばり・突っ張り…142　腫れ…143　随伴症状…144　生活歴・既往歴・家族歴…144

13．神経 ……………………147
　一般的な質問…147　意識障害・失神…148　痙攣…148　認知障害…150　脳神経障害…152　運動障害…153　感覚障害…156　自律神経障害…157　随伴症状…157　既往歴・家族歴…158

14．皮膚 ……………………159
　一般的な質問…159　発疹…159　ほくろ…164　頭髪・体毛…164　爪…166

15．精神・心理 ………………168
　一般的な質問…168　睡眠障害…168　ストレス…169　不安・恐怖…171　抑うつ状態…173　躁状態…176　アルコール依存…177　摂食障害…180　妄想…181　幻覚・性格変化…182　職歴・学歴・既往歴・家族歴…184

● 健診異常 ……………………186

■ 既往歴 ………………………187
● これまでの健康状態 …………187
● かかりつけの医師 ……………187
● 既往症 ………………………187
● 事故・怪我 …………………192
● 入院 …………………………192
● 手術 …………………………193
● 血液型・輸血歴 ………………194
● 補完代替医療 …………………194
● 薬歴 …………………………194
● アレルギー …………………195
● 妊娠・授乳 …………………197
● 予防接種 ……………………198

- ●健診・人間ドック ……………198
- ●海外渡航歴 ……………………199
- ■家族歴 …………………………200
- ●家族構成 ………………………200
- ●家族の病気 ……………………200
- ■生活習慣・活動 ………………202
- ●睡眠 ……………………………202
- ●食習慣 …………………………202
- ●便通 ……………………………204
- ●喫煙・飲酒・麻薬 ……………205
  喫煙…205 飲酒…205 麻薬…206
- ●趣味・運動 ……………………207
  趣味…207 運動…207
- ●ペット …………………………208
- ■問診の最後に …………………209

## Chapter 4　身体の診察　　　211

- ■診察前 …………………………212
- ■身体計測・バイタルサイン …212
- ●身体計測 ………………………212
- ●バイタルサイン ………………213
- ■系統別診察 ……………………217
- ●頭頸部(頭頸・眼・耳鼻咽喉)の診察 ………………………………217
  頭頸…217 眼…217 耳鼻咽喉…219
- ●胸背部・乳房の診察 …………222
  胸背部…222 乳房…223
- ●腹部(消化器・鼠径)の診察 …224
  消化器…224 鼠径…225
- ●直腸診・生殖器の診察 ………225
  直腸診…225 生殖器…226
- ●骨格(上肢・下肢・脊柱)の診察
  ……………………………………227
  上肢…227 下肢…227 脊柱…228
- ●神経の診察 ……………………229
  意識状態・大脳高次機能…229 脳神経…229 運動機能…231 感覚機能…232 小脳機能…232 髄膜刺激症状…233
- ■診察の終了 ……………………234

## Chapter 5　診察が終わって　　　237

- ■検査の説明 ……………………238
- ●検査の必要がないとき ………238
- ●検査が必要なとき ……………238
  当日検査…239 予約検査…240
- ■診断の説明 ……………………245
- ●検査結果の説明 ………………245
- ●診断内容 ………………………246
  異常がないとき…246 一般的な説明…246 深刻な説明…247
- ■治療の説明 ……………………254
- ●治療の必要がないとき ………254
- ●治療が必要なとき ……………254
  投薬・注射…254 外科的処置…256 リハビリテーション…257 入院…258 手術…258
- ■専門医への紹介 ………………260
- ■次回の診察予約 ………………263

## Chapter 6　検査　269

- ■検査一般 …………………270
- ●インフォームド・コンセント …270
- ●検査前に …………………271
  - 検査日以前…271　検査当日…272
- ●検査後に …………………272

- ■各種検査 …………………275
- ●血液検査 …………………275
- ●尿検査 ……………………276
- ●心電図検査 ………………276
- ●トレッドミル負荷心電図検査 …………………………277
  - 検査日以前…277　検査当日…277
- ●ホルター心電図検査 ………278
  - 検査日以前…278　検査当日…279
- ●X線検査 …………………280
- ●CT/MRI検査 ……………282
- ●超音波検査(エコー) ………283
- ●内視鏡検査 ………………285
- ●呼吸機能検査 ……………286
- ●マンモグラフィ検査 ………287
- ●乳房の自己検診 …………288
- ●視力検査 …………………289
- ●聴力検査 …………………290

## Chapter 7　薬剤投与　297

- ■薬の処方箋 ………………298
- ■薬剤の服用歴 ……………300
- ●使用中の薬 ………………300
- ●補完代替医薬品(サプリメント) …………………………301
- ●処方する薬について ………301
- ●アレルギーについて ………302

- ■用法・用量 ………………303
- ●一般的な説明 ……………303
- ●内服薬 ……………………303
- ●舌下錠 ……………………306
- ●うがい薬 …………………307
- ●吸入薬 ……………………307
- ●点眼・点耳・点鼻薬 ………308
- ●坐薬 ………………………309
- ●軟膏・クリーム・ローション …………………………310
- ●湿布薬 ……………………311
- ●注射薬 ……………………312

- ■服薬・使用上の注意 ………313
- ●一般的な注意 ……………313
- ●飲み忘れ・飲みすぎ ………314
- ●妊娠・授乳 ………………314
- ●医師・看護師への相談 ……315
- ●緊急用カード・携行品 ……316

- ■保管上の注意 ……………317

- ■副作用 ……………………318
- ●緊急を要する場合 …………319
- ●副作用の一般的な症状 ……320

## Chapter 8　手術　323

- ■ インフォームド・コンセント ……………………………324
- ■ 手術の説明 …………………325
- ■ 麻酔の説明 …………………327
- ■ 手術当日 ……………………330
- ● 手術直前 ……………………330
- ● 手術直後 ……………………330
- ■ 手術後 ………………………331
- ■ 自宅ケア ……………………333

## Chapter 9　入院　337

- ■ 入院前 ………………………338
- ■ 入院当日 ……………………342
- ● あいさつ ……………………342
- ● 病室・病棟案内 ……………347
- ● 病院生活 ……………………349
- ■ 患者さんへの指示（安静度・移動）……………………………352
- ■ 患者さんへの対応 …………353
- ● 投薬・処置 …………………353
- ● 患者さんのケア ……………354
- ● 患者さんから呼ばれて ……355
- ■ 退院 …………………………359

## Chapter 10　妊娠・分娩　363

- ■ 妊娠歴・分娩歴・その他の病歴 ……………………………364
- ● 妊娠歴 ………………………364
- ● 分娩歴 ………………………364
- ● その他の病歴 ………………366
- ■ 妊娠 …………………………367
- ● 問診 …………………………367
- ● 検査 …………………………369
- ● 診察 …………………………370
- ● 診察が終わって ……………372
- ■ 分娩 …………………………375
- ● 診察室で ……………………375
- ● 陣痛室で ……………………375
- ● 分娩室で ……………………376
- ● 出産後 ………………………377

## Chapter 11　小児　379

- ■ 子供のプロフィール ………380
- ● 年齢 …………………………380
- ● 家族 …………………………380
- ● 現在の健康状態 ……………380
- ■ 現病歴 ………………………382
- ● 主訴 …………………………382
- ● 機嫌・意識 …………………382
- ● 食欲・体重 …………………383

- ●系統別の病歴 ……………384
  皮膚…384　耳・鼻…384　眼…385　呼吸器…385　心・血管…386　消化器…386　泌尿器・生殖器…387　筋・骨格…387　感染症…388　事故…388
- ■栄養 ………………………389
- ■成長発達 …………………390
- ●運動・動作・生活習慣 …390
- ●言語 ………………………390
- ●社会性 ……………………391
- ●個人特性 …………………391
- ■既往歴 ……………………392
- ●出生前・出生時情報 ……392
- ●既往症 ……………………394
- ●薬歴 ………………………396
- ■薬剤投与 …………………397
- ■家族歴・ペット …………397
- ■予防接種・健診 …………398
- ●予防接種 …………………398
- ●健診 ………………………398

## Chapter 12　リハビリテーション　401

- ■リハビリテーションの案内 …402
- ■リハビリテーション専門医の診察 ……………………403
- ■理学療法 …………………404
- ●平行棒を使った歩行訓練 …404
- ■作業療法 …………………406
- ●ペグボードを使った機能回復訓練 ……………………406
- ■言語聴覚療法 ……………407
- ●顔面筋肉訓練 ……………407

## Chapter 13　医療福祉相談　411

- ■相談室の案内 ……………412
- ■相談当日 …………………414
- ■相談内容 …………………415
- ●受診 ………………………415
- ●入院生活 …………………416
- ●退院後の生活 ……………417
  退院後の転出先…417　退院後の在宅介護…418　社会復帰…420　その他…420
- ●経済問題 …………………421
  医療費…421　生活費…424
- ●その他の心配事 …………425

インフォームド・コンセントのサンプル ……………………427
問い合わせ手紙文のサンプル ………………………………428
紹介状サンプル(1) ………429
紹介状サンプル(2) ………431
患者満足度アンケート(例) …432
参考文献 ……………………435

索引 …………………………437

## コラム

- ●宗教を尋ねる意味……………10
- ●名前につける敬称……………15
- ●訊きにくい／尋ねにくい質問
  …………………………………116
- ●悪い知らせの伝え方 …………249
- ●視力の測り方の違い …………291
- ●死の伝え方 ……………………360
- ●妊娠週数・月数の数え方 ……368

## 用語・表現ファイル

- ■患者さんの話を聞き取るためのヒント……………………………19
- ■病歴をとるためのヒント………22
- ■痛みの表現………………………31
- ■診療部門…………………………52
- ■病院関係者………………………89
- ■病名 その1 主要な病気 …189
- ■数字の読み方 …………………214
- ■単位の換算表(概算) …………216
- ■病院会話のヒント その1 診察中に安心感を与える表現 ……235
- ■病院会話のヒント その2 確認，励まし，慰め，慰労 ……242
- ■専門医 …………………………261
- ■日常生活への指示 ……………265
- ■病院会話のヒント その3 場所の表現 ……………………………274
- ■検査項目 ………………………292
- ■頻度の表現 ……………………321
- ■病院会話のヒント その4 相づち ……………………………335
- ■病院会話のヒント その5 入院患者さんへのあいさつ ……340
- ■病院案内 ………………………343
- ■病院会話のヒント その6 一般的な話題(患者さんの気持ちを和らげるために)……………………357
- ■病名 その2 小児に多い病気
  ……………………………………395
- ■予防接種 ………………………400
- ■呼吸法 …………………………408

## 名句・ことわざ

- ◆Do (to others) as you would be done by. ……………………………………6
- ◆Practice makes perfect. ……………………………………………………9
- ◆The Hospital is the only proper College in which to rear a true disciple of Aesculapius. ……………………………………………………………15
- ◆While there's life, there's hope. …………………………………………20
- ◆In the case of our habits we are only masters of the beginning, their growth by gradual stages being imperceptible, like the growth of disease.
  …………………………………………………………………………………51

xv

- ◆The eyes are the window of the soul. ……………………………59
- ◆Smoking or health：the choice is yours. …………………………83
- ◆There is no royal road to learning. …………………………………91
- ◆Feed by measure and defy the physician. ………………………102
- ◆The best doctors in the world are Dr. Diet, Dr. Quiet, and Dr. Merryman.
  ……………………………………………………………………133
- ◆頭寒足熱 ………………………………………………………138
- ◆A sound mind in a sound body. ……………………………………185
- ◆Habit is a second nature. …………………………………………188
- ◆風邪は万病のもと ……………………………………………208
- ◆Art is long, life is short. ……………………………………………209
- ◆情けは他人の為ならず ………………………………………234
- ◆To study the phenomena of disease without books is to sail an uncharted sea, while to study books without patients is not to go to sea at all. …241
- ◆医は生涯の業にて，とても上手名人には至らざるものと見ゆ．己れ上手と思わば，はや下手になる兆としるべし． ……………………248
- ◆Physician, heal [cure] thyself. ……………………………………262
- ◆A disease known is half cured. ……………………………………264
- ◆笑う門には福来たる …………………………………………267
- ◆Bitter pills may have blessed effects. ……………………………299
- ◆An apple a day keeps the doctor away. ……………………………302
- ◆Charity begins at home. ……………………………………………311
- ◆Sleep is better than medicine. ……………………………………315
- ◆Knowledge comes, but wisdom lingers. …………………………319
- ◆All is well that ends well. …………………………………………332
- ◆It may seem a strange principle to enunciate as the very first requirement in a Hospital that it should do the sick no harm. ……………………341
- ◆Tomorrow is another day. …………………………………………342
- ◆If Winter comes, can Spring be far behind? ………………………358
- ◆All the world's a stage, And all the men and women merely players; They have their exits and their entrances; And one man in his time plays many parts, ... ……………………………………………………………371
- ◆All we know is still infinitely less than all that still remain unknown.
  ……………………………………………………………………396
- ◆Prevention is better than cure. ……………………………………399
- ◆We should all know that diversity makes for a rich tapestry, ... ………413
- ◆Health is better than wealth. ………………………………………421

chapter **1**

# 患者さんのプロフィール

## Patient Profile

個人に関する一般情報　2
婚姻歴・家族　5
学歴・職歴　7
宗教　10
健康保険・支払い　11

## 個人に関する一般情報

| | |
|---|---|
| いくつか質問をいたします. | ☐ Can you tell me a little about yourself?<br>☐ I'd like to ask you some questions. |
| この用紙に書き込んで下さい. | ☐ Please fill out this form. |
| 活字体で書いて下さい. | ☐ Write in block letters, please. |

### ➲ 名前・年齢

| | |
|---|---|
| お名前をお聞かせ下さい. | ☐ What's your name, please? ★1<br>☐ May I have [ask] your name? ★2 |
| お名前はどうつづるのですか. | ☐ How do you spell your name? ★3 |
| 姓のほうのお名前はどう発音しますか. | ☐ How do you pronounce your family [last] name? |
| 年はおいくつですか. | ☐ How old are you? |
| 生年月日はいつですか. | ☐ What's your birthdate [date of birth]?<br>☐ When were you born? |

### ➲ 出生地・国籍

| | |
|---|---|
| ご出身はどちらですか. | ☐ Where are you from? |
| どこで生まれましたか. | ☐ Where were you born?<br>☐ What's your birthplace? |
| 国籍はどちらですか. | ☐ What's your nationality? |

---

★1 上昇調でいう.
★2 より丁寧な表現.
★3 姓は family [last] name, 個人名は first name.

| | |
|---|---|
| —アメリカ人〔カナダ人／オーストラリア人／インド人／イギリス人／フィリピン人／ガーナ人〕ですか. | — Are you American〔Canadian/Australian/Indian/British/Filipino/Ghanaian〕?★4 |
| いつ日本へ来ましたか. | ☐ When did you come to Japan? |
| 日本に住んでどのくらいになりますか. | ☐ How long have you stayed in Japan? |
| これからどのくらい滞在しますか. | ☐ How long are you going to stay here? |

## ● 住所・電話番号・E メールアドレス

| | |
|---|---|
| どこにお住まいですか. | ☐ Where do you live? |
| 住所はどちらですか. | ☐ What's your (home) address? |
| 本籍地〔勤務先の住所〕はどちらですか. | ☐ What's your permanent address〔business address〕? |
| 自宅〔勤務先〕のお電話は何番ですか. | ☐ What's your phone number〔business phone number〕? |
| E メールアドレスは何ですか. | ☐ What's your email address? |
| 緊急連絡先は何番ですか. | ☐ What's your emergency contact number? |
| 緊急連絡先はどなたですか. | ☐ Who is the person to be contacted in an emergency? |
| —その方の名前, ご関係を教えて下さい. | — Can you tell me his〔her〕name and the relationship? |

---

★4 イギリス (the United Kingdom; U. K.) 国籍のイギリス人の場合は,一括して British (イギリス人,英国人) というが,出身地別に English (イングランド人), Scottish (スコットランド人), Irish (アイルランド人), Welsh (ウエールズ人) ともいう. うっかり "Are you English?" と訊ねると,"No, I'm Scottish." という答えがかえってくるかもしれないので注意.

## ➲ 日本語能力

| | |
|---|---|
| 日本語が話せますか. | ☐ Do you speak some Japanese? ★ |
| 日本語の読み書きはできますか. | ☐ Do you read and write Japanese? ★ |
| 誰か日本語を話す人がいますか. | ☐ Is there anyone who speaks Japanese? |
| ―どなたですか. | ― Who is he〔she〕? |
| あなたの母語は何ですか. | ☐ What's your native language? |
| 通訳が必要ですか. | ☐ Do you need an interpreter? |
| 通訳が必要ならば，医療ソーシャルワーカーに相談して手配してもらって下さい. | ☐ If you need an interpreter, check with a medical social worker to arrange the interpreter service. |

☞「医療福祉相談」(411 ページ)

---

★ Can you...? は相手の言語能力を訊ねるという響きがあるので避けたい．"Do you..." のほうがより丁寧な表現．

## 婚姻歴・家族

### ● 同居人

| | |
|---|---|
| お一人でお住まいですか. | ☐ Do you live alone? |
| どなたとご一緒にお住まいですか. | ☐ Who do you live with? |
| 一緒にお住まいの方は奥さん〔ご主人／ご両親／子ども／友達／パートナー／親戚／日本人の家族〕ですか. | ☐ Do you live with your wife 〔your husband/your parents [father and mother]/your children/ your friend/your partner/your relatives/a Japanese (host) family〕? |
| 困ったとき近くに助けてくれる人がいますか. | ☐ In time of crisis, do you have anyone nearby who can help you? |
| ―例えば，家族，友人，近所の人などがいますか. | ― Your family, friends, or neighbors? |

### ● 婚姻歴

あなたは…
1. 独身ですか.
2. 結婚していますか.
3. 別居していますか.
4. 離婚していますか.
5. 配偶者が亡くなられましたか.
6. 独身で，現在パートナーと暮らしていますか.

☐ Are you ...
1. single?
2. married?
3. separated?
4. divorced?
5. widowed?
6. single, but living with a partner?

| | |
|---|---|
| これまでに結婚したことがありますか. | ☐ Have you ever been married before? |
| 結婚してどのくらいになりますか. | ☐ How long have you been married? |

chapter 1 患者さんのプロフィール

## ⊃ 子供・両親

| | |
|---|---|
| お子さんはいらっしゃいますか． | ☐ Do you have any children? |
| —お子さんは何人いますか． | — How many children do you have? |
| —お子さんは男〔女／両方〕ですか． | — Are they boys 〔girls/both boys and girls〕? |
| —何歳ですか． | — How old are they? |
| ご両親はご健在ですか． | ☐ Are your parents still living? |
| ご家族はぜんぶで何人ですか． | ☐ How many people are there in your family? |
| 皆さんお元気ですか． | ☐ Are they all in good health? |

名句・ことわざ

**Do (to others) as you would be done by.**
**己の欲する所を人に施せ**

聖書由来のことわざで「黄金律 (the golden rule)」として有名．同様の趣旨の教えを孔子も残しているが，孔子は「己の欲せざる所は人に施す勿れ」，すなわち「人が嫌がることはするな」と否定表現を用いているのに対し，聖書では「人が喜ぶことをせよ」と積極的な行動を求めている．

## 学歴・職歴

### ● 最終学歴

学校教育はどのくらい受けましたか.
- [ ] How much schooling did you have?

最終学歴は高校〔大学／大学院／専門学校〕ですか.
- [ ] Did you finish [graduate from] high school [college [university]/graduate school/professional school]?

### ● 職業

現在何をしているかを教えて下さい.
—お勤め〔パート勤め／自営業／退職者／家庭の主婦〔夫〕／学生〕ですか.
- [ ] Can you tell me your current position?
— Are you employed [employed part-time/self-employed/retired/a home maker/a student]?

ご職業は何ですか.
—教師〔会社員／店員／ウエイター〔ウエイトレス〕／工場労働者／工事作業員〕ですか？
- [ ] What's your occupation?
— Are you a teacher [an office worker/a salesperson/a waiter [waitress]/a factory worker/ a construction worker]?

どんなお仕事ですか.
- [ ] What type of work do you do?

この仕事についてどのくらいになりますか.
- [ ] How long have you had this job?

(失業中の人に) 今, 失業中ですか.
—1年以上〔1年以内〕ですか.
- [ ] Are you now out of work?
— For more than 1 year [For less than 1 year]?

—働くことができないのですか.
— Are you not able to work?

(家庭の主婦〔夫〕に) 結婚前のお仕事は何でしたか.
- [ ] What did you do before your marriage?

| | |
|---|---|
| （退職している人に）退職前のお仕事は何でしたか． | ☐ What did you do before your retirement? |
| あなたの国でのお仕事は何でしたか． | ☐ What did you do in your country? |
| 今までどんなお仕事につかれたかを話して下さい． | ☐ What other jobs have you had?<br>☐ Tell me about jobs you have had in the past. |

## ● 仕事の環境

| | |
|---|---|
| いつも遅くまで仕事をしますか．<br>—どのくらい遅くまで仕事をするのですか．<br>—1日〔週〕何時間働いていますか． | ☐ Do you usually work late?<br>— How late do you work?<br>— How many hours a day〔week〕do you work? |
| きつい肉体労働ですか． | ☐ Is it heavy physical work? |
| 仕事中コンピュータをかなり使いますか． | ☐ Do you use a computer extensively in your work? |
| 仕事先では化学薬品〔動物／放射性物質／有害物質〕を扱いますか． | ☐ Do you work with any chemicals〔animals/radiation/toxic substances〕? |
| 仕事中に粉塵〔ガス／極度の高温／極度の低温〕にさらされますか．<br>—どのくらい長くですか．<br>—そのための予防措置を講じていますか．<br>—どんな措置ですか． | ☐ Are you exposed to dust〔gases/extremely high temperatures/extremely low temperatures〕?<br>— For how long?<br>— Do you use any precautionary measures?<br>— What measures? |
| 今のお仕事に満足していますか．<br>—（特に不満がある場合）それはなぜですか． | ☐ Are you happy with your work?<br>— Why? |

| | |
|---|---|
| 仕事によるストレスを感じていますか. | ☐ Do you feel 〔Have you felt〕 stress in your work? |

### ● 家族の仕事

| | |
|---|---|
| ご家族のどなたかが働いていますか. | ☐ Does anyone else in the family work? |
| あなたの奥さん〔ご主人〕は（家の）外で働いていますか. | ☐ Does your wife 〔husband〕 work outside the home? |
| どんなお仕事をなさっていますか. | ☐ What kind of work does she 〔he〕 do? |
| パートで働いていますか. | ☐ Does she 〔he〕 work part-time? |

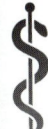

---

名句・ことわざ

**Practice makes perfect.**

実践が完璧さを生む

「練習は継続することで完璧になる」という意味で，上達の秘訣は繰り返し練習すること．日本のことわざでは「習うより慣れよ」に相当する．

## 宗教

宗教心をおもちですか.
- [ ] Do you consider yourself a religious person?

宗教は何ですか.
- [ ] What's your religious background?

カトリック〔プロテスタント／ユダヤ教／イスラム教／ヒンズー教／仏教／その他〕ですか.
- [ ] Is your religion Catholic 〔Protestant/Jewish/Muslim/Hindu/Buddhism/something else〕?

宗教上の要望や制約が何かありますか.
- [ ] Do you have any religious needs or restrictions?

宗教上の理由で食べられないものはありますか.
- [ ] Are there any kinds of food that you can't eat for religious reasons?

---

**コラム**

### 宗教を尋ねる意味

宗教と病気は無関係のように思われるが，食事や輸血などの治療に配慮が必要な場合があるし，また危篤状態になったとき宗旨によっては特別な儀式を行うので，前もって尋ねておくほうがよい．「エホバの証人」は "Jehovah's Witness" という．

# 健康保険・支払い

## ● 保険

保険についておうかがいします．
- [ ] Let me ask you about your insurance.

日本の健康保険〔海外旅行保険／他の公的〔私的〕援助〕がありますか．
- [ ] Do you have Japanese health insurance〔overseas travel insurance/other public〔private〕assistance〕?

保険証をもっていますか．
―それを見せて下さい．
―次回に必ず持参して下さい．
- [ ] Do you have an insurance card?
― Please show it to me.
― Please be sure to bring it next time you come.

保険がないと自費診療になります．
- [ ] If you don't have insurance, you'll have to pay all your medical charges.

申し訳ありませんが，当院では外国の保険は扱えません．
- [ ] I'm sorry that we can't accept foreign insurance at our hospital.

## ● 支払い

病院の費用は何でお支払いになりますか．
―現金〔カード〕ですか．
- [ ] How will you pay hospital charges?
― Cash〔Credit card〕?

会社からの払い戻しはありますか．
- [ ] Does your company reimburse you?

―それでは，次回のとき保険申請書をもってきて下さい．
― Then, please bring your company's insurance claim form next time you come.

chapter 2

# 診察室に患者さんを迎える

## Consultation

受付で 14
診察室でのあいさつ 16
主訴を訊く 18

## 受付で

| | |
|---|---|
| グリーンさん,おはようございます〔こんにちは〕. | ☐ Good morning〔Hello〕, Mr.〔Mrs./Ms./Miss〕Green. |
| この書類に記入して下さい. | ☐ Please fill out this form. |
| 熱は測ってきましたか. | ☐ Did you take your temperature at home? |
| ―何度ありましたか. | ― How high was it? |
| この体温計で熱を測って下さい. | ☐ Please take your temperature with this thermometer. |
| ―ピーッと鳴るまでわきの下にはさんで下さい. | ― Please keep it under your arm until it beeps. |
| ☞「発熱」(24 ページ). | |
| マスクをして下さい. | ☐ Please put on a mask. |
| (感染症や結核の患者さんに)―マスクをしていて下さい. | ― Please wear a mask. |
| 医師がまもなく診察いたします. | ☐ The doctor will see you soon. |
| お呼びするまでここでお待ち下さい. | ☐ Please wait here until we call you. |
| ご気分が悪いようでしたら,おっしゃって下さい. | ☐ Please let us know if you feel sick. |
| グリーンさん,診察室 5 番にお入り下さい. | ☐ Mr.〔Mrs./Ms./Miss〕Green, please come into room 5. |
| こちらへどうぞ. | ☐ This way, please. |
| 足元にお気をつけ下さい. | ☐ Please watch your step. |

### コラム

## 名前につける敬称

　大人の患者さんの場合は，相手がファーストネームで呼んでほしいと言わない限り，Mr., Mrs., Ms., Miss, Dr. をつけて姓で話しかける．再診のとき，ファーストネームで呼びかけたほうが親しみがわくと判断したときには，"May I call you Tom ?" などと訊いてからにする．

---

### 名句・ことわざ

**The Hospital is the only proper College in which to rear a true disciple of Aesculapius.**

**病院は医神アスクレピオスの真の弟子を育てるに相応しい唯一の大学である**

英国の著名な外科医で，解剖学者・生理学者でもあるアバネーシィ(John Abernethy, 1764-1831) の名言．アスクレピオスはギリシャ神話とローマ神話に登場する名医で，医術によって死者すら蘇らせたという．彼が手にする蛇の巻きついた杖は医学・医療のシンボルマークになっている．アバネーシィは名講義をしたことで有名(William Osler, *Aequanimitas*).

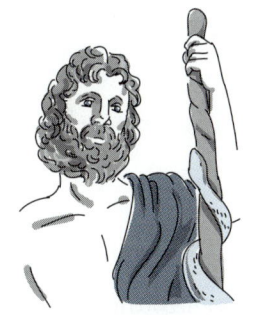

## 診察室でのあいさつ

### ➡ 初診のあいさつ

| | |
|---|---|
| こんにちは．私は医師の田中です．★ | ☐ Hello, I'm 〔my name is〕 Dr. Tanaka. |
| 看護師の佐藤です．★ | ☐ I'm 〔My name is〕 Ms. 〔Mr.〕 Sato, a nurse. |
| ジェイムズ・グリーンさんですね． | ☐ Are you Mr. James Green? |
| グリーンさん，おはようございます． | ☐ Good morning, Mr. Green. |
| （子供の患者さんに）こんにちは．ピーター君ですね． | ☐ Hi 〔Hello〕, are you Peter? |
| お待たせしてすみません． | ☐ I'm sorry to have kept you waiting. |
| お座り下さい． | ☐ Please sit down. |
| まず少しお話を聞かせて下さい． | ☐ We can talk a little bit first. |
| どなたのご紹介ですか．<br>—紹介状をお持ちですか． | ☐ Who sent [referred] you here?<br>— Do you have a referral letter? |
| 佐藤先生からの紹介状を読ませていただきました． | ☐ I've just read a referral letter from Dr. Sato. |

---

★医師や看護師は自己紹介し，患者さんに名前を知ってもらうことが重要である．それによって信頼関係が生まれる．その際，握手をしてもよい．

## ● 再診のあいさつ

|  |  |
|---|---|
| グリーンさん，おはようございます． | ☐ Good morning, Mr. Green. |
| ピーター君，こんにちは． | ☐ Hi [Hello], Peter. |
| またお会いしてうれしく思います． | ☐ Nice to see you again. |
| お座り下さい． | ☐ Please sit down. |
| 今日はいかがですか． | ☐ How are you today?<br>☐ How do you feel today? |
| 具合はいかがですか． | ☐ How are you feeling? |
| お腹〔背中〕の調子はいかがですか． | ☐ How's your stomach [back]? |
| この前診察してから具合はいかがですか． | ☐ How have you been since I last saw you? |
| 手術後の経過について教えて下さい． | ☐ Tell me how things are going after the surgery. |
| 前回の治療〔薬〕は効果がありましたか． | ☐ Did the last treatment [medication] work well? |

## 主訴を訊く

どうなさいましたか.★
- [ ] How can I help you today?
- [ ] What can I do for you today?
- [ ] Can you tell me about your problem?
- [ ] What seems to be the problem [trouble]?
- [ ] Tell me why you came today.

あなたのご心配〔悩み〕は何ですか.
- [ ] What kind of concerns [difficulties] are you having?

看護師から背中が痛むと聞きましたが,どんな様子ですか.
- [ ] The nurse tells me you have a pain in your back. Tell me about it.

そのほか何かありますか.
- [ ] Anything else?

(子供の親や付き添いへの質問) エイミーはどうしましたか.
- [ ] What kind of problem is Amy having?

---

★この他にもさまざまな言い方があるので,自分の好みの表現を覚えておくとよい.

# 用語・表現ファイル
## 患者さんの話を聞き取るためのヒント

### 1. 確認するための表現

| | |
|---|---|
| すみませんが，もう一度言って下さい． | I beg your pardon?<br>Pardon me?<br>Could you please say it again? |
| 繰り返していただけますか． | Could you repeat that, please? |
| いま何とおっしゃいましたか． | What did you say, please? |
| すみません，よく聞こえなかったのですが． | I'm sorry I couldn't hear you. |
| もっとゆっくり話して下さい． | Could you speak more slowly, please? |
| もっとゆっくり発音して下さい． | Could you pronounce it more slowly? |
| ——とおっしゃるのはどういう意味ですか． | What do you mean when you say____?<br>Tell me what you mean by____. |
| お話を録音してもいいですか．メモをとらなくてすみますので． | Is it all right if I record what you tell me? Then, I don't have to take notes while we're talking. |
| それをこの紙に書いて下さい． | Could you write it on this paper? |

### 2. 患者さんの発言を促すための表現

| | |
|---|---|
| それで？ | Yes? / And? / Uh huh?/ Mmm, hmmm./Go on. |
| 他に何かありますか． | And what else? /Anything else? |
| もう少し詳しく話して下さい． | Tell me more about it. |

## 用語・表現ファイル（つづき）

### 3. 関心や共感を示す表現

| | |
|---|---|
| そうですか［なるほど］． | I see. |
| わかりました． | I understand. |
| （患者さんの言葉を繰り返す）背中がとてもかゆいのですね． | （患者さん）My back feels really itchy.<br>→ Your back feels really itchy? |
| （患者さんの言葉を言い換える）具合がよくないのですね． | （患者さん）I feel really awful.<br>→ So you're really not feeling well, are you? |

---

### 名句・ことわざ

**While there's life, there's hope.**
**命さえあれば望みがある**

古代ローマの政治家で雄弁家として有名なキケロ(Marcus Tullius Cicero, 106- 43 B.C., *Ad Atticum*) に由来する名言．"The sick person, while he hath life, hath hope." (病人は命のある間は，望みがある) ということわざもある．

chapter **3**

# 病歴を訊く

## History of Present Illness

**現病歴** 24
  **主要症状** 24
    発熱 24　痛み（頭痛・胸痛・腹痛・腰背部痛）　27
    全身倦怠感 42　めまい 43　浮腫 46
    腫瘤・腫脹・リンパ節腫大 48　外傷 50
  **系統別レビュー** 54
    眼 54　耳鼻咽喉・頸部 60　歯・口腔 70
    呼吸器 76　心・血管 84　消化器 92
    腎・泌尿器 103　男性生殖器 110
    乳房・女性生殖器 117　代謝・内分泌 127
    血液 134　筋・骨格 139　神経 147　皮膚 159
    精神・心理 168
  **健診異常** 186
**既往歴** 187
**家族歴** 200
**生活習慣・活動** 202
**問診の最後に** 209

## 用語・表現ファイル

### 病歴をとるためのヒント

**1. 一般的な質問**

| | |
|---|---|
| 目〔呼吸／胃／皮膚〕に何か問題がありますか. | (Do you have) any problems with your eyes〔breathing/stomach/skin〕? |

**2. 症状について**

1) 症状の特徴

| | |
|---|---|
| どんな具合か. | What is the problem like? |
| | What does it feel like? |
| どんな種類か. | What kind of problem is it? |
| 程度はどれくらいか. | How severe is it? |

2) 症状の部位

| | |
|---|---|
| 場所はどこか. | Where is it? |
| 放散〔移動〕するか. | Does it radiate〔move〕? |

3) 経過

① 発症時刻, 時期

| | |
|---|---|
| いつ発症したか. | When did it start? |
| 最初に気づいたのはいつか. | When did you first notice it? |

② 症状の起こり方

| | |
|---|---|
| どんな起こり方か. | How does it occur? |
| 夜〔朝〕などの特に決まった時間帯か. | At a specific time at night〔in the morning〕? |
| 突然か, 徐々に[ゆっくり]か. | Suddenly or gradually [slowly]? |
| 一過性か, 持続性か. | Does it come and go, or does it stay? |

③ 持続時間, 期間

| | |
|---|---|
| どのくらい続いているか. | How long have you had it? |
| 毎回どのくらい続くか. | How long does it last each time? |

④ 頻度

| | |
|---|---|
| 起こる頻度はどのくらいか. | How often does it occur? |
| | How often do you have it? |

## 用語・表現ファイル（つづき）

⑤症状の変化
軽快傾向か，悪化傾向か，変化なしか．
Is it getting better, getting worse, or the same?

⑥同様の症状の経験
同じような症状を経験したことがあるか．
Have you had this kind of symptom [this problem] before?
いつ〔どこで／誰から／どんな〕治療を受けたか．
When [Where/By whom/How] was it treated?

4) 症状の誘発因子，増悪因子，緩和因子
何が原因で起こるか〔起こったか〕．
What brings [brought] it on?
思い当たる誘因は何か．
What do you think is [was] causing it?
Is there any cause you can identify?
悪化させるものは何か．
What makes it worse?
緩和させる〔消す〕ものは何か．
What makes it better [go away]?

5) 随伴症状
ほかに徴候や症状があるか．
Do you have any other signs or symptoms (with it)?

## 現病歴

☞ 主訴は「主訴を訊く」(18 ページ).

## → 主要症状

### 発熱

**症状の特徴**

最近,熱が出ましたか.

熱っぽい〔熱っぽかった〕ですか.

1. 微熱です〔でした〕か.
2. 高熱で〔でした〕か.

熱〔体温〕を測りましたか.
— 何度あります〔ました〕か.
1. 38℃以下.
2. 38℃以上.

熱は…
1. 1日中出ていましたか.
2. 1日のうちで上下しましたか.
3. 2, 3日ごとに出ましたか.
4. 決まった時間帯に出ましたか.

朝〔日中／夕方〕ですか.

**時間経過**

いつ熱が出始めましたか.

☐ Have you had a fever recently? ★1
☐ Do 〔Did〕 you feel feverish?
☐ Do 〔Did〕 you feel as though you have 〔had〕 a fever?
  1. A slight fever?
  2. A high fever?

☐ Did you take your temperature?
— How high is 〔was〕 it?
  1. 38℃ [100.4°F] or lower? ★2
  2. 38℃ [100.4°F] or higher?

☐ Did the fever...
  1. continue all day long?
  2. rise and fall within a day?
  3. recur [come and go] every few days?
  4. occur at a certain time of day?

☐ In the morning [During the day/In the evening]?

☐ When did the fever start?

---

★1 fever は正常より高い「発熱」をさす.
★2 温度　華氏 °F = (°C × 1.8) + 32
　　　　　摂氏 °C = (°F − 32) × 5/9
　摂氏 °C は degrees Celsius [centigrade], 華氏 °F は degrees Fahrenheit と読む.
　☞「単位の換算表」(216 ページ).

熱は何日続いていますか.

—1日〔3日以上／2, 3週間〕ですか.

### 随伴症状
熱のほかに徴候や症状がありますか.
—それは何ですか.
1. 寒気, 頭痛, 鼻水, 鼻づまり, くしゃみ, のどの痛み, 耳の痛み.

2. 咳, 痰, 血痰, 息切れ, 胸痛.

3. 腹痛, 嘔吐, 下痢.

4. 頻尿, 尿の変色・混濁, 排尿痛, 腰痛, 背部痛.

5. 頸部硬直, 痙攣, 意識低下.

6. 動悸, 不整脈.

7. 発疹, 腫れ〔腫脹〕.
8. 関節痛, 筋痛, 筋力低下.

9. その他.

### その他
熱の原因は何だと思いますか.

—家庭, 学校, 職場で同じ症状の人はいますか.

☐ How many days have you had the fever?
— For a day 〔For 3 days or more/ For a few weeks〕?

☐ Do you have any other signs or symptoms?
— What are they?
1. Chills, a headache, a runny nose, a stuffy nose, sneezing, a sore throat, or an earache?

2. Cough, coughing up sputum [phlegm], coughing up blood, shortness of breath, or chest pain?

3. Abdominal pain, vomiting, or diarrhea?

4. Frequent urination, discolored or cloudy urine, pain in urination, low back pain, or back pain?

5. Stiff neck, seizures [convulsions], or drowsiness [impaired consciousness]?

6. Palpitations or irregular pulse?

7. Rash or swelling?
8. Joint pain [aches], muscle pain [aches], or muscle weakness?

9. Any other signs or symptoms?

☐ What do you think is causing your fever?

— Does anyone around you have similar symptoms at home, at school, or in your place of work?

―その人との接触はありましたか. — Have you been exposed to him〔her〕?

―直射日光や高温のところにいましたか. — Have you been exposed to strong direct sunlight or high temperatures?

最近,手術や怪我をしましたか. ☐ Have you recently had any surgery or injury?

最近,日本の国外へ出てどこかへ旅行しましたか. ☐ Have you recently traveled anywhere out of Japan?
―いつ,どこの国へ行きましたか. — When and which country〔countries〕?

結核,心臓病,マラリアなどの病気にかかったことはありますか. ☐ Have you ever had a disease, such as tuberculosis, heart disease, malaria, or any other disease?

鳥,犬,猫などのペットを飼っていますか. ☐ Do you have pets, such as birds, a dog, a cat, or any other pets?

インフルエンザ,BCGなどの予防接種を受けましたか. ☐ Have you had vaccinations, such as a flu shot, a BCG shot, or any other vaccinations?

☞「予防接種」(400ページ).

熱を下げる薬を飲みましたか. ☐ Did you take any drugs or medications for your fever to bring it down?

―例えば,アセトアミノフェン,アスピリン,イブプロフェンなど. — Acetaminophen, aspirin, ibuprofen, or any other medications?

―その他に,熱が出る前後に薬を飲んでいましたか.何ですか. — Did you take any drugs or medications before or after your fever? What is it?

―薬を持っていれば見せて下さい. — May I see if you have it now?

痛み

### ▶ 頭痛

☞「痛みの表現」(31 ページ).

**症状の特徴**

|  |  |
|---|---|
| 頭痛がしますか. | ☐ Do you have a headache? |
| どこが痛みますか. | ☐ Where is the pain?<br>☐ Where do you feel the pain?<br>☐ Where does it hurt? |
| 1. 額にかけて. | 1. Across your forehead? |
| 2. 目の周りと目の奥. | 2. Around and behind your eyes? |
| 3. こめかみに沿って. | 3. Along your temples? |
| 4. ほお骨の後ろ. | 4. Behind your cheekbones? |
| 5. 後頭部. | 5. In the back of your head? |
| 6. 頭全体. | 6. All over your head? |
| 7. 片側. | 7. On one side of your head? |
| 8. その他の部位. | 8. Anywhere else? |
| どんな痛みですか. | ☐ What is the pain like?<br>☐ Can you describe the pain for me? |
| 1. 軽い. | 1. Mild? |
| 2. 鈍痛. | 2. Dull ache? |
| 3. 中程度. | 3. Moderate? |
| 4. 激しい. | 4. Severe? |
| 5. 割れるように激しい. | 5. Splitting? |
| 6. ずきずきする. | 6. Throbbing? |
| 7. 刺すような. | 7. Stabbing? |
| 8. バンドで頭を締め付けられるような. | 8. Like a band squeezing your head? |
| 9. ピリピリッとくる［電撃性の］. | 9. Electric shock-like? |
| 10. （表面が）ビーンと走るような. | 10. Shooting? |
| 11. （表面が）ヒリヒリする. | 11. Burning? |
| 12. 我慢できないほどの痛み. | 12. An unbearable pain? |

chapter 3 現病歴（主要症状—痛み）

13. これまでに経験したことのない激しい痛み.

その痛みは…
1. ずっと続いていますか.
2. 痛んだり痛まなかったりしますか.
3. 反復性ですか,周期性ですか？

痛みが起こるのはいつですか.

1. 朝.
2. 日中.
3. 夜.
4. 月経前〔月経中〕.

痛みの起こり方は…ですか.
1. 突然
2. 徐々に〔ゆっくり〕

どういうときに痛みますか.
1. 疲れたとき.
2. 運動をした後で.
3. 飲酒をした後で.

痛みは毎回どのくらい長く続きますか.

頭痛を悪化させるものがありますか.
―それは何ですか.
―運動,姿勢,飲酒,ストレス,咳,ある種の食べ物ですか.

13. An extreme pain which you've never experienced before?

☐ Is the pain...
　1. constant?
　　 Does it hurt all the time?
　2. intermittent?
　　 Does it come and go?
　3. recurrent or periodic?
　　 Does it come repeatedly or at regular intervals?

☐ When do you usually get it?
☐ When does it occur?
　1. In the morning?
　2. During the day?
　3. At night?
　4. Before 〔During〕 your menstrual period?

☐ Does it come on...
　1. suddenly?
　2. gradually 〔slowly〕?

☐ In what situations do you get it?
　1. When you are tired?
　2. After you exercised?
　3. After you drank alcohol?

☐ How long does it last each time?

☐ Is there anything that makes the headache worse?
— What is it?
— Physical activity, posture, alcohol, stress, coughing, or certain foods?

| | |
|---|---|
| 頭痛を軽くするものがありますか. | ☐ Is there anything that relieves the headache? |
| —それは何ですか. | — What is it? |
| —入浴, 睡眠, 安静ですか. | — Taking a bath, sleeping, or resting? |
| —横になると痛みがとれますか. | — Does it go away when you lie down? |

**時間経過**

初めて痛んだのはいつですか.

☐ When did you first get this pain?
☐ When did this pain start?

どのくらい長く痛んでいますか.
1. 2, 3 〔5, 6〕時間.
2. 2, 3 日.
3. 2, 3 週間.
4. もっと長く.

☐ How long have you had it?
1. A few 〔Several〕 hours?
2. A few days?
3. A few weeks?
4. Longer?

どのくらいの頻度で痛みますか.
1. 頻繁に.
2. さほど頻繁ではなく.
3. めったに痛まない.
4. 1 か月に 1 回〔2 回／2, 3 回〕.

☐ How often do you have it?
1. Often [Frequently]?
2. Not so often [Infrequently]?
3. Rarely?
4. Once 〔Two times/A few times〕a month?

その痛みは…
1. 軽くなっていますか.
2. だんだん悪化していますか.
3. 変わりませんか.

☐ Is it...
1. getting better?
2. getting worse?
3. the same?

**随伴症状**

頭痛のほかに徴候や症状がありますか.
—それは何ですか.
1. 発熱.
2. 鼻汁.
3. 鼻閉.
4. 肩こり.
5. 吐き気.

☐ Do you have any other signs or symptoms?
— What are they?
1. Fever?
2. Discharge from the nose?
3. Stuffy nose?
4. Stiff shoulders?
5. Nausea?

| | |
|---|---|
| 6. 嘔吐. | 6. Vomiting? |
| 7. めまい. | 7. Dizziness? |
| 8. 首の硬直. | 8. Stiff neck? |
| 9. 神経症状〔感覚障害／運動障害／言語障害〕. | 9. Neurological symptoms 〔Sensory problem/Motor problem/Verbal problem〕? |
| 10. かすみ目［霧視］. | 10. Blurred vision? |
| 11. 光がまぶしい［羞明］. | 11. Sensitivity to light? |
| 12. 流涙. | 12. Increased tearing? |
| 13. 結膜充血. | 13. Redness of the conjunctiva? |
| 14. 閃輝性暗点. | 14. Blind spot containing flashing lights? |
| 15. 視力障害. | 15. Vision problem? |
| 16. 不安. | 16. Anxiety? |
| 17. 緊張. | 17. Tension or strain? |
| 18. 抑うつ. | 18. Depression? |
| 19. その他. | 19. Any other symptoms? |

**その他**

| | |
|---|---|
| 頭痛の原因は何だと思いますか. | ☐ What do you think is causing your headache? |
| 痛み止めを飲んでいますか.<br>―何を飲んでいますか．効き目がありますか. | ☐ Are you taking anything for it?<br>— What are you taking? Does it help? |
| これまでにこのような頭痛を経験したことがありますか. | ☐ Have you ever had this kind of headache before? |
| これまでに…にかかったことがありますか. | ☐ Have you ever had… |
| 1. 頭部外傷 | 1. a head injury? |
| 2. 高血圧 | 2. high blood pressure? |
| 3. 耳の病気 | 3. problems with ears? |
| 4. 副鼻腔炎など鼻の病気 | 4. problems with nose such as sinusitis? |
| 5. 緑内障など目の病気 | 5. problems with eyes such as glaucoma? |
| 6. 歯の病気 | 6. problems with teeth? |

| 家族に同様の症状を持っている人はいますか？ | ☐ Does anyone in your immediate family have a similar symptom? |

## 用語・表現ファイル

### 痛みの表現

#### 1. 痛みの程度を示す表現

no pain（無痛）
↓
mild（軽い痛み，少しの痛い）
↓
tolerable（我慢できるほどの痛み）
↓
moderate（中程度の痛み）
↓
severe（激しい痛み，強い痛み）
↓
worst possible（経験したことがないほどの激痛）

#### 2. 痛みの起こり方，持続を示す表現

| | |
|---|---|
| 突然の | sudden |
| 急性の | acute |
| 慢性の | chronic |
| 瞬時の | momentary |
| 短い | brief |
| 規則的に繰り返す［周期性の］ | periodic |
| 発作的に繰り返す［間欠性の］ | intermittent |
| ずっと続く［持続性の］ | constant［persistent］ |

#### 3. 痛みの領域を示す表現

| | |
|---|---|
| 表面的な［表在の］ | superficial［external］ |
| 深部の | deep［internal］ |
| 限局性の | localized |
| 広範性の | generalized |
| 他の部分へ放散する［放散性の］ | radiating |
| 他の部分へ移動する［移動性の］ | moving |

## ▶ 胸痛

☞「痛みの表現」(31 ページ).

### 症状の特徴

これまでに胸の痛みや不快感がありましたか.
—それについて話して下さい.
—今,胸が痛みますか.
—心臓のあたりが痛むことがありますか.

どこが痛みますか.
—指でさして教えて下さい.

—痛みはほかの場所へ広がりますか〔移動しますか〕.
—どこへですか.
  1. あご〔のど〕に.
  2. 首の後ろ.
  3. 背中に.
  4. 肩に.
  5. 左腕に.
  6. お腹に.

どんな痛みですか.

  1. 鋭い [ナイフで刺すような].
  2. 鈍い.
  3. 胸が締め付けられるような.
  4. 胸が圧迫されるような.
  5. 焼け付くような.
  6. チクチクするような.
  7. チクンとするような.
  8. (表面が)ビーンと走るような.
  9. 圧迫すると痛む.
—胸が詰まったような感じがしますか.

☐ Have you ever had any pain or discomfort in your chest?
— Please tell me about it.
— Do you have chest pain now?
— Do you ever have pain around your heart?

☐ Where is the pain?
— Please point to it with one finger.

— Does it radiate 〔move〕 to another place?
— To where?
  1. To your jaw 〔throat〕?
  2. To the back of your neck?
  3. To your back?
  4. To your shoulders?
  5. To your left arm?
  6. To your abdomen?

☐ What is the pain like?
☐ Can you describe the pain for me?
  1. Sharp [Stabbing like a knife]?
  2. Dull ache?
  3. Sqeezing [Crushing/Tight]?
  4. Pressure-like?
  5. Burning?
  6. Tingling?
  7. Prickly?
  8. Shooting?
  9. Tender?
— Do you have a sense of fullness in your chest?

その痛みは…
1. ずっと続いていますか.
2. 痛んだり痛まなかったりしますか.

痛みはいつ起こります〔ました〕か.
1. 早朝.
2. 起床時.
3. 朝.
4. 日中.
5. 夜.

痛みの起こり方は…ですか.
1. 突然
2. 徐々に［ゆっくり］

どういうときに痛みますか.

1. 安静にしているとき.
2. 眠っているとき.
3. 体の位置を変えるとき.
4. 歩いているとき.
5. 運動しているとき.
6. 普通に呼吸をするとき.
7. 深呼吸するとき.
8. 咳をするとき.
9. くしゃみをするとき.
10. 食べるとき.
11. 胃にもたれる食事をした後で.
12. 排便するとき.
13. 気が動転しているとき.
14. 心配事があるとき.
15. 心臓がドキドキするとき.
16. 寒いとき.

☐ Is the pain...
1. constant?
   Does it hurt all the time?
2. intermittent?
   Does it come and go?

☐ When does〔did〕it start?
1. Early in the morning?
2. When you wake〔woke〕up?
3. In the morning?
4. During the day?
5. At night?

☐ Does it come on...
1. suddenly?
2. gradually［slowly］?

☐ In what situations do you get it?
☐ When does it occur?
1. When you are resting?
2. When you are sleeping?
3. When you change your position?
4. When you are walking?
5. When you are exercising?
6. When you breathe normally?
7. When you breathe deeply?
8. When you cough?
9. When you sneeze?
10. When you eat?
11. After you eat a heavy meal?
12. When you have a bowel movement?
13. When you are upset?
14. When you are worried?
15. When your heart beats fast?
16. When it is cold?

痛みの発作はどのくらい長く続きますか.
1. 一瞬.
2. 2,3〔5,6〕秒.
3. 2,3分.
4. 2,3時間.
5. 2,3日.

☐ How long does this attack〔pain〕last?
1. An instant?
2. A few〔Several〕seconds?
3. A few minutes?
4. A few hours?
5. A few days?

胸の痛みを…がありますか.
1. 軽くするもの［こと］
2. 悪化させるもの［こと］
—それは何ですか.
—階段を上がったり，坂道を登ったりするとき，痛みは増しますか.
—深呼吸をすると，痛みは増しますか.
—体を休めると痛みがとれますか.

☐ Is there anything that makes the chest pain...
1. better?
2. worse?
— What is it?
— Does it increase when you go up stairs or slopes?
— Does it increase when you take a deep breath?
— Does it go away when you rest?

ニトログリセリンは有効でしたか.

☐ Did the nitroglycerin help〔work well〕?

## 時間経過
痛むようになったのは…ですか.
1. つい最近
2. かなり前

☐ Did you have the pain...
1. just recently?
2. some time ago?

初めて痛んだのはいつですか.

☐ When did you first get it?
☐ When did it start?

痛み始めてからどのくらいですか.
1. 2,3〔5,6〕時間.
2. 2,3日.
3. 2,3週間.
4. 2,3か月.
5. 2,3年.

☐ How long have you had it?
1. A few〔Several〕hours?
2. A few days?
3. A few weeks?
4. A few months?
5. A few years?

どのくらいの頻度で痛みますか.
1. 頻繁に.
2. さほど頻繁ではなく.

☐ How often do you have it?
1. Often〔Frequently〕?
2. Not so often〔Infrequently〕?

3. 時々.
  4. 1か月に1〔2／2,3〕回.

その痛みは…
  1. 軽くなっていますか.
  2. だんだん悪化していますか.
  3. 変わりませんか.

**随伴症状**
胸痛のほかに徴候や症状がありますか.
―それは何ですか.
  1. 息切れ.
  2. 冷や汗.
  3. 吐き気, 嘔吐.
  4. 意識消失.
  5. その他.

胸が痛むとき, 顔が青白くなると人から言われたことがありますか.

**その他**
これまでにこのような胸の痛みを経験したことがありますか.

これまでに…にかかったことがありますか.
  1. 心臓病
  2. 高血圧
  3. 脂質異常症
  4. 脳血管疾患

  3. Occasionally [Once in a while]?
  4. Once [Two times/A few times] a month?

☐ Is it...
  1. getting better?
  2. getting worse?
  3. the same?

☐ Do you have any other signs or symptoms?
— What are they?
  1. Shortness of breath?
  2. Cold sweat?
  3. Nausea and [or] vomiting?
  4. Loss of consciousness? Have you blacked out?
  5. Any other symptoms?

☐ Have you ever been told that you turn pale or bluish when you have chest pain?

☐ Have you ever had this kind of chest pain before?

☐ Have you ever had...
  1. heart disease?
  2. high blood pressure?
  3. dyslipidemia?
  4. cerebrovascular disease?

### ▶ 腹痛

☞「痛みの表現」(31 ページ).

#### 症状の特徴

| | |
|---|---|
| お腹に痛みや不快感がありますか. | ☐ Do you have any pain or discomfort in your stomach or abdomen? |
| —それについて話して下さい. | — Please tell me about it. |
| どこが痛みますか. | ☐ Where is the pain? |
| 1. お腹全体. | 1. All over? |
| 2. みぞおち. | 2. In the pit of your stomach? |
| 3. おへその周り. | 3. Around your navel? |
| 4. おへその右〔左〕側. | 4. On the right〔left〕side of your navel? |
| 5. 下腹部. | 5. In your lower abdomen? |
| —指でさして教えて下さい. | — Please point to it with one finger. |
| —痛みはほかの場所へ広がりますか〔移動しますか〕. | — Does it radiate〔move〕to another place? |
| —どこからどこへですか. | — From where to where? |
| どんな痛みですか. | ☐ What is the pain like? |
| | ☐ Can you describe the pain for me? |
| 1. 鈍い. | 1. Dull ache? |
| 2. 鋭い. | 2. Sharp? |
| 3. チクチクする. | 3. Pricking? |
| 4. きりきりする. | 4. Squeezing? |
| 5. 焼けるような. | 5. Burning? |
| 6. しくしくする. | 6. Nagging? |
| 7. 重苦しい. | 7. Heavy? |
| 8. 差し込むような. | 8. Colicky〔Griping〕?★ |
| 9. (表面が)ビーンと走るような. | 9. Shooting? |
| 10. 圧迫すると痛む. | 10. Tender? |

---

★激しい腹痛・生理痛は cramps という.

| | |
|---|---|
| お腹が張っていますか． | ☐ Do you feel your abdomen distended? |
| —（ガスで）お腹が張っていますか． | — Do you feel your abdomen bloated (with gas)? |
| —お腹がゴロゴロしますか． | — Does your stomach rumble? |
| —ガスがよく出ますか． | — Do you pass a lot of gas? |
| その痛みは… | ☐ Is the pain... |
| 1. ずっと続いていますか． | 1. constant? Does it hurt all the time? |
| 2. 痛んだり痛まなかったりしますか． | 2. intermittent? Does it come and go? |
| 3. 反復性ですか，周期性ですか． | 3. recurrent or periodic? Does it come repeatedly or at regular intervals? |
| 痛みの起こり方は…ですか． | ☐ Does it come on... |
| 1. 突然 | 1. suddenly? |
| 2. 徐々に［ゆっくり］ | 2. gradually [slowly]? |
| どういうときに痛みますか． | ☐ In what situations do you get it? |
| | ☐ When does it occur? |
| 1. 空腹時． | 1. When you are hungry? |
| 2. 食事後． | 2. After you eat? |
| 3. 寝ている間． | 3. When you are asleep? |
| 4. 便をする前． | 4. Before you move your bowels? |
| 5. 咳やくしゃみをするとき． | 5. When you cough or sneeze? |
| 6. ストレスを受けたとき． | 6. When you are under stress? |
| 7. 月経のとき． | 7. When you have menstrual periods? |
| 痛みを悪化させるものがありますか． | ☐ Is there anything that makes the pain worse? |
| —それは何ですか． | — What is it? |
| —どんなものを食べたり飲むと痛みがひどくなりますか． | — What kind of foods or drinks make it worse [aggravate it]? |
| 1. 酒類． | 1. Alcohol? |
| 2. タバコ． | 2. Cigarettes? |
| 3. コーヒー． | 3. Coffee? |

4. 牛乳〔乳製品〕.
5. 脂っこいもの.
6. 香辛料のきいたもの.
7. その他.
―体を動かしたり，体の位置を変えたりすると悪くなりますか.

痛みを軽くするものがありますか.

―それは何ですか.
―痛みは食事をすると治りますか.
―痛みは体位によって楽になりますか.
　1. 横になる.
　2. 座る.
　3. 体を曲げる.
　4. その他.

**時間経過**
初めて痛んだのはいつですか.

どのくらい長く痛んでいますか.

いつから.

どのくらいの頻度で痛みますか.

その痛みは…
　1. 軽くなっていますか.
　2. だんだん悪化していますか.
　3. 変わりませんか.

**随伴症状**
腹痛のほかに徴候や症状がありますか.
―それは何ですか.
　1. 食欲低下.
　2. 吐き気，嘔吐.

4. Milk〔Milk products〕?
5. Fatty foods?
6. Spicy foods?
7. Something else?
— Does it get worse when you move your body or you change your position?

☐ Is there anything that makes the pain better?
— What is it?
— Does it go away after meals?
— Is it relieved by changing your body position?
　1. Lying down?
　2. Sitting up?
　3. Bending over?
　4. Any other position?

☐ When did you first get this pain?
☐ When did this pain start?

☐ How long have you had it?

☐ Since when?

☐ How often do you have it?

☐ Is it...
　1. getting better?
　2. getting worse?
　3. the same?

☐ Do you have any other signs or symptoms?
— What are they?
　1. Poor appetite?
　2. Nausea and〔or〕vomiting?

| | |
|---|---|
| 3. 便通異常．便秘．下痢． | 3. Problems with your bowel movement? Constipation? Diarrhea? |
| 4. 冷や汗． | 4. Cold sweat? |
| 5. 血尿． | 5. Bloody urine? |
| 6. その他． | 6. Any other symptoms? |

### その他

| | |
|---|---|
| これまでにこのような痛みを経験したことがありますか． | ☐ Have you ever had this kind of pain before? |
| これまでに…にかかったことがありますか． | ☐ Have you ever had... |
| 1. 胃潰瘍． | 1. gastric ulcer? |
| 2. 十二指腸潰瘍． | 2. duodenal ulcer? |
| 3. 虫垂炎． | 3. appendicitis? |
| 4. 胆石． | 4. gallstone(s)? |
| 5. 尿路結石． | 5. urinary stone(s)? |
| お腹の手術をしたことがありますか． | ☐ Have you ever had surgery on your stomach or abdomen? |
| 常用または最近服用している薬はありますか．鎮痛薬など． | ☐ Do you take any drugs or medications regularly? Any pain killer? |
| 最終月経はいつですか． | ☐ When was your last menstrual period? |
| ―妊娠していますか． | ― Are you pregnant? |
| ―妊娠の可能性はありますか． | ― Could you be pregnant? |

### ▶ 腰背部痛

☞「痛みの表現」(31 ページ).

### 症状の特徴

| | |
|---|---|
| これまでに背中〔腰〕に痛みや不快感がありましたか． | ☐ Have you ever had any pain or discomfort in your back〔lower back〕? |
| ―それについて話して下さい． | ― Please tell me about it. |

| | |
|---|---|
| どこが痛みますか. | ☐ Where is the pain? |
| 1. 真ん中. | 1. In the middle? |
| 2. 片側性. | 2. Only on one side? |
| 　右側あるいは左側. | 　On the right side or on the left side? |
| ―痛みはほかの場所へ広がりますか〔移動しますか〕. | ― Does it radiate〔move〕to another place? |
| ―どこへですか. | ― To where? |
| 1. 臀部に. | 1. To your hips and buttocks? |
| 2. 大腿部に. | 2. To your thighs? |
| 3. 下腿部に. | 3. To your lower leg(s)? |
| 4. 下腹部に. | 4. To your lower abdomen? |
| どんな痛みですか. | ☐ What is the pain like? |
| | ☐ Can you describe the pain for me? |
| 1. 鋭い［ナイフで刺すような］. | 1. Sharp [Stabbing like a knife]? |
| 2. 鈍い. | 2. Dull ache? |
| その痛みは… | ☐ Is the pain... |
| 1. ずっと続いていますか. | 1. constant? |
| | 　Does it hurt all the time? |
| 2. 痛んだり痛まなかったりしますか. | 2. intermittent? |
| | 　Does it come and go? |
| 痛みの起こり方は…ですか. | ☐ Does it come on... |
| 1. 突然 | 1. suddenly? |
| 2. 徐々に［ゆっくり］ | 2. gradually [slowly]? |
| どういうときに痛みますか. | ☐ In what situations do you get it? |
| | ☐ When does it occur? |
| 1. 安静にしているとき. | 1. When you are resting [lying down]? |
| 2. 動き始めるとき. | 2. When you start to move? |
| 3. 同じ姿勢でいるとき. | 3. When you hold the same posture? |
| 4. 前かがみになるとき. | 4. When you bend forward? |
| 5. 背筋を伸ばしたとき. | 5. When you straighten your back? |

| | |
|---|---|
| 6. 重いものを持つとき. | 6. When you carry a heavy object? |

| | |
|---|---|
| 姿勢を変えるとよくなりますか. | ☐ Does it get better when you change your position? |
| —体を休めると痛みがとれますか. | — Does it go away when you rest? |

**時間経過**

| | |
|---|---|
| 痛むようになったのは…ですか.<br>1. つい最近<br>2. かなり前 | ☐ Did you have the pain...<br>1. just recently?<br>2. some time ago? |
| 何かきっかけはありましたか.<br>1. スポーツ.<br>2. 重いものを持った,持ち上げた.<br>3. 急に動いた. | ☐ What do you think triggered it?<br>1. Did you play some sport?<br>2. Did you carry or lift a heavy object?<br>3. Did you move abruptly? |
| 初めて痛んだのはいつですか. | ☐ When did you first get it?<br>☐ When did it start? |
| 痛み始めてからどのくらいになりますか.<br>1. 2, 3〔5, 6〕時間.<br>2. 2, 3 日.<br>3. 2, 3 週間.<br>4. 2, 3 か月.<br>5. 2, 3 年. | ☐ How long have you been having it?<br>1. A few〔Several〕hours?<br>2. A few days?<br>3. A few weeks?<br>4. A few months?<br>5. A few years? |
| どのくらいの頻度で痛みますか.<br>1. 頻繁に.<br>2. さほど頻繁ではなく.<br>3. 時々. | ☐ How often do you have it?<br>1. Often [Frequently]?<br>2. Not so often [Infrequently]?<br>3. Occasionally [Once in a while]? |

**随伴症状**

| | |
|---|---|
| 腰痛〔背部痛〕のほかに徴候や症状がありますか.<br>—それは何ですか.<br>1. 筋力低下. | ☐ Do you have any other signs or symptoms?<br>— What are they?<br>1. Muscle weakness? |

| | |
|---|---|
| 2. 歩行障害. | 2. Walking difficulty? |
| 3. 感覚障害〔しびれ〕. | 3. Sensory disturbance [Numbness]? |
| 4. 血尿. | 4. Bloody urine? |
| 5. その他. | 5. Any other symptoms? |

### 全身倦怠感

**症状の特徴**

体がだるい，または脱力感がありますか.
1. いつもですか.
2. 時々そうなるのですか.

☐ Do you feel tired or do you feel excessive fatigue? ★
1. Constantly [All the time]?
2. Does it come and go? Intermittently?

―以前とくらべて疲れますか.

― Do you get tired more easily than you used to?

―だるいのは全身ですか，体の一部のみですか.

― Do you feel tired all over or in one part of your body?

だるさ〔疲労〕を感じるのはいつですか.
1. 朝.
2. 1日の終わり頃.
3. 1日中.

☐ When do you feel tired [fatigued]?
1. In the morning?
2. Later in the day?
3. All day long? All the time?

どんな動作〔活動〕をすると疲れますか.

1. 洋服を着替える，歯を磨く，髪をとかす，など日常動作.
2. 歩く.
3. 運動する.
4. 仕事をする.
5. 家事をする.
6. その他の動作.

☐ What kind of movement [activity] causes you to feel tired?

1. Activities of daily living, such as dressing, brushing your teeth, or combing your hair?
2. Walking?
3. Exercising?
4. Doing your work?
5. Doing your housework?
6. Any other movement?

---

★脱力感は a feeling of exhaustion ともいう.

|  |  |
|---|---|
| その症状のため就寝が必要ですか. | ☐ Is bed rest necessary (because of your problem)? |
| —仕事〔学業〕に差し支えますか. | — Does your problem interfere with your job 〔schoolwork〕? |
| —仕事〔学校〕を休みましたか. どのくらいの期間ですか. | — Did you lose time from work 〔school〕? If so, how long? |
| —休息すると疲れがとれますか. | — Does rest relieve your tiredness? |
| —睡眠はよくとれていますか. | — Do you get enough sleep? |
| —何時間寝ていますか. | — How many hours do you sleep? |
| —睡眠薬を常用していますか. | — Are you taking sleeping pills regularly? |
| —毎朝,元気が回復していますか. | — Do you feel rested every morning? |

### 時間経過

| | |
|---|---|
| 初めて気づいたのはいつですか. | ☐ When did you first notice it? |
| —その状態はどのくらい続いていますか. | — How long have you felt this way? |

### 随伴症状

| | |
|---|---|
| だるさ〔疲労〕のほかに徴候や症状がありますか. | ☐ Do you have any other signs or symptoms? |
| —それは何ですか. | — What are they? |
| 1. 発熱. | 1. Fever? |
| 2. 体重減少. | 2. Weight loss? |
| 3. 咽頭痛. | 3. Sore throat? |
| 4. 咳. | 4. Coughing? |
| 5. 吐き気,嘔吐. | 5. Nausea and 〔or〕 vomiting? |
| 6. 下痢. | 6. Diarrhea? |
| 7. その他. | 7. Any other symptoms? |

> めまい

### 症状の特徴

| | |
|---|---|
| めまいがしますか. | ☐ Do you ever feel dizzy? |
| —めまいの発作を起こしますか. | — Do you have attacks of dizziness?★ |

---

★回転性めまいはとくに vertigo という.

どんなめまいですか.
- □ What is your dizziness like?
- □ Can you describe it for me?

1. 部屋の中の物が動いたり, ぐるぐる回る.
2. 自分自身がぐるぐる回る.
3. 回転する感じがする.
4. 頭がふわっとする.
5. 不安定感がある.
6. 体がふらふらする.
7. 気を失いそうな感じがする.
8. 目の前が真っ暗になる.
9. その他.

1. Do objects in the room move or spin around?
2. Do you feel like spinning around?
3. Do you have sensations of rotating?
4. Do you feel lightheaded?
5. Do you have sensations of unsteadiness?
6. Do you feel groggy?
7. Do you feel like fainting?
8. Do you black out?
9. Anything else?

めまいの程度はどのくらいですか.
軽い〔中程度／激しい〕ですか.
—日常生活ができますか.
—立ち上がるのが難しいですか.
—その間, 寝たきりになりますか.

- □ How is your dizziness?
- □ Mild〔Moderate/Severe〕?
- — Can you cope with everyday matters?
- — Do you have difficulty standing up?
- — Do you have to be in bed during the attack?

めまいの起こり方は … ですか.
1. 突然
2. 徐々に［ゆっくりと］

- □ Does it come on...
  1. suddenly?
  2. gradually [slowly]?

めまいは反復性ですか, 発作性ですか.
—発作が起こりそうな予兆がありますか.

- □ Does it come repeatedly or does it come in attacks?
- — Do you have any warning that an attack is about to begin?

どんなときめまいが起こりますか.
1. 首をひねったり, 上をむいたりするとき.
2. 急に立ち上がったり, 身を起こしたりするとき.

- □ In what situations do you get it?
  1. When you twist your neck or look upward?
  2. When you rise abruptly from a sitting or lying position?

3. 長時間立ち続けるとき.
4. 身をかがめるとき.
5. （肉体的〔精神的〕）疲労時に.
6. 思い当たる原因もなく.

毎回, どのくらい続きますか.
1. 2, 3〔5, 6〕分.
2. 2, 3 時間.
3. 何日にもわたって.

## 時間経過

初めてめまいに気づいたのはいつですか.
―最近, いつ起こりましたか.
―起こったのは 2 回以上ですか.

―どのくらいの頻度で起こりますか.
1. 頻繁に起こる. 週に 1 回以上.
2. 月に 1 回.
3. 月に 1 回以上.
4. めったに起こらない.

めまいは…
1. 軽くなっていますか.
2. だんだん悪化していますか.
3. 変わりませんか.

## 随伴症状

めまいのほかに徴候や症状がありますか.
―それは何ですか.
1. 耳鳴り, 耳閉感, 聴力低下.

2. 頭痛.

3. When you keep standing for a long time?
4. When you bend over?
5. When you're tired (physically〔mentally〕)?
6. For no obvious reason?

☐ How long does it last each time?
1. For a few〔several〕minutes?
2. For a few hours?
3. For a period of days?

☐ When did you first notice your dizziness?
— When did this happen recently?
— Has it happened two times or more?

— How often do you have your dizzy spells?
1. Often [Frequently]? More than once a week?
2. Once a month?
3. More than once a month?
4. Rarely?

☐ Is it...
1. getting better?
2. getting worse?
3. the same?

☐ Do you have any other signs or symptoms?
— What are they?
1. Ringing in your ear(s), sensations of fullness or pressure in your ear(s), or hearing loss?

2. Headaches?

3. 発熱.
4. 吐き気, 嘔吐.
5. 言語障害.
6. 視野の障害.
7. 体の一部のしびれ感, チクチク感, 筋力低下, 知覚低下.
8. 意識障害 [混乱].
9. その他

3. Fever?
4. Nausea and [or] vomiting?
5. Difficulty speaking?
6. Disturbed vision?
7. Numbness, tingling sensations, muscle weakness, or decreased sensation in any part of your body?
8. Confusion?
9. Any other symptoms?

### その他

これまでに…にかかったことがありますか.
1. 内耳疾患
2. 頭頸部外傷
3. 高血圧
4. 低血圧
5. 心臓疾患
6. 貧血

☐ Have you ever had...
1. inner ear disease?
2. injury to your head or neck?
3. high blood pressure?
4. low blood pressure?
5. heart disease?
6. anemia?

睡眠をよくとっていますか.

☐ Are you getting enough sleep?

最近, 働きすぎですか.

☐ Have you overworked recently?

### 浮腫

#### 症状の特徴

体のどこかがむくんでいる感じがしますか.

☐ Does any area of your body feel swollen?
☐ Do you have any swelling in any area of your body? ★

―どこですか.
1. 足.
2. 足首.
3. 足首から下の部分.
4. 手.
5. 顔 [瞼].

― Where?
1. Your legs?
2. Your ankles?
3. Your feet?
4. Your hands?
5. Your face [Your eyelids]?

---

★ swelling, edema (浮腫, むくみ) は, 腫脹 (腫れ) の意味にも用いられる.

| | |
|---|---|
| 6. 体全体. | 6. All over your body? |
| ―片側性ですか. | — Is the swelling on one side? |
| ―靴や指輪がきつい感じがしますか. | — Do your shoes or rings feel tight? |
| ―押すとへこんだままですか. | — Does a dent remain in the area if you press on it? |

最近,体重が増えましたか. ☐ Have you noticed any weight gain recently?
―どのくらい増えましたか. — How much have you gained?
―1週間で何キロ〔ポンド〕増えましたか. — How many kilos〔pounds〕did you gain within a week?
―1日のなかで体重の変動はありますか. — Does your weight change within a day?

☞「単位の換算表」(216 ページ).

## 時間経過

どのくらい長くむくみを感じていますか. ☐ How long have you noticed this swelling?
―いつから. — Since when?

むくみ始めたのは…ですか. ☐ Did it come on...
 1. 突然 1. suddenly?
 2. 徐々に[ゆっくり] 2. gradually [slowly]?

朝と夕方とではどちらがひどいですか. ☐ Which does it get worse, in the morning or in the late afternoon?

月経前にむくみますか. ☐ Do you have it before your menstrual periods?

## 随伴症状

むくみのほかに徴候や症状がありますか. ☐ Do you have any other signs or symptoms?
―それは何ですか. — What are they?
 1. 息切れ. 1. Shortness of breath?
 2. 風邪,インフルエンザ症状. 2. Cold or flu symptoms?
 3. 血尿. 3. Bloody urine?
 4. その他. 4. Any other symptoms?

**その他**

…を指摘されたことがありますか.

1. 心臓疾患
2. 腎障害
3. 肝障害
4. 検診での蛋白尿

最近服用した薬があればすべて教えて下さい.

—それは何ですか.

☐ Have you ever been told by a doctor that you have...

1. heart disease?
2. a kidney problem?
3. a liver problem?
4. proteinuria at your checkup?

☐ Please tell me all the medications you have taken recently.

— What are they?

## 腫瘤・腫脹・リンパ節腫大

### ▶ 腫瘤・腫脹

体のどこかに, しこりや腫れがありますか.

—どこですか.
1. 頭.
2. 首〔前頸部／側頸部〕.

3. 顔.
4. 皮下.
5. 乳房.
6. 脇の下.
7. 鼠径部.
8. その他.

☐ Do you have any lumps [bumps] or swellings on any area of your body?★

— Where?
1. On your head?
2. On your neck〔On the front of your neck/On one or both sides of your neck〕?
3. On your face?
4. Under the skin?
5. In your breast(s)?
6. Under your armpit(s)?
7. In your groin(s)?
8. Any other part of your body?

☞乳房腫瘤については「乳房・女性生殖器」(117 ページ).
☞前頸部腫瘤については「代謝・内分泌」(127 ページ).

初めて腫れに気づいたのはいつですか.

—どのくらい長く腫れているのですか. いつからですか.

☐ When did you first notice it?

— How long have you had it? Since when?

---

★bump は打撲によるものをさす.

しこり〔腫れ〕は
1. 大きくなっていますか.
2. ひいてきていますか.
3. 変化なしですか.

- [ ] Is it...
  1. growing [getting bigger]?
  2. decreasing [getting smaller]?
  3. the same?

痛みますか.

- [ ] Does it hurt?
- [ ] Is it painful?

―そこを押すと痛みますか.

— Is the area tender?

家族に同様の症状を持っている人はいますか.

- [ ] Is there anyone in your immediate family who has a similar symptom?

### ▶ リンパ節腫大

リンパ節が腫れていますか.

- [ ] Do you have swollen lymph nodes?

―どこですか.
1. 首.
2. 脇の下.
3. 鼠径部.
4. その他.

— Where?
1. In your neck?
2. Under your armpit(s)?
3. In your groin(s)?
4. In any other part of your body?

―リンパ節の腫れは両方ですか, それとも片方ですか.

— Does the swelling appear on both sides or only on one side?

痛みますか.

- [ ] Does it hurt?
- [ ] Is it painful?

―そこを押すと痛みますか.

— Is the area tender?

初めて腫れに気づいたのはいつですか.

- [ ] When did you first notice the swelling?

―どのくらい長く腫れているのですか. いつからですか.

— How long have you had it? Since when?

腫れは
1. 大きくなっていますか.
2. ひいてきていますか.
3. 変化なしですか.

- [ ] Is it...
  1. growing [getting bigger]?
  2. decreasing [getting smaller]?
  3. the same?

| | |
|---|---|
| 腫れのほかに徴候や症状がありますか. | ☐ Do you have any other signs or symptoms? |
| —それは何ですか. | — What are they? |
| 1. 発熱. | 1. Fever? |
| 2. 咽頭痛. | 2. Sore throat? |
| 3. 体重減少. | 3. Weight loss? |
| 4. 寝汗. | 4. Sweating at night? |
| 5. 関節痛. | 5. Joint pains? |
| 6. 発疹. | 6. Rash? |
| 7. その他. | 7. Any other symptoms? |
| 風邪やインフルエンザ症状はありましたか. | ☐ Have you had cold or flu symptoms? |
| 虫歯はありますか. | ☐ Do you have tooth decay? |
| 最近,手や足に傷ができましたか. | ☐ Have you recently had injuries to your arms or legs? ★ |
| ペットを飼っていますか. | ☐ Do you have pets? |

### 外傷

| | |
|---|---|
| 怪我〔事故〕の受傷時刻を教えて下さい. | ☐ Tell me when the injury 〔accident〕 occurred. |
| —いつですか. | — When did it happen? |
| 怪我〔事故〕の受傷状況を教えて下さい. | ☐ Please describe how the injury 〔accident〕 occurred. |
| —どうしたのですか[何が起こったのですか]. | — What happened? |
| —転倒しましたか. | — Did you fall? |
| —どんなふうに転びましたか. | — How did you fall? |
| —交通事故にあったのですか. | — Did you have [get involved in] a traffic accident? |

---

★ arm は肩から手首まで,hand は手首より先,leg はももの付け根から足首まで,foot は足首から先を指す.なお,arm は上肢全体,leg は下肢全体を表す言葉として用いられることもある.

| | |
|---|---|
| ―その時意識を失いましたか．どのくらい長い間でしたか． | ― Did you lose consciousness? For how long? |
| 火傷ですか． | ☐ Did you get burned? |
| 打撲傷ですか． | ☐ Did you have bruises? |
| 裂傷ですか． | ☐ Did you have lacerations? |
| 切り傷ですか． | ☐ Did you have cuts? |
| 今痛むところをすべて教えて下さい．<br>1. 頭．<br>2. 顔．<br>3. 首．<br>4. 胸部．<br>5. 腹部．<br>6. 背部．<br>7. 腰部．<br>8. 上肢．<br><br>9. 下肢． | ☐ Tell me all the places where it hurts now.<br>1. Your head?<br>2. Your face?<br>3. Your neck?<br>4. Your chest?<br>5. Your abdomen?<br>6. Your back?<br>7. Your lower back?<br>8. Your arms?<br>    Your upper limbs?<br>9. Your legs?<br>    Your lower limbs? |

---

### 名句・ことわざ

**In the case of our habits we are only masters of the beginning, their growth by gradual stages being imperceptible, like the growth of disease.**

習慣に関しては，われわれはまだ初心者にすぎないが，病気が拡がるのと同様に，習慣は徐々に形成され知覚できぬものである

古代ギリシャの哲学者アリストテレス（Aristotle, 384-322 B.C., *Ethics*）の名言．私たちは日々繰り返す習慣によって作られる――この言葉は現代の生活習慣病を予言している．

# 用語・表現ファイル

## 診療部門

| 診療科 | Clinical Division [Department] |
|---|---|
| 総合診療科 | General Medicine |
| 内科 | Internal Medicine |
| 　一般内科 | General Internal Medicine |
| 　呼吸器内科 | Pulmonology |
| 　循環器内科 | Cardiology |
| 　消化器内科 | Gastroenterology |
| 　代謝・内分泌内科 | Metabolism and Endocrinology |
| 　腎臓内科 | Nephrology |
| 　神経内科 | Neurology [Neuroscience] |
| 　血液内科 | Hematology |
| 　リウマチ内科 | Rheumatology |
| 　老年内科 | Geriatrics |
| 　心療内科 | Psychosomatic Medicine |
| 　腫瘍内科 | Oncology |
| 外科 | Surgery |
| 　一般外科 | General Surgery |
| 　心臓血管外科 | Cardiovascular Surgery |
| 　呼吸器外科 | Thoracic Surgery |
| 　消化器外科 | Gastroenterological Surgery |
| 　乳腺・内分泌外科 | Breast and Endocrine Surgery |
| 　脳神経外科 | Neurosurgery |
| 　整形外科 | Orthopedics |
| 　形成外科 | Plastic Surgery |
| 　小児外科 | Pediatric Surgery |
| 小児科 | Pediatrics |
| 産科 | Obstetrics |
| 婦人科 | Gynecology |
| 泌尿器科 | Urology |
| 精神科 | Psychiatry |
| 眼科 | Ophthalmology |
| 耳鼻咽喉科 | Otorhinolaryngology ENT (Ear, Nose, and Throat) |

## 用語・表現ファイル（つづき）

| | |
|---|---|
| 皮膚科 | Dermatology |
| 緩和ケア科 | Palliative Care |
| 放射線科 | Radiology |
| 麻酔科 | Anesthesiology |
| 病理診断科 | Diagnostic Pathology |
| 歯科 | Dentistry |
| 口腔外科 | Oral (and Maxillofacial) Surgery |
| 遺伝子診療部 | Medical Genetics |
| 救急部 | Emergency and Critical Care |
| リハビリテーション科 | Rehabilitation |
| **健診センター** | Health Screening Center |

## 系統別レビュー

### 1 眼

☞「眼の診察」(217 ページ).

#### 一般的な質問

目の具合が悪いのですか.
- ☐ (Do you have) any problems with your eyes?
- ☐ (Is there) anything wrong with your eyes?

―どんな問題ですか.
― What kind of problems?

それはどのくらい続いていますか.
- ☐ How long have you had the problems?

―いつからですか.
― Since when?

このような問題は以前にもありましたか.
- ☐ Have you had these problems before?

☞「病歴をとるためのヒント」(22 ページ).

#### 視力・視野

最近, 物が見えにくいですか.
- ☐ Have you had difficulty looking at things recently?

―どちらの目ですか.
1. 右目.
2. 左目.
3. 両目.

― Which eye?
1. Right?
2. Left?
3. Both eyes?

あなたは…見えますか.
1. 物がぼやけて
2. 目がかすんで
3. 物が二重に
4. 物がゆがんで

- ☐ Is your vision...
  1. cloudy?
  2. blurred [blurry]?
  3. double?
  4. distorted?

…が見えにくいですか.
1. 近くの物
2. 遠くの物

- ☐ Do you have difficulty seeing...
  1. things close at hand?
  2. things at a distance?

| 近視ですか〔近視と言われたことがありますか〕. | ☐ Are you〔Have you ever been told that you are〕near-sighted? |

| 遠視ですか〔遠視と言われたことがありますか〕. | ☐ Are you〔Have you ever been told that you are〕far-sighted? |

| 乱視ですか〔乱視と言われたことがありますか〕. | ☐ Do you have〔Have you ever been told that you have〕astigmatism? |

あなたは…を使用していますか.
1. 眼鏡
2. コンタクトレンズ
    a. ハードレンズ
    b. ソフトレンズ
―どの程度使用していますか.
1. いつも.
2. 必要におうじて.
    a. 細かい作業のため.
    b. 読書用に.
    c. 遠くを見るため.
    d. 運転用に.
    e. その他の目的のため.
―どのくらい長く使用していますか. いつから.
―最近, 眼鏡が合わなくなったと感じますか.

☐ Do you wear...
1. glasses?
2. contact lenses?
    a. hard contact lenses?
    b. soft contact lenses?
— How much do you wear them?
1. All the time?
2. For certain activities?
    a. For close work?
    b. For reading?
    c. For distance?
    d. For driving?
    e. For other purposes?
— How long have you worn them? Since when?
— Do you recently feel that your glasses don't work for you any more?

最近では, いつ視力検査を受けましたか.

☐ When was the last time you had a vision test?

視野が狭くなっていますか.

☐ Has your visual field narrowed?

あなたは…にある物が見えにくいですか.
1. 右側
2. 左側
3. 中心部
4. 周辺部

☐ Do you have difficulty seeing things that are ...
1. to the right?
2. to the left?
3. in the middle?
4. in the area around your eyes?

5. その他

目の前に…が見えますか．

1. 浮遊性の斑点［ゴミの糸くずのようなもの］
2. 黒い点
3. 電灯の周囲に虹のような輪
4. ぱっと走るような光
5. ちらちらする光

物が小さく見えますか．

夜見えにくいですか．

### 目の痛み

☞「痛みの表現」(31 ページ)．

目が痛みますか．

どんな痛みですか．

1. ずきずきする（拍動性の）．
2. 針で刺すような．
3. 焼けるような．

目の奥が痛みますか．

頻繁に頭痛や肩こりがありますか．

### 目のかゆみ・目やに・涙

目が…

---

5. in other areas?

☐ Do you see...in front of your eyes?
1. floaters [specks like waste threads]
2. a dark spot
3. rainbow-like halos around lights
4. flashing lights
5. flickering lights

☐ Do things appear small?

☐ Do you have difficulty seeing at night?

☐ Do you have any pain in your eyes?

☐ What is the pain like?
☐ Can you describe the pain for me?
1. Throbbing?
2. Stinging?
3. Burning?

☐ Do you feel pain at the back of your eyes?

☐ Do you have frequent headaches or stiff shoulders?

☐ Do your eyes feel...

1. かゆいですか．
2. ひりひりしますか．
3. 焼けるようですか．

1. itchy?
2. irritated?
3. burning?

目やにが出ますか．

☐ Do you have any discharge from your eyes?

涙がたくさん出ますか．

☐ Do your eyes water a lot?
Do you have watery [teary] eyes?

目が乾いている感じですか．

☐ Do your eyes feel dry?

その症状はある決まった季節に起こりますか．
1. 春．
2. 夏．
3. 秋．
4. 冬．

☐ Does the problem usually occur in specific seasons of the year?
1. In the spring?
2. In the summer?
3. In the fall?
4. In the winter?

### 目の中の異物

目に何かが入ったのですか．

☐ Have you got something in your eye(s)?

今，目の中に異物がある感じがしますか．

☐ Do you feel as if something is in your eye(s)?

目がごろごろしますか．

☐ Does your eye [Do your eyes] feel gritty?

### その他の症状

目の動きを調節しにくいですか．

☐ Do you have difficulty controlling your eye movements?

1. 目を開けにくい．
2. 目を閉じにくい．

1. Difficulty opening your eyes?
2. Difficulty closing your eyes?

| 光がまぶしいですか. | ☐ Do you have problems with glare? |
| --- | --- |
| | ☐ Does light [sun] bother your eyes? |
| 目の疲れがありますか. | ☐ Have you got eyestrain? |
| 目がすぐ疲れますか. | ☐ Do your eyes get tired easily? |
| 色の区別がつきにくいですか. | ☐ Do you have difficulty discerning colors? |
| まぶたが腫れていますか. | ☐ Do you have swelling in your eyelids? |

そのほかの徴候や症状がありますか.
―それは何ですか.
  1. 頭痛.
  2. めまい.
  3. 吐き気.
  4. その他.

☐ Do you have any other signs or symptoms?
― What are they?
  1. Headache?
  2. Dizziness?
  3. Nausea?
  4. Any other symptoms?

### 既往歴・家族歴

これまでに目の病気にかかったことがありますか.
―どのような異常でしたか.
―いつですか.
―どんな治療を受けましたか.

☐ Have you ever had an eye disease?
― What kind of problem was it?
― When did it occur?
― How was it treated?

これまでに…にかかったことがありますか.
  1. 花粉症
  2. 糖尿病
  3. 高血圧

☐ Have you ever had...
  1. hay fever?
  2. diabetes?
  3. high blood pressure?

これまでに目の怪我や手術をしたことがありますか.

☐ Have you ever had an eye injury or eye surgery?

―どのような怪我〔手術〕でしたか. ― What kind of injury 〔surgery〕 was it?

―いつですか. ― When did it occur?

―どんな治療を受けましたか. ― How was it treated?

家族の中に目の病気の人はいますか. ☐ Does anyone in your immediate family have eye diseases?
―それは何ですか. ― What are they?
　1. 緑内障.　　　　　　　　　　　1. Glaucoma?
　2. 白内障.　　　　　　　　　　　2. Cataract?
　3. 盲目.　　　　　　　　　　　　3. Blindness?
　4. 色覚異常.　　　　　　　　　　4. Color blindness?

家族の中で，あなたと同じ症状の人はいますか. ☐ Does anyone in your immediate family have similar symptoms?

---

### 名句・ことわざ

#### The eyes are the window of the soul.

#### 目は心の窓

"The eye is the window of the heart [mind]." あるいは "The face is the index of the mind." ともいう．日本では「目は心の鏡」という中国由来の名句がある．

## 2 耳鼻咽喉・頸部

☞「めまい」(43 ページ).

### 一般的な質問

| | |
|---|---|
| 耳〔鼻／のど／口／頸〕の具合が悪いのですか. | ☐ (Do you have) any problems with your ears〔nose/throat/mouth/neck〕? |
| | ☐ (Is there) anything wrong with your ears〔nose/throat/mouth/neck〕? |
| ―どんな問題ですか. | ― What kind of problems? |
| それはどのくらい続いていますか. | ☐ How long have you had the problems? |
| ―いつからですか. | ― Since when? |
| このような問題は以前にもありましたか. | ☐ Have you ever had these problems before? |

☞「病歴をとるためのヒント」(22 ページ).

### 耳

☞「耳の診察」(219 ページ).

#### ▶ 聴力

| | |
|---|---|
| 聴力に何か問題がありますか. | ☐ Do you have difficulty hearing? |
| ―どちら側［どちらの耳］ですか. | ― Which side〔ear〕? |
| 　1. 右. | 　1. Right? |
| 　2. 左. | 　2. Left? |
| 　3. 両側［両耳］. | 　3. Both sides〔ears〕? |
| 耳が遠くなりましたか. | ☐ Are you hard of hearing? |
| ―どういう音が聞こえにくいですか. | ― What kind of sounds do you have difficulty hearing? |
| 　1. かん高い音［高音］のみ. | 　1. Only high-pitched sounds? |
| 　2. 低音のみ. | 　2. Only low-pitched sounds? |
| 　3. あらゆる音. | 　3. All sounds? |

| | |
|---|---|
| 耳がふさがった〔つまった〕感じですか. | ☐ Do you feel as if your ears are blocked up〔clogged up〕? |
| 自分の声が響く感じがしますか. | ☐ Do you feel that your own voice vibrates? |
| 補聴器をつけていますか.<br>—どのくらい長くつけていますか.<br>　いつから. | ☐ Do you wear a hearing aid?<br>— How long have you worn it? Since when? |
| 最近では, いつ聴力検査を受けましたか. | ☐ When was the last time you had a hearing test? |
| 騒音にさらされた経験がありますか. | ☐ Have you ever been exposed to loud noise? |
| いつも大きい音の音楽を聴いていますか. | ☐ Do you regularly listen to loud music? |
| 服用している, または最近服用した薬はありますか. | ☐ Are you taking or have you recently taken any drugs or medications? |

### ▶ 耳鳴

| | |
|---|---|
| 耳鳴りがしますか.<br><br>—どんな音ですか.<br>　1. 警笛, キーという音などの高音ですか.<br>　2. 遠くで聞こえる雷, 怒って唸る犬の声などの低音ですか. | ☐ Do you have ringing in your ear(s)?<br>— What is it like?<br>　1. High-pitched sounds, such as whistling or screeching?<br>　2. Low-pitched sounds, such as a far-away thunder or growling of a dog? |
| 雑音は気になりますか. | ☐ Does noise bother you? |

### ▶ 耳痛・耳漏・かゆみ

| | |
|---|---|
| 耳や耳の周囲が痛みますか. | ☐ Do you have earaches or pain in or around your ear(s)? |

―物を噛むとき痛みますか. — Does it hurt you when you chew something?

☞「痛みの表現」(31 ページ).

耳だれがありますか. ☐ Do you have any discharge from your ear (s)?

耳がかゆいですか. ☐ Are your ears〔Is your ear〕itchy?

### ▶ 既往歴

これまでに耳の病気にかかったことがありますか.
―どんな異常でしたか.
―いつですか.
―どんな治療を受けましたか.

☐ Have you ever had an ear problem [disease]?
— What kind of problem was it?
— When did it occur?
— How was it treated?

よく風邪をひきますか. ☐ Do you often have colds?

最近, 風邪やインフルエンザの症状はありましたか. ☐ Have you recently had cold or flu symptoms?

鼓膜が破れたことがありますか. ☐ Have you ever had a ruptured eardrum?

水泳後に耳の感染症にかかったことがありますか. ☐ Have you ever had swimmer's ear?

耳栓をしましたか. ☐ Have you had tubes in your ears?

最近, 飛行機に乗りましたか. ☐ Have you recently ridden an airplane?

耳に, 思い当たるような傷を負ったことがありますか.
 1. 耳掻き.
 2. 平手で叩かれる.

☐ Have you ever had any ear injury that you can identify?
 1. Picking your ear (s)?
 2. Having your ear (s) slapped?

3. 耳に尖った物を入れる.

3. Sticking a sharp object in your ear(s)?

### 鼻

☞「鼻の診察」(220 ページ).

#### ▶ 鼻汁・鼻閉

鼻水がたくさん出ますか.

- [ ] Does your nose run a lot?
- [ ] Do you have a lot of discharge from your nose?

—どんな鼻汁ですか.
1. 水っぽい［水様性］.
2. 薄くてサラサラしている.
3. 粘液性でネバネバしている.
4. 膿のよう.

— What is it like?
1. Watery?
2. Thin?
3. Thick?
4. Like pus?

—どんな色をしていますか.
1. 透明.
2. 白色.
3. 黄色.
4. 緑色.
5. 血性.
6. その他の色.

— What color is it?
1. Clear［Colorless］?
2. White?
3. Yellow?
4. Green?
5. Bloody?
6. Any other color?

—悪臭がしますか.

— Is there any bad smell coming from your nose?

鼻汁は喉のほうにたれますか.

- [ ] Does nasal mucus drain into your throat?
- [ ] Do you have postnasal drip?

鼻はかゆい，あるいはむずむずしますか.

- [ ] Does your nose feel itchy or irritated?

くしゃみがよく出ますか.

- [ ] Do you sneeze a lot?

その症状はある決まった季節に起こりますか.
1. 春.
2. 夏.

- [ ] Does the problem usually occur in specific seasons of the year?
1. In the spring?
2. In the summer?

| | |
|---|---|
| 3. 秋. | 3. In the fall? |
| 4. 冬. | 4. In the winter? |
| 5. 梅雨期. | 5. In the rainy season? |

よく鼻がつまりますか.

☐ Do you often have a stuffy nose?
☐ Does your nose get stuffy frequently?

鼻で息をするのが苦しいですか.

☐ Do you have difficulty breathing through your nose?

### ▶ 鼻出血

鼻血が出ますか.
1. いつも決まった側からですか.
2. 両側からですか.

☐ Do you have nosebleeds?
1. Always from the same side?
2. From both sides?

鼻血は毎回どのくらい続きますか.

1. 1分以内.
2. 2, 3分.
3. もっと長く.

How long do they last each time?
1. Less than a minute?
2. A few minutes?
3. Longer?

どのくらいの頻度で起こりますか.
1. 頻繁に.
2. それほど頻繁ではなく.
3. めったに起こらない.

How often do you have them?
1. Often [Frequently]?
2. Not so often [Infrequently]?
3. Rarely?

何か思い当たる誘因はありますか.

☐ What do you think is causing them?
☐ Is there any cause that you can identify?

1. 鼻をほじる.
2. 鼻をかむ.
3. 飲酒.
4. 風邪をひいた.
5. 外傷.

1. Picking your nose?
2. Blowing your nose?
3. Drinking alcohol?
4. Having had a cold?
5. Having had an injury to your nose?

| 高血圧，肝疾患などの既往がありますか． | ☐ Do you have a history of high blood pressure, liver disease, or any other health problems? |

出血傾向がありますか． ☐ Do you bleed easily?

### ▶ 鼻の痛み・潰瘍

鼻が痛みますか． ☐ Do you have any pain in your nose?

鼻の中に潰瘍〔傷〕ができていますか．
—どんなものですか．

1. やわらかい．
2. 硬い．
3. かさぶた状．

☐ Do you have any ulcers 〔lesions〕 in your nose?
— What are they like?
Can you describe them for me?
1. Soft?
2. Hard?
3. Crusty?

### ▶ 嗅覚

においはよくわかりますか．

☐ Can you smell things accurately?
☐ Do you have a good sense of smell?

最近，嗅覚に変化がありましたか．

—どんな変化ですか．
1. 嗅覚を失った［においがわからなくなった］．
2. 変な〔不快な〕においがする．

☐ Have you recently had any changes in your sense of smell?
— What kind of change is it?
1. Have you lost your sense of smell?
2. Do you have a sensation of odd〔unpleasant〕odors?

### ▶ 既往歴

これまでに鼻の病気にかかったことがありますか．
—どんな異常でしたか．
1. 鼻アレルギー．

☐ Have you ever had a nose problem [disease]?
— What kind of problem was it?
1. Nasal allergy?

| | |
|---|---|
| 2. 副鼻腔炎. | 2. Sinusitis? |
| 3. 花粉症. | 3. Hay fever? |
| —いつですか. | — When did it occur? |
| —どんな治療を受けましたか. | — How was it treated? |

よく風邪をひきますか.　　☐ Do you often have colds?

### 咽喉頭

☞「咽喉の診察」(220 ページ).

#### ▶ 咽頭痛・不快感

のどが痛みますか.

☐ Do you have a sore throat?

痛むのは…ですか.
1. いつも
2. 食べたり飲んだりするとき
3. 話すとき
4. 息をするだけでも

☐ Does it hurt...
1. all the time?
2. when you eat or drink?
3. when you talk?
4. even on breathing?

どんな痛みですか

☐ What is the pain like?
☐ Can you describe the pain for me?

1. ひりひりする.
2. 焼けるような.
3. 針で刺すような.
4. チクチクうずく.
5. 圧迫されたときの痛み.

1. Pricking?
2. Burning?
3. Stinging?
4. Tingling?
5. Tenderness?

のどに不快感がありますか.

☐ Do you feel discomfort in your throat?
☐ Does your throat feel uncomfortable?

—どんな感じがしますか.

— What is it like?
　Can you describe it for me?

1. つかえたような.
2. むずがゆい.
3. 乾燥した.
4. いがらっぽい.

1. Tight?
2. Itchy?
3. Dry?
4. Irritated?

| | |
|---|---|
| 何か思い当たる誘因はありますか. | ☐ What do you think is causing it? |
| | ☐ Is there any cause that you can identify? |
| 1. 風邪をひいている. | 1. A cold? |
| 2. 魚の骨や，鶏肉の骨がのどに突き刺さった，ひっかかった. | 2. A fish bone or a chicken bone stuck or got caught in your throat? |
| 3. タバコを吸いすぎた. | 3. Smoking heavily? |

### ▶ 嗄声

| | |
|---|---|
| 声がかれますか. | ☐ Do you get hoarse? |
| —声が出ないことがありますか. | — Do you ever lose your voice? |
| —話をするのがつらいですか. | — Do you have difficulty speaking? |
| 声がれはどのくらい続いていますか. | ☐ How long has your voice been hoarse? |
| 声を使い過ぎていますか. | ☐ Have you been using your voice excessively? |
| 声に変化がありましたか. | ☐ Has your voice changed? |
| —どんな変化ですか. | — What kind of change is it? |
| 1. いつもより高い. | 1. Higher? |
| 2. いつもより低い. | 2. Lower? |
| 3. いつもより声が弱い. | 3. Weaker? |
| 4. 声がしわがれる. | 4. Hoarse [Husky]? |
| 5. かすれる. | 5. Scratchy? |
| 6. その他. | 6. Any other change? |
| 最近，風邪をひきましたか. | ☐ Have you recently had a cold? |
| 声をよく使う職業ですか. | ☐ Do you use your voice a lot in your work? |
| タバコを吸いますか. | ☐ Do you smoke? |
| —どのくらい長く吸ってきましたか. | — How long have you been smoking? |
| —何年間〔何歳から〕ですか. | — For how many years〔Since you were how old〕? |

chapter 3　現病歴（耳鼻咽喉・頸部）

| | |
|---|---|
| ― 1 日に何本〔何箱〕吸いますか. | ― How many cigarettes〔packs of cigarettes〕do you smoke a day? |

### 頸部

☞「頭頸の診察」(217 ページ).

| | |
|---|---|
| 首にしこりや腫れているところがありますか. | ☐ Do you have any lumps or swellings on your neck? |
| ―どこですか. | ― Where? |
| 　1. 首の両側. | 　1. On both sides of the neck? |
| 　2. 首の前側. | 　2. On the front of the neck? |
| ―腫脹は反復性,再発性ですか. | ― Is it recurrent? Does it clear up and then recur〔come back〕? |
| 腫れは… | ☐ Is the swelling... |
| 　1. 大きくなっていますか. | 　1. growing〔getting bigger〕? |
| 　2. ひいてきていますか. | 　2. decreasing〔getting smaller〕? |
| 　3. 変化なしですか. | 　3. the same? |
| 痛みはありますか. | ☐ Do you have any pain? |
| ―そこを押すと痛みますか. | ― Is the area tender? |
| 食事との関連はありますか. | ☐ Is the swelling affected by meals? |
| ―食後悪化する傾向がありますか. | ― Does it often get worse after eating? Is it likely to get worse after meals? |
| しこりや腫れのほかに徴候や症状がありますか. | ☐ Do you have any other signs or symptoms? |
| ―それは何ですか. | ― What are they? |
| 　1. 熱. | 　1. Fever? |
| 　2. 動悸. | 　2. Palpitations? |
| 　3. 頻脈. | 　3. Rapid heart rate? |
| 　4. 多汗. | 　4. Profuse sweating? |
| 　5. 手指の震え. | 　5. Trembling and shaking of hands and fingers? |

6. 倦怠感.
7. むくみ.
8. 便秘.
9. 寒がり.

6. Sense of fatigue?
7. Edema?
8. Constipation?
9. Sensitivity to (the) cold?

## 3 歯・口腔

☞口腔内の症状は「耳鼻咽喉・頸部」(60 ページ).
☞「咽喉の診察」(220 ページ).

### 一般的な質問

歯〔顎／口〕の具合が悪いのですか.
- □ (Do you have) any problems with your teeth〔jaw/mouth〕?
- □ (Is there) anything wrong with your teeth〔jaw/mouth〕?

—どんな問題ですか. — What kind of problems?

それはどのくらい続いていますか.
- □ How long have you had the problems?

—いつからですか. — Since when?

このような問題は以前にもありましたか.
- □ Have you had these problems before?

☞「病歴をとるためのヒント」(22 ページ).

### 歯痛・炎症

☞「痛みの表現」(31 ページ).

歯が痛みますか.
—どの歯が痛みますか.
—歯茎が痛みますか.
- □ Do you have a toothache?
- — Which tooth hurts?
- — Do you have pain in your gums?

痛み始めたのはいつですか.
- □ When did you first get this pain?
- □ When did this pain start?

どんな痛みですか.
- □ What is the pain like?
- □ Can you describe the pain for me?

1. 鈍痛.
2. 軽い.
3. 強い [激しい].
4. ずきずきする.
5. 鋭く走るような.

1. Dull ache?
2. Mild?
3. Severe?
4. Throbbing?
5. Shooting?

6. その他.

6. Any other kind of pain?

歯は…痛み〔しみ〕ますか.
1. 冷たいものを飲むとき
2. 熱いものを飲むとき
3. 甘いものを食べるとき
4. 噛むとき
5. 歯を磨くとき

☐ Does it hurt〔smart〕...
1. when you drink cold liquids?
2. when you drink hot liquids?
3. when you eat sweets?
4. when you chew?
5. when you brush your teeth?

虫歯がありますか.

☐ Do you have tooth decay?

ぐらぐらする歯がありますか.

☐ Does any of your teeth feel loose?

歯茎がただれていますか.

☐ Are your gums sore?

歯茎がどこか腫れていますか.

☐ Are the gums around any of your teeth swollen?

歯を磨くと歯茎から出血しますか.

☐ Do your gums bleed when you brush your teeth?

### 顎の痛み

顎が痛みますか.

☐ Do you have pain in your jaw?

初めて気づいたのはいつですか.

☐ When did you first notice the pain?

どんな痛みですか.

☐ What is the pain like?
☐ Can you describe the pain for me?

―口を開けると痛みますか.

― Does it hurt when you open your mouth?

―物を噛むとき痛みますか.

― Does it hurt when you chew something?

口を開けにくいですか.

☐ Do you have difficulty opening your mouth?

| | |
|---|---|
| あごを動かすとコキンという音がしますか. | ☐ Do you notice your jaw clicking? |

## 口腔

### ▶ 口腔粘膜・舌の炎症

| | |
|---|---|
| 口の中や周りに斑点〔潰瘍／傷／腫れ〕がありますか. | ☐ Do you have patches〔ulcers/lesions/a swelling〕in or around your mouth? |
| ―どこですか. | ― Where? |
| 　1. 口の中. | 　1. Inside your mouth? |
| 　2. 口角. | 　2. On the corners of your mouth? |
| 　3. 舌. | 　3. On your tongue? |
| 　4. 唇やその周辺. | 　4. On or around your lips? |
| 　5. 歯茎. | 　5. On your gums? |
| ―潰瘍は再発性ですか. | ― Is the ulcer recurrent? Does the ulcer clear up and then recur〔come back〕? |
| ―場所は一定ですか. | ― Is it always in the same place? |
| | |
| 痛みますか. | ☐ Is it painful? |
| ―どんな痛みですか. | ― What is the pain like? |
| ―食べたり飲んだりするのがつらいですか. | ― Do you have difficulty eating or drinking? |
| ―口を開けると痛みますか. | ― Does it hurt when you open your mouth? |
| | |
| 未治療の虫歯，治療したばかりの歯はありますか. | ☐ Do you have untreated tooth decay or teeth that have been recently treated? |
| | |
| 口〔舌〕は…いますか〔ですか〕. | ☐ Does your mouth〔tongue〕feel... |
| 　1. 乾燥して | 　1. dry? |
| 　2. しびれて | 　2. numb? |
| 　3. 苔がはえているよう | 　3. furry? |
| 　4. ひりひり痛む感じ | 　4. burning? |
| 　5. ざらざらして［荒れて］ | 　5. sandy［rough］? |

唇は…いますか．
1. 乾燥して
2. 荒れて

☐ Are your lips...
1. dry?
2. rough?

規則正しい食生活をしていますか．
―バランスのとれた食事をしていますか．

☐ Do you eat at regular times?
― Do you eat well-balanced meals?

服用している，または最近服用した薬はありますか．

☐ Are you taking or have you recently taken any drugs or medications?

▶ 味覚

味覚に何か変化が起きましたか．

―どんな変化ですか．
1. 味がわからなくなっている．
2. 実際には食べていない物の味がする．
3. ふだん食べ慣れた物の味が変だったり，違ったりする．

☐ Have you had any changes in your taste?
― What kind of change is it?
1. Do you think you are losing your sense of taste?
2. Do you taste foods you are not eating?
3. Do you find foods that normally taste good to be unpleasant or different?

あなたは…がわかりますか．
1. 甘い味
2. 苦い味
3. 酸っぱい味
4. 塩味

☐ Can you tell...taste?
1. sweet
2. bitter
3. sour
4. salty

規則正しい食生活をしていますか．
―バランスのとれた食事をしていますか．

☐ Do you eat at regular times?
― Do you eat well-balanced meals?

服用している，または最近服用した薬はありますか．

1. 抗リウマチ薬．
2. 抗パーキンソン薬．

☐ Are you taking or have you recently taken any drugs or medications?
1. Antirheumatics?
2. Antiparkinsons?

| | |
|---|---|
| 3. 血圧降下薬. | 3. Antihypertensives? |
| 糖尿病はありますか. | ☐ Do you have diabetes? |

### ▶ 唾液

唾液の量が，以前と比べて…
1. 増えましたか.
2. 減りましたか.

☐ Do you have...than you used to?
1. more saliva
2. less saliva

口〔舌〕は乾燥していますか.

☐ Does your mouth〔tongue〕feel dry?

のどはよく渇きますか.

☐ Are you often thirsty?

虫歯がありますか.

☐ Do you have tooth decay?

目も乾燥しやすいですか.
―ごろごろしやすいですか.

☐ Do your eyes often feel dry, too?
— Do they often feel sandy?

服用している，または最近服用した薬はありますか.

1. 抗ヒスタミン薬.
2. 利尿薬.
3. 抗不安薬.
4. 抗うつ薬.
5. 抗パーキンソン薬.

☐ Are you taking or have you recently taken any drugs or medications?

1. Antihistamines?
2. Diuretics?
3. Antianxiety drugs?
4. Antidepressants?
5. Antiparkinsons?

### ▶ 口臭

口臭が気になりますか.

☐ Do you worry about having bad breath?

―自分で感じるのですか.
―人から指摘されたのですか.

— Do you smell it yourself?
— Have you been told that you have bad breath?

虫歯や歯周病などはありますか.

☐ Do you have tooth decay or periodontitis?

| | |
|---|---|
| 鼻や副鼻腔の病気を指摘されたことはありますか. | ☐ Have you ever been told that you have a nose disease or sinusitis? |
| 気道や肺の病気はありますか. | ☐ Do you have airway or lung diseases? |
| 胃腸は弱いほうですか. | ☐ Do you have poor digestion [stomach problems]? |

### その他

| | |
|---|---|
| 歯科医へ定期的に通っていますか. | ☐ Do you go to a dentist regularly? |
| 最近では，いつ歯科医に行きましたか. | ☐ When did you last see your dentist? |
| 最近，歯を抜きましたか. | ☐ Have you had any of your teeth pulled recently? |
| ―いつのことですか. | ― When was it? |
| 最近，歯をぶつけましたか. | ☐ Have you bumped your teeth recently? |
| 入れ歯をしていますか. | ☐ Do you wear dentures? |
| ―入れ歯が合わないと感じますか. | ― Do you feel that your dentures don't fit you any more? |
| 口内炎はよくできますか．どこですか． | ☐ Do you often have inflammation of the mouth? Where? |
| ―場所を指でさして教えて下さい． | ― Please point to the place. |
| 睡眠中歯ぎしりをすると言われたことがありますか． | ☐ Have you ever been told that you grind your teeth during sleep? |
| 歯の麻酔はしたことがありますか． | ☐ Have you ever had dental anesthesia? |
| ―その時何か異常〔アレルギー〕はありましたか． | ― Did you have any problem [Were you allergic to it] then? |

## 4 呼吸器

☞「胸痛」(32 ページ).
☞「胸背部の診察」(222 ページ).

### 一般的な質問

呼吸をするのに何か問題がありますか.
- ☐ (Do you have) any problems with your breathing?
- ☐ (Is there) anything wrong with your breathing?

―どんな問題ですか.
― What kind of problems?

それはどのくらい続いていますか.
- ☐ How long have you had the problems?

―いつからですか.
― Since when?

このような問題は以前にもありましたか.
- ☐ Have you had these problems before?

☞「病歴をとるためのヒント」(22 ページ).

### 咳・痰

咳が出ますか.
- ☐ Do you cough a lot?

どんな咳ですか.
- ☐ What does your cough sound like?
  1. Dry?
  2. Productive?
  3. Wheezy?
  4. Hacking?
  5. Barking?
  6. Spasmodic?

  1. 空咳.
  2. 痰がからむ咳.
  3. ゼイゼイする咳.
  4. コンコンする空咳.
  5. 犬が吠えるような咳.
  6. 発作的な咳.

咳の程度はどうですか.
  1. ものすごく激しい.
  2. 激しい.
  3. ほどほどの [中程度].
  4. 軽い.
  5. 少々の.
- ☐ How bad is your cough?
  1. Violent?
  2. Severe?
  3. Moderate?
  4. Mild?
  5. Slight?

1日のある決まった時間帯に出ますか．それはいつですか．
1. 朝．
2. 日中．
3. 夜．
4. 睡眠中．
5. 明け方近く．

☐ Do you usually cough at a certain time of day?  What time of day do you cough?
1. In the morning?
2. During the day?
3. At night?
4. During sleep?
5. Toward daybreak?

どういうときに出ますか，ひどくなりますか．
1. 外出時，帰宅時などの温度変化時．
2. 仕事中．
3. 会話中．
4. 食事中．
5. 運動中．

☐ In what situations is your cough brought on or made worse?
1. At the time of temperature change, such as when going out or coming home?
2. During work?
3. During a conversation?
4. During a meal?
5. During exercise?

咳はどのくらい長く続いていますか．
1. 2, 3〔5, 6〕日．
2. 2, 3 週間．
3. 2, 3 か月．
4. 2, 3 年．

☐ How long have you had the cough?
1. A few〔Several〕days?
2. A few weeks?
3. A few months?
4. A few years?

どのくらいの頻度で咳が出ますか．
1. 頻繁に．
2. さほど頻繁ではなく．
3. 時々．

☐ How often do you cough?
1. Often [Frequently]?
2. Not so often [Infrequently]?
3. Occasionally [Once in a while]?

咳をすると痰が出ますか．

☐ Do you cough up sputum [phlegm]?

痰の量は1日にどのくらい出ますか．
1. 多量．
2. ごく少量．

☐ How much do you cough up each day?
1. A lot [Abundant]?
2. A little bit [A small amount]?

それはどんな痰ですか．
1. どろどろした．
2. さらさらした．
3. ねばねばした［粘性の］．
4. 泡状の．
5. 膿のような．
6. 線状の血が混じっている．

どんな色をしていますか．
1. 透明か白い．
2. 緑色の．
3. 黄色味を帯びている．
4. ピンクがかっている．
5. 赤さび色の．
6. 赤い．
7. 灰色の．

どんなにおいの痰ですか．悪臭がしますか．

血痰が出ますか．

1. 鮮血．
2. 暗赤色．
—血液はどんな混じり方ですか．

1. 点状．
2. 線状．
3. 全体．

咳や痰のほかに徴候や症状がありますか．
—それは何ですか．
1. 胸痛．
2. 胸焼け．
3. 鼻水，鼻づまりなど副鼻腔の症状．
4. 発熱．
5. 喘鳴．

☐ What kind of sputum is it?
1. Thick?
2. Thin?
3. Sticky [Viscous]?
4. Frothy [Foamy]?
5. Like pus?
6. Blood-streaked?

☐ What color is it?
1. Clear or white?
2. Green?
3. Yellowish?
4. Pinkish?
5. Reddish brown?
6. Red?
7. Gray?

☐ How does it smell? Is it foul-smelling?

☐ Do you cough up bloody sputum?
1. Bright red blood?
2. Dark-colored blood?
— How is the blood mixed in with the sputum?
1. Stained?
2. Streaky?
3. All over?

☐ Do you have any other signs or symptoms?
— What are they?
1. Chest pain?
2. Heartburns?
3. Sinus troubles, such as a runny nose or a stuffy nose?
4. Fever?
5. Wheeziness?

| 最近，風邪やインフルエンザの症状がありましたか． | ☐ Have you recently had cold or flu symptoms? |

血圧の薬を常用していますか．
―それは何ですか．

☐ Are you taking any medications for your blood pressure?
― What are they?

### 息切れ

息切れしますか．

☐ Do you get short of breath?
☐ Do you have shortness of breath?

息をするのが苦しいですか．

☐ Do you have difficulty breathing?

息切れしないで健康な人と同じスピードで階段を上がる〔歩く〕ことができますか．

―休まないで何メートル歩けますか．

☐ Can you climb stairs〔walk〕at the same speed as other healthy people without getting short of breath?
― How many meters can you walk without taking any rest?

仰向けに寝るとひどくなりますか．

―座ると楽になりますか．

―昨晩は横になって眠れましたか，それとも，座ったままか，枕を背に当てて寝ましたか．

☐ Do you find breathing more difficult lying flat on your back?
― Do you find breathing easier sitting upright?
― Were you able to sleep lying in bed last night, or did you sleep sitting up or propped up by pillows in an upright position?

家庭や仕事上のストレスが呼吸に影響していますか．

☐ Does stress at home or work affect your breathing?

息切れが起こるのはたいていいつですか．
  1. 早朝．
  2. 日中．
  3. 夜間．

☐ What time of day do you usually get short of breath?
  1. Early in the morning?
  2. During the day?
  3. During the night?

chapter 3 現病歴（呼吸器）

どんなとき息切れしますか.

1. 座っているとき.
2. 立っているとき.
3. 横になっているとき.
4. 歩いているとき.
5. 階段〔坂〕を登っているとき.
6. 走っているとき.
7. 入浴しているとき.
8. 運動しているとき.
9. 休息しているとき.
10. 気が動転しているとき.

息切れし始めたのは…ですか.

1. つい最近
2. かなり前から

息切れは…
1. よくなっていますか.
2. 悪化していますか.
3. 変わりませんか.

息切れのほかに徴候や症状がありますか.
—それは何ですか.
1. 胸痛.
2. 血痰や泡状の痰が出る.
3. 唇, 爪など皮膚が青みを帯びる.
4. むくみ.
5. 喘鳴.
6. 意識がもうろうとする.
7. 手足のしびれ.

☐ In what situations do you get short of breath?
1. When you are sitting?
2. When you are standing?
3. When you are lying down?
4. When you are walking?
5. When you are climbing stairs 〔slopes〕?
6. When you are running?
7. When you are taking a bath?
8. When you are exercising?
9. When you are resting?
10. When you are upset?

☐ Have you had your shortness of breath...
1. just recently?
2. since some time ago?

☐ Is it...
1. getting better?
2. getting worse?
3. the same?

☐ Do you have any other signs or symptoms?
— What are they?
1. Chest pain?
2. Coughing up bloody or frothy sputum [phlegm]?
3. Bluish color of the skin, such as blue lips or blue fingernails?
4. Swelling?
5. Wheeziness?
6. Feeling confused?
7. Numbness in your arms and legs?

### いびき・睡眠時無呼吸

いびきをかくと人から言われたことがありますか.

☐ Have you ever been told that you snore?

睡眠中の無呼吸を指摘されたことがありますか.

☐ Have you ever been told that you stop breathing while you sleep?

―どのくらい無呼吸は続きますか.
 1. 10秒くらい.
 2. 1分くらい.
 3. もっと長く.

― How long does it continue?
 1. About 10 seconds?
 2. About 1 minute?
 3. Longer?

―飲酒や疲労で悪化しますか.

― Is it made worse by alcohol or fatigue?

最近（若いときにくらべて）体重は増えましたか.

☐ Have you noticed any weight gain recently (compared with your weight when you were young)?

―首周りのサイズは大きくなりましたか.

― Has your collar size become larger?

仕事中に居眠りが多いですか.

☐ Do you often nod off to sleep at work?

居眠り運転で事故を起こした, あるいは起こしそうになったことがありますか.

☐ Have you ever had an accident or a near-miss accident related to falling asleep while driving?

高血圧と言われたことがありますか.

☐ Have you ever been told that you have high blood pressure?

### 既往歴・生活習慣・家族歴

これまでに…のような肺の病気にかかったことがありますか.
 1. 喘息
 2. 慢性閉塞性肺疾患
 3. 肺炎

☐ Have you had any lung disease, such as...
 1. asthma?
 2. COPD [chronic obstructive pulmonary disease]?
 3. pneumonia?

| | |
|---|---|
| 4. 肺結核 | 4. tuberculosis? |
| 5. 肺がん | 5. lung cancer? |

これまでに心臓に何か異常がありましたか. — Have you ever had any trouble with your heart?

貧血だと言われたことがありますか. — Have you ever been told that you have anemia?

アレルギーは何かありますか. — Do you have allergies?
1. アトピー性皮膚炎. — 1. Atopic eczema?
2. アレルギー性鼻炎. — 2. Allergic rhinitis?
3. 結膜炎. — 3. Conjunctivitis?
4. 花粉症. — 4. Hay fever?

副鼻腔に異常がありますか. — Do you have any trouble with your sinuses?

症状を詳しく話して下さい. — Please tell me more about your problem.
—いつ診断されましたか. — When was it diagnosed?
—どんな治療を受けましたか. — How was it treated?

胸のX線写真を最後に撮ったのはいつですか. — When was your last chest X-ray?
—結果はどうでしたか. — What was the result?

ツベルクリン検査を最後に受けたのはいつですか. — When was your last tuberculin skin test?
—その結果は…でしたか. — Was the result...
1. 陽性 — 1. positive?
2. 陰性 — 2. negative?
—陽性になったのはいつですか. — When did you turn positive?
—BCG接種を受けたことがありますか. — Have you ever had a BCG shot [tuberculosis vaccination]?
—結核にかかっている人に接触したことがありますか. それはいつですか. — Have you ever been exposed to anyone with tuberculosis? When?

タバコを吸いますか. — Do you smoke?

| | |
|---|---|
| —どのくらい長く吸ってきましたか. | — How long have you been smoking? |
| —何年間〔何歳から〕ですか. | — For how many years〔Since you were how old〕? |
| —1日に何本〔何箱〕吸いますか. | — How many cigarettes〔packs of cigarettes〕do you smoke a day? |
| ペットを飼っていますか. | ☐ Do you have pets? |
| 仕事場で化学薬品や粉塵を吸いますか. | ☐ Do you breathe in chemicals or dust at work? |
| ご家族の中に…のような肺の病気にかかった人がいますか. | ☐ Has anyone in your immediate family had any lung problems, such as... |
| 1. 喘息 | 1. asthma? |
| 2. 慢性閉塞性肺疾患 | 2. COPD [chronic obstructive pulmonary disease]? |
| 3. 肺炎 | 3. pneumonia? |
| 4. 肺結核 | 4. tuberculosis? |
| 5. 肺がん | 5. lung cancer? |

---

### 名句・ことわざ

**Smoking or health：the choice is yours.**

**喫煙か健康か，選択はあなた次第**

世界保健機関（WHO）による禁煙デー（1980年）のスローガン．毎年5月31日を禁煙デーとし，世界各地で様々なキャンペーンを行っている．

## 5 心・血管

☞「胸痛」,「全身倦怠感」,「めまい」,「浮腫」(32, 42, 43, 46 ページ).
☞「咳・痰」,「息切れ」(76, 79 ページ).
☞「胸背部の診察」(222 ページ).

### 一般的な質問

心臓の具合が悪いのですか.
- ☐ (Do you have) any problems with your heart?
- ☐ (Is there) anything wrong with your heart?

—どんな問題ですか.
— What kind of problems?

それはどのくらい続いていますか.
- ☐ How long have you had the problems?

—いつからですか.
— Since when?

このような問題は以前にもありましたか.
- ☐ Have you had these problems before?

☞「病歴をとるためのヒント」(22 ページ).

### 動悸

心臓の鼓動に何か問題がありますか.
—どんな感じですか.
1. 非常に激しい.
2. 非常に速い.
3. 不規則.

- ☐ Do you have any problem with your heart beat?
— What does it feel like?
  1. Particularly strong [Pounding]?
  2. Particularly rapid [Racing]?
  3. Irregular [Skipping beats]?

どういうときその症状が起こりますか.

1. 休んでいるとき.
2. 活動している間.
3. 運動した後.
4. 階段や坂を登った後.
5. 食事をした後.

- ☐ When do you have the symptom?
- ☐ When does the symptom occur?
  1. While resting?
  2. During an activity?
  3. After exercise?
  4. After going up stairs or slopes?
  5. After eating?

—ストレスを受けると心臓がドキドキしますか.
—動悸がするとき意識が遠のきますか.
—動悸がして意識を失ったことがありますか.

発作はどのくらい長く続きますか.
1. 2, 3〔5, 6〕秒.
2. 2, 3 分.
3. 2, 3 時間.
4. 2, 3 日.

どのくらいの頻度で起こりますか.
1. 頻繁に.
2. さほど頻繁ではなく.
3. 時々.

始まるのは…ですか.
1. 突然
2. 徐々に〔ゆっくり〕

おさまるのは…ですか.
1. 突然
2. 徐々に〔ゆっくり〕

ほかに徴候や症状がありますか.

—それは何ですか.
1. 手指の震え.
2. 多汗.

— Does your heart pound after stress?
— Do you feel faint when your heart is pounding?
— Have you ever lost consciousness with attacks of palpitations?

☐ How long do the attacks last?
1. A few〔Several〕seconds?
2. A few minutes?
3. A few hours?
4. A few days?

☐ How often do you have them?
1. Often〔Frequently〕?
2. Not so often〔Infrequently〕?
3. Occasionally〔Once in a while〕?

☐ Do they come on...
1. suddenly?
2. gradually〔slowly〕?

☐ Do they go away...
1. suddenly?
2. gradually〔slowly〕?

☐ Do you have any other signs or symptoms?
— What are they?
1. Trembling or shaking of your hands and fingers?
2. Profuse sweating?

### 四肢の冷感・疼痛・腫脹

| | |
|---|---|
| 手足が冷たくなることがありますか. | ☐ Do your hands or feet ever feel cold?★ |
| 手足が痛むことがありますか. | ☐ Do you ever have pain in your hands or feet? |
| しびれるか,知覚異常がありますか. | ☐ Do you have numbness or sensory abnormality? |
| 足に潰瘍やただれができていますか. | ☐ Do you have any ulcers or sores on your legs? |
| 手足が腫れていますか. | ☐ Do you have swellings on or in your hands or feet? |
| 足がつることがありますか. | ☐ Do you ever have cramps in your legs? |

皮膚の色に変化がありますか.
1. 蒼白.
2. 発赤.
3. 紫.

☐ Has your skin changed its color?
1. Pale?
2. Red [Flushed (red)]?
3. Purple?

その症状に初めて気づいたのはいつですか.

☐ When did you first notice the symptom?

どういう時に症状が起きますか.

1. 安静時.
2. 運動時.
3. 寒いとき.
4. 夕方,夜間.

☐ In what situations does it come on?

1. When you are at rest?
2. When you are exercising?
3. When it is cold?
4. In the evening or during the night?

―休むとよくなりますか.

― Does it disappear with rest?

---

★ foot は足首から先までをいう.

### 既往歴・家族歴

…といった問題がありますか.
1. 高血圧
2. 脂質異常症
3. 糖尿病
4. 静脈瘤
5. その他

☐ Do you have any problems, such as...
1. high blood pressure?
2. dyslipidemia?
3. diabetes?
4. varicose veins?
5. any other problem?

これまでに心臓に異常がありましたか.
1. 不整脈.
2. 狭心症.
3. 先天性心臓病.
4. 心雑音.
5. 心電図異常.

☐ Have you had any heart trouble before?
1. Irregular pulse?
2. Angina pectoris?
3. Congenital heart disease?
4. Heart murmur?
5. Abnormal ECG?

これまでに…にかかったことがありますか.
1. リウマチ熱
2. 溶連菌感染症
3. 川崎病
4. 脳血管疾患

☐ Have you ever had...
1. rheumatic fever?
2. a strep infection?
3. Kawasaki disease?
4. cerebrovascular disease?

そう診断されたのはいつですか.

☐ When was the disorder diagnosed?

―どんな治療を受けていますか〔受けましたか〕.

― How is〔was〕it treated?

タバコを吸いますか.
―どのくらい長く吸ってきましたか.
―何年間〔何歳から〕ですか.

―1日に何本〔何箱〕吸いますか.

☐ Do you smoke?
― How long have you been smoking?
― For how many years〔Since you were how old〕?

― How many cigarettes〔packs of cigarettes〕do you smoke a day?

| | |
|---|---|
| 定期的に運動していますか. | ☐ Do you exercise routinely? |
| —どんな種類の運動ですか. | — What kind of exercise do you do? |
| —週に何回くらいですか. | — How often do you exercise a week? |
| —1回の運動時間はどのくらいですか. | — How long do you spend exercising each time? |
| 何か不安や心配事がありますか. | ☐ Are you nervous or anxious about anything? |
| ご家族に心臓病の人がいますか. | ☐ Does anyone in your immediate family have a heart disease? |
| 1. 不整脈. | 1. Irregular pulse? |
| 2. 狭心症. | 2. Angina pectoris? |
| 3. 心筋梗塞. | 3. Heart attack [Myocardial infarction]? |
| ご家族に脳血管疾患の人がいますか. | ☐ Does anyone in your immediate family have a cerebrovascular disease? |
| ご家族に原因不明で突然亡くなられた人がいますか. | ☐ Has anyone in your immediate family died suddenly of an unknown cause? |

# 用語・表現ファイル

## 病院関係者

### 1. 専門職

| | |
|---|---|
| 医師 | physician [doctor] |
| 　内科医 | internist [physician] |
| 　外科医 | surgeon |
| 　専門医 | specialist |
| 　一般医 | generalist |
| 　研修医 | resident, house physician [doctor] |
| 　担当医 [受持ち医] | attending physician [doctor in charge] |

☞各専門医の名称は「専門医」(261 ページ).

| | |
|---|---|
| 歯科医 | dentist |
| 口腔外科医 | oral [dental] surgeon, maxillofacial surgeon |
| 看護師 | nurse |
| 助産師 | midwife |
| 保健師 | public health nurse [PHN] |
| 薬剤師 | pharmacist |
| 栄養士 | dietician [nutritionist] |
| 医療ソーシャルワーカー | medical social worker [MSW] |
| 精神保健福祉士 | psychiatric social worker [PSW] |
| 臨床心理士 | clinical psycologist |
| 作業療法士 | occupational therapist [OT] |
| 理学療法士 | physical therapist [PT] |
| 言語聴覚士 | speech-language-hearing therapist [ST] |
| 聴能訓練士 | audiologist |
| 視能訓練士 | orthoptist [ORT] |
| ストーマ療法士 | enterostomal therapist [ET], stoma therapist |
| 義肢装具士 | prosthetist and orthotist [PO] |
| 診療放射線技師 | medical radiation [radiologic] technologist [MRT] |
| 臨床検査技師 | clinical laboratory technician |
| 聴覚検査技師 | audiometrist |

## 用語・表現ファイル（つづき）

| | |
|---|---|
| 検眼士［視力検査技師］ | optometrist |
| 臨床工学技士 | clinical engineer［CE］, medical engineer［ME］ |
| 救急救命士 | paramedic, emergency medical technician［EMT］ |
| 歯科衛生士 | dental hygienist |
| 歯科技工士 | dental technician |

### 2. サービス職

| | |
|---|---|
| 介護員 | hospital attendant, (男性の)orderly |
| 看護助手 | nursing assistant［nurse's aide］ |
| 警備員 | guard |
| 清掃員 | the cleaning［housekeeping］staff, cleaning man〔woman〕 |
| 用務員 | janitor |

### 3. 事務職

| | |
|---|---|
| 一般事務（職員） | (general office) clerk |
| 受付事務（職員） | receptionist |
| 会計事務（職員） | cashier |
| 病棟事務（職員） | unit clerk |

### 4. 管理職

| | |
|---|---|
| 院長 | president［hospital administrator］ |
| 副院長 | vice president |
| 診療部長 | medical director for physicians |
| 科長（…科の） | the head (of the __ Department) |
| 看護部長 | director of nursing |
| 看護師長 | nursing supervisor |
| 看護主任［主任看護師］ | charge［head］nurse |
| 薬剤部長 | director of pharmacy |
| 事務長 | director of the administration department |

## 用語・表現ファイル（つづき）

### 5. その他

| | |
|---|---|
| 医学生 | medical student |
| 看護学生 | nursing student |
| 医療通訳 | medical interpreter |
| ボランティア | volunteer |
| （病院付きの）牧師 | chaplain |

chapter 3　現病歴（心・血管）

### 名句・ことわざ

**There is no royal road to learning.**

学問に王道なし

古代ギリシャの数学者・天文学者ユークリッド（Euclid, 300? B.C., *Elements*）に由来する名言．エジプトの王に幾何学を教えていたとき，王が「幾何学を学ぶのに近道はないのか」と訊いたところ，ユークリッドは "There's no royal road to geometry." （幾何学に王道なし）と答えたという．

## 6 消化器

☞「腹痛」(36 ページ).
☞「消化器の診察」(224 ページ).

### 一般的な質問

| | |
|---|---|
| 胃腸の具合が悪いのですか. | ☐ Do you have any problems with your stomach or bowels? |
| —どんな問題ですか. | — What kind of problems? |
| それはどのくらい続いていますか. | ☐ How long have you had the problems? |
| —いつからですか. | — Since when? |
| このような問題は以前にもありましたか. | ☐ Have you had these problems before? |

☞「病歴をとるためのヒント」(22 ページ).

### 嚥下障害

| | |
|---|---|
| 物が飲み込みにくいですか. | ☐ Do you have difficulty swallowing? |
| 食べ物がよくのどにつかえますか. | ☐ Do you often choke on food?<br>☐ Does food often get stuck in your throat? |
| 食事中に，よくむせますか. | ☐ Do you often choke and cough while having a meal? |
| 何かがのどにつかえている感じがありますか. | ☐ Do you feel as if something is sticking in your throat? |
| どんなときにのどにつかえますか.<br>　1. 固い食べ物を食べるとき.<br>　2. 水を飲み込むとき.<br>　3. つば［唾液］を飲み込むとき.<br>　4. いつも. | ☐ When do you choke?<br>　1. When you eat solid food?<br>　2. When you swallow water?<br>　3. When you swallow saliva?<br>　4. All the time? |

| | |
|---|---|
| 飲み込むとき痛みますか. | ☐ Do you have pain when you swallow? |
| ―どこが痛みますか. | ― Where? |
| そのほかに徴候や症状がありますか. | ☐ Do you have any other signs or symptoms? |
| ―それは何ですか. | ― What are they? |
| 最近,体重が減少しましたか. | ☐ Have you recently lost weight? |

### 消化不良

消化の具合が悪いのですか.　　☐ Do you have problems with your digestion?

胸焼けしますか.　　☐ Do you have heartburn?

胃が重苦しいですか.　　☐ Do you have a heavy feeling in your stomach?

胃［食べ物］がもたれますか.　　☐ Does food sit heavy on your stomach?

消化不良を起こしますか.　　☐ Do you have indigestion?
―いつ起こりますか.　　― When does it occur?
―どんなものを食べたり飲んだりした後で起こりますか.　　― What kind of foods or drinks cause it?

### 吐き気・嘔吐

頻繁に…　　☐ Do you often...
　1. 吐き気がしますか.　　　1. feel nauseated［feel like vomiting］?
　2. 吐きますか.　　　2. vomit［throw up］?
　3. ゲップが出ますか.　　　3. belch［burp］?

吐きましたか.　　☐ Did you vomit?

いつ吐きましたか.　　☐ When did it occur?
　1. 食後すぐですか.　　　1. Immediately after eating?

| | |
|---|---|
| 2. 食後 2, 3 時間経ってからですか. | 2. A few hours after eating? |
| 3. 食事とは無関係ですか. | 3. Not related to when you ate? |
| 4. 朝ですか. | 4. In the morning? |

何回吐きましたか.
1. 2, 3 回.
2. 5, 6 回.
3. もっと多く.

☐ How many times did you vomit?
1. A few times?
2. Several times?
3. More?

どのくらいの量を吐きましたか.
—少量ですか, 多量ですか.

1. コップ半分.
2. コップ1杯.
3. もっと多い量.

☐ How much did you vomit?
— A small amount or a large amount?

1. Half a cup?
2. A cup?
3. More?

吐いたものは何でしたか.

1. 直前に食べた未消化のもの.
2. 透明な液体.
3. 鮮血.
4. 暗赤色の [黒っぽい] 血.
5. コーヒーかす状の液体.

—どんな色をしていましたか.
1. 透明.
2. 黄色.
3. 緑色.
4. 濃い茶色 [コーヒーかすの色].
5. 黒色.

—どんな味でしたか.
1. 酸っぱい味.
2. 苦い味.

—吐いた物に血が混じっていましたか. 血の量はどのくらいでしたか.

—便の臭いがしましたか.

☐ What did you vomit?
☐ What did the vomit look like?
1. Undigested food that you had just eaten?
2. Clear liquid?
3. Bright red blood?
4. Dark-colored blood?
5. Liquid like coffee grounds?

— What color was it?
1. Clear?
2. Yellow?
3. Green?
4. Dark brown [Color of coffee grounds]?
5. Black?

— What did it taste like?
1. Acidic in taste?
2. Bitter in taste?

— Did you notice any blood in the vomit? How much blood was there in it?

— Did it have a fecal odor?

| | |
|---|---|
| 吐いた後は楽になりましたか. | ☐ Did you feel better after you had vomited? |
| 何か思い当たる誘因はありますか. | ☐ What do you think is causing it?<br>☐ Is there any cause that you can identify? |
| 1. アレルギー物質を含む食品, 腐った食品. | 1. Eating food to which you may be allergic, or food that may have been contaminated? |
| 2. お酒の飲みすぎ. | 2. Drinking a large amount of alcohol? |
| 3. 周囲に同じような症状の人がいる. | 3. Having someone around you who has a similar symptom? |
| 4. 不快な臭気, 味. | 4. Experiencing unpleasant smells or tastes? |
| 5. 薬の内服. | 5. Taking any drugs or medications? |
| 6. 不安感. | 6. Suffering from anxiety? |
| 妊娠していますか. その可能性はありますか.<br>—最終月経はいつでしたか. | ☐ Are you pregnant? Could you be pregnant?<br>— When was your last menstrual period? |
| お腹の手術をしたことがありますか. | ☐ Have you ever had surgery on your stomach or abdomen? |
| そのほかに徴候や症状がありますか.<br>—それは何ですか. | ☐ Do you have any other signs or symptoms?<br>— What are they? |
| 1. 腹痛. | 1. Pain in your stomach or abdomen? |
| 2. 便秘, 下痢などの便通異常. | 2. Problems with your bowel movement, such as constipation or diarrhea? |
| 3. 頭痛. | 3. Headache? |
| 4. 発熱. | 4. Fever? |
| 5. 体重減少. | 5. Weight loss? |

chapter 3 現病歴(消化器)

便通異常（血便・便秘・下痢）

## 排便の状況

便通は規則的にありますか.

—便通の回数はどのくらいですか.

1. 毎日1回.
2. 毎日1回以上.
3. 1日おき.
4. 3日に1回.
5. もっと回数が多い〔少ない〕.

便通の習慣に変化がありましたか.

—どう変化しましたか.
1. 便の回数が増えた.
2. 便の回数が減った.

便の硬さや形はどんなですか.
1. 硬い.
2. やわらかい.
3. ゆるい.
4. 水のような.
5. 泥状の.
6. 鉛筆状の.
7. 固まっている.

—便の色はどうですか.
1. 茶色.
2. 緑色がかった.
3. 黒い.
4. タール様.
5. 白い.
6. 赤っぽい.

—どんな臭いですか.
1. 腐敗臭.
2. 酸っぱい臭い.

☐ Do you have regular bowel movements?
— How often do you move your bowels?
1. Once a day?
2. More than once a day?
3. Every other day?
4. Once every three days?
5. More〔less〕frequently?

☐ Have you noticed any change in your bowel habits?
— How has it changed?
1. Bowel movements more frequent?
2. Bowel movements less frequent?

☐ What do your stools look like?
1. Hard?
2. Soft?
3. Loose?
4. Watery?
5. Muddy?
6. Pencil-like?
7. Formed?

— What color are they?
1. Brown?
2. Greenish?
3. Black?
4. Tarry?
5. White?
6. Reddish?

— What do they smell like?
1. Foul-smelling?
2. Acidic?

便をするとき痛みがありますか.

☐ When you move your bowels, do you have any pain?

便をした後,まだ便意が残っていますか.

☐ When you finish, do you feel as if you still have to move your bowels?

## 血便
血便が出ますか.

☐ Do you have blood in your stools?

―出血の量はどのくらいですか.
1. 多い.
2. 少ない.
3. すじ状につく程度.
4. トイレットペーパーに付着する程度.

― How much do you bleed?
1. Heavy?
2. Slight?
3. Streaks?
4. Blood on the toilet paper?

―血はどんな色をしていますか.
1. 黒い.
2. 黒ずんでいる.
3. コーヒーかすの様な濃い茶色.
4. 真っ赤[鮮やかで赤い].

― What color is it?
1. Black?
2. Dark?
3. Dark brown like coffee grounds?
4. Bright red?

―血は便の表面についていますか.

― Is the blood on the surface of your stools?

―血は便に混じっていますか.

― Is the blood mixed in with your stools?

―血の塊に気づきましたか.

― Have you noticed any clots of blood?

## 便秘
便秘していますか.

☐ Are you constipated?
☐ Do you have constipation?

―最後に便をしたのはいつですか.

― When did you last move your bowels?

―便が出にくいですか.

― Do you have difficulty moving your bowels?

下痢と便秘を交互に繰り返しますか.

☐ Do you have diarrhea alternating with constipation?

| | |
|---|---|
| 腹痛や吐き気がありますか，嘔吐がありましたか． | ☐ Do you have any abdominal pain or any nausea? Have you vomited? |
| 薬を服用していますか，あるいは最近服用しましたか． | ☐ Are you taking or have you recently taken any drugs or medications? |
| お腹の手術をしたことがありますか． | ☐ Have you ever had surgery on your stomach or abdomen? |

### 下痢

| | |
|---|---|
| 下痢をしていますか． | ☐ Do you have diarrhea? |
| ― 1日に何回下痢をしますか． | ― How many times a day do you have diarrhea? |
| ―下痢の量はどうですか． | ― How much is it? |
| 　1．多い． | 　1．A large amount? |
| 　2．少ない． | 　2．A small amount? |
| ―下痢はどんな色をしていますか． | ― What color is it? |
| ―どんな下痢ですか． | ― What does it look like? |
| 　1．水様． | 　1．Watery? |
| 　2．血が混じった． | 　2．Bloody? |
| 　3．脂肪が混じった． | 　3．With fat [Fatty]? |
| 　4．粘液が混じった． | 　4．With mucus [Mucousy]? |
| 　5．膿が混じった． | 　5．With pus [Pussy]? |
| 　6．米のとぎ汁様． | 　6．Cloudy like water in which rice has been washed? |
| 　7．イチゴゼリー状． | 　7．Blood-stained like strawberry jelly? |
| 下痢の原因となるようなものを食べましたか． | ☐ Have you eaten anything that may have caused your diarrhea? |
| 最近，抗生物質などの薬を服用しましたか． | ☐ Have you recently taken any drugs or medications, such as antibiotics? |
| 最近，（仕事上や家庭で）ストレスの多い生活でしたか． | ☐ Have you recently been under particular strain [stress] (at work or at home)? |

| | |
|---|---|
| 周囲に同じような症状の人がいますか. | ☐ Does anyone around you have a similar symptom? |
| 下痢のほかに徴候や症状がありますか. | ☐ Do you have any other signs or symptoms? |
| —それは何ですか. | — What are they? |
| 　1. 痛み〔腹痛〕. | 　1. Pain 〔Abdominal pain〕? |
| 　2. 腹部の張り. | 　2. Distension 〔Bloating〕? |
| 　3. ガス. | 　3. Gas? |
| 　4. 吐き気,嘔吐. | 　4. Nausea and 〔or〕 vomiting? |
| 　5. 発熱. | 　5. Fever? |
| 　6. 体重減少. | 　6. Weight loss? |
| 　7. その他. | 　7. Any other symptoms? |
| 最近,日本の国外へ出てどこかへ旅行しましたか. | ☐ Have you recently traveled anywhere out of Japan? |
| —いつ,どこの国へ行きましたか. | — When and which country 〔countries〕? |

### 食欲

| | |
|---|---|
| 食欲はありますか. | ☐ Do you have a good appetite? |
| —食欲はどうですか. | — How is your appetite? |
| 　1. よい. | 　1. Good? |
| 　2. まあまあ. | 　2. Fair? |
| 　3. ない. | 　3. Poor? |
| 最近,食欲が変化しましたか. どんな変化ですか. | ☐ Have you had a change in your appetite recently? What kind of change? |
| —いつもよりお腹が… | — Are you... |
| 　1. すきますか. | 　1. more hungry than usual? |
| 　2. すきませんか. | 　2. less hungry than usual? |
| —食べる量は…ですか. | — Do you eat... |
| 　1. いつもより多い | 　1. more than usual? |
| 　2. いつもより少ない | 　2. less than usual? |
| 　3. いつも通り | 　3. the same as usual? |
| ダイエットしていますか. | ☐ Are you on a diet? |

☞「食習慣」(202 ページ).

### 体重変化

☞「単位の換算表」(216 ページ).

| | |
|---|---|
| 体重はどのくらいありますか. | ☐ How much do you weigh now? |
| —昨年,体重はどのくらいありましたか. | — How much did you weigh last year? |
| —最高の体重はいくらですか. | — What is the most you've weighed? |
| —最低の体重はいくらですか. | — What is the least you've weighed? |

最近,体重に変化がありましたか. ☐ Has your weight changed recently?

  1. 増えましたか. 　1. Have you gained weight?
  2. 減りましたか. 　2. Have you lost weight?
—どのくらい増え〔減り〕ましたか. — How much did you gain〔lose〕?
—何か月の間にですか. — Over how many months?

体重を増やしたいですか. ☐ Do you want to gain weight?
—現在の体重を維持したいですか. — Do you want to maintain your present weight?
—体重を減らしたいですか. — Do you want to lose weight?

### 黄疸

あなたは…に気づきましたか. ☐ Have you ever noticed...
  1. 皮膚や白目の部分の黄色 　1. a yellow color to your skin or the whites of your eyes?
  2. 皮膚の痒み 　2. itching of your skin?
  3. 尿の色の変化 　3. a change in the color of your urine?
  4. 便の色の変化.灰白色 　4. a change in the color of your stools?  Light gray?

最近,風邪の症状がありましたか. ☐ Have you recently had cold symptoms?

| | |
|---|---|
| 肝機能異常を指摘されたことがありますか. | ☐ Have you ever been told that you have a liver function disorder? |
| B型肝炎, C型肝炎などの肝炎を指摘されたことがありますか. | ☐ Have you ever been told that you have hepatitis, such as hepatitis B or hepatitis C? |
| お酒を飲みますか.<br>―かなりの量を飲んでいますか.<br>―1日どのくらいの量を飲みますか. | ☐ Do you drink alcohol?<br>― Have you been drinking excessively?<br>― How much do you drink a day? |
| 薬を服用していますか, 最近, 服用しましたか. | ☐ Are you taking or have you recently taken any drugs or medications? |
| 輸血をしたことがありますか. | ☐ Have you ever had a blood transfusion? |
| 不特定多数の人と性交渉をもちましたか. | ☐ Have you had sexual intercourse with many unknown partners? |
| 最近, 日本の国外へ出てどこかへ旅行しましたか.<br>―いつ, どこの国へ行きましたか. | ☐ Have you recently traveled anywhere out of Japan?<br>― When and which country 〔countries〕? |
| 柑橘類を好んで食べますか. | ☐ Do you particularly like eating citrus fruits? |

### 既往歴・家族歴

| | |
|---|---|
| これまでに…に異常がありましたか.<br>  1. 胃<br>  2. 腸<br>  3. 胆嚢などの腹部臓器 | ☐ Have you ever had any trouble with your...<br>  1. stomach?<br>  2. intestine?<br>  3. abdominal organs, such as your gallbladder? |

―どのような異常でしたか．
―診断を受けたのはいつですか．
―どんな治療を受けましたか．
―手術を受けましたか．

— What was it?
— When was it diagnosed?
— How was it treated?
— Did you have surgery on it?

摂食障害になったことがありますか．
1. 拒食症．
2. 過食症．

☐ Have you ever had any eating disorder?
1. Anorexia nervosa?
2. Bulimia [Binging and purging]?

ご家族のどなたかが…にかかったことがありますか．
1. 胃腸の病気
2. 大腸がん〔ポリープ〕
3. 肝炎
4. 肝臓がん
5. その他

☐ Has anyone in your immediate family had...
1. a GI tract disorder?
2. colon cancer〔polyps〕?
3. hepatitis?
4. liver cancer?
5. any other disorders?

---

### 名句・ことわざ

**Feed by measure and defy the physician.**
**ほどほどの食事で医者無用**

"A good meal, a bad meal, and a middling meal preseves a man in health."（健康を保つには，朝たっぷり，昼ちょっぴり，夜は中くらい食べる）ということわざもある．日本の「腹八分に医者いらず」に相当する．

## 7　腎・泌尿器

### 一般的な質問

腎臓か膀胱の具合が悪いのですか.
☐ (Do you have) any problems with your kidneys or bladder?

―どんな問題ですか.
― What kind of problems?

排尿に問題がありますか.
☐ (Do you have) any problems urinating?

―尿を出すときの感じを話して下さい.
― Please tell me how it feels when you urinate.

それはどのくらい続いていますか.
☐ How long have you had the problems?

―いつからですか.
― Since when?

このような問題は以前にもありましたか.
☐ Have you had these problems before?

☞「病歴をとるためのヒント」(22 ページ).

### 尿の性状

どんな尿が出ますか.
―尿は…
1. 澄んでいますか.
2. 濁っていますか.

☐ What is your urine like?
― Does it appear…
1. clear?
2. cloudy?

尿はどんな色をしていますか.
1. 淡い黄色.
2. 濃い黄色.
3. 赤みがかった.
4. その他.

☐ What color is it?
1. Light yellow?
2. Dark yellow?
3. Reddish?
4. Any other color?

尿に…が混じりますか.
1. 血
2. 膿
3. 血の塊
4. 小さな石または砂

☐ Have you noticed any … in your urine?
1. blood
2. pus
3. blood clots
4. small stones or sand

―その量はどのくらいですか.
1. ごく少量.
2. 多量.

― How much is it〔are they〕?
1. A little bit〔A small amount〕?
2. Abundant〔A lot〕?

### 排尿回数・尿量

排尿回数は…ですか.
1. いつもより多い
2. いつもより少ない

☐ Do you have to urinate...
1. more frequently than usual?
2. less frequently than usual?

1日に何回排尿しますか.

☐ How many times a day do you urinate?

―24時間で10回以上ですか.

― More than 10 times over 24 hours?

―夜,排尿のために何回起きますか.

― How many times do you wake up to urinate at night?

尿量はどのくらいですか.
1. いつもより多い.
2. いつもより少ない.
3. いつもと同じ.
―夜間に尿量は多いですか.

☐ How much do you urinate?
1. In larger volumes than usual?
2. In smaller volumes than usual?
3. The same volume?
― Do you have to urinate a lot at night?

水分を飲む量は多いですか,少ないですか.

☐ Do you tend to drink large amounts of liquid or small amounts of liquid?

―水分は1日にどのくらい飲みますか.

― How much liquid do you drink a day?

―どんなものを飲みますか.

― What kind of liquid do you drink?

―夜,水分をたくさん飲みますか.

― Do you drink large amounts of liquid at night?

排尿回数や尿量のほかに徴候や症状がありますか.
―それは何ですか.

☐ Do you have any other signs or symptoms?
― What are they?

1. 頭痛，視力障害，脱毛，無月経.
2. 筋力低下.
3. 浮腫.
4. 体重増加.
5. その他.

1. Headache, visual problems, loss of hair, or absence of menstrual periods?
2. Muscle weakness?
3. Swelling of the body?
4. Weight gain?
5. Any other symptoms?

糖尿病はありますか．

☐ Do you have diabetes?

高血圧や心臓疾患に対する利尿薬などの薬を服用していますか，最近服用しましたか．

☐ Are you taking or have you recently taken any drugs or medications, such as diuretics for high blood pressure or heart diseases?

### 尿失禁

排尿のコントロールが難しいですか．

☐ Do you have difficulty controlling your urine?

尿意をがまんすることができますか．

☐ Can you hold your urine?

尿を漏らすことがありますか．
—それはどういう時に起きますか．
1. くしゃみをするとき．
2. 咳をするとき．
3. 運動中．
4. 尿意を感じるとき．
5. 睡眠中．

☐ Do you ever drip [leak] urine?
— When does it occur?
1. When you sneeze?
2. When you cough?
3. While you exercise?
4. When you feel the urge to urinate?
5. While you sleep at night?

妊娠したことがありますか．
—これまでに何回出産しましたか．

☐ Have you ever been pregnant?
— How many babies have you had?

### 排尿困難

尿が出にくいことがありますか.
- [ ] Do you have difficulty urinating?

—排尿し始めが出にくいですか.
— Do you have difficulty starting to urinate?

—排尿終了までいつもより時間がかかりますか.
— Does it take longer than usual to finish urinating?

—排尿途中で尿線が途切れますか.
— Do you have an interrupted urinary stream?

尿線が〔に〕…
- [ ] Have you noticed any decrease in...
  1. 細くなりますか.
  2. 勢いがなくなりますか.
  1. the size of your stream?
  2. the force of your stream?

尿は最後にしたたるように出ますか.
- [ ] Does your urine continue to dribble at the end of urination?

排尿するのにいきみますか.
- [ ] Do you strain when urinating?

夜, 排尿のために何回起きますか.
- [ ] How many times do you get up to urinate during the night?

残尿感がありますか.
- [ ] After you urinate, do you feel that your bladder is not empty?

尿意を突然もよおすことがありますか.
- [ ] Do you have a feeling of urgency to urinate?

### 排尿痛

☞「痛みの表現」(31 ページ).

排尿時に痛み〔焼けつくような感じ〕がありますか.
- [ ] Do you have pain〔a burning sensation〕when you urinate?

どこが痛みますか.
1. 尿道の出口付近.
- [ ] Where is the pain?
  1. Around the area of the urethral opening?

2. 下腹部.
3. 腰.

―痛みは広がり〔移動し〕ますか.

―どこからどこへですか.

どんな痛みですか.

1. 焼けるような.
2. 鈍い.
3. 鋭く,刺すような.
4. きりきりする.
5. 重苦しい.

それは排尿時のいつ起こりますか.

1. 最初.
2. 排尿中ずっと.
3. 最後.

初めて痛んだのはいつですか.

分泌物が出ることがありますか.

―尿道口からですか.

そのほかに徴候や症状がありますか.
―それは何ですか.
1. 腹痛.
2. 腰痛.
3. 発熱.
4. のどの渇き.

2. In the lower abdomen?
3. In the lower back?

—Does the pain radiate 〔move〕 to another area?

—From where to where?

☐ What is the pain like?
☐ Can you describe the pain for me?
1. Burning?
2. Dull ache?
3. Sharp and stabbing?
4. Squeezing?
5. Sensation of heaviness?

☐ When do you have it on urination?
1. At the start?
2. The whole time?
3. At the end?

☐ When did you first get it?
☐ When did it start?

☐ Have you noticed any discharge?

— From the opening where you urinate?

☐ Do you have any other signs or symptoms?
— What are they?
1. Pain in the stomach or abdomen?
2. Low back pain?
3. Fever?
4. Increased thirst?

### 既往歴・生活習慣・家族歴

これまでに…に異常がありましたか.
1. 腎臓
2. 膀胱
3. 性器
4. 尿道
5. 前立腺

― どのような異常でしたか.
1. （検診での）血尿や蛋白尿.
2. 腎障害.
3. 感染症.
4. 結石.
5. 外傷.
6. 奇形.

― いつですか.
― どんな治療を受けましたか.
― その後も感染症や結石は繰り返していますか.

これまでに…にかかったことがありますか.
1. 高血圧
2. 脳血管障害
3. 脊髄疾患
4. 糖尿病
5. 高尿酸血症〔痛風〕
6. 性感染症
7. その他

カテーテルを留置したことがありますか.

☐ Have you ever had any trouble with your...
1. kidneys?
2. bladder?
3. genitals [genitalia]?
4. urethra?
5. prostate gland?

― What kind of trouble was it?
1. Bloody urine or proteinuria (found at the time of general checkup)?
2. Kidney disorder?
3. Infections?
4. Stones?
5. Injury?
6. Birth defect?

― When did you have it?
― How was it treated?
― Have you been suffering from recurrent episodes of the infections or stones?

☐ Have you ever had...
1. high blood pressure?
2. a cerebrovascular disorder?
3. a spinal cord disease?
4. diabetes?
5. hyperuricemia [gout]?
6. a sexually transmitted infection?
7. any other disorders?

☐ Have you ever been catheterized?

| | |
|---|---|
| 薬を服用していますか，最近，服用しましたか． | ☐ Are you taking or have you recently taken any drugs or medications? |
| 1. 利尿薬． | 1. Diuretics? |
| 2. 抗コリン薬． | 2. Anticholinergic drugs? |
| | |
| 特別な食事療法をしていますか． | ☐ Are you on a special diet? |
| —どんな食事療法ですか． | — What kind of diet is it? |
| —塩分の制限をしていますか． | — Are you limiting the intake of salt? |
| | |
| ご家族のどなたかが腎臓の病気にかかったことがありますか． | ☐ Has anyone in your immediate family had kidney disease? |
| —どなたですか． | — Who is it? |
| —それは何でしたか． | — What was the problem? |

## 8 男性生殖器

### 一般的な質問

性器〔ペニスか陰囊〕に何か問題がありますか.
□ (Do you have) any problems with your male organs〔penis or scrotum〕?

―どんな問題ですか.
― What kind of problems?

それはどのくらい続いていますか.
□ How long have you had the problems?

―いつからですか.
― Since when?

このような問題は以前にもありましたか.
□ Have you had these problems before?

☞「病歴をとるためのヒント」(22 ページ).

### 痛み

☞「痛みの表現」(31 ページ).

…に痛みや不快感がありますか.
□ Do you feel any pain or discomfort...

1. ペニス
2. 睾丸
3. 陰囊のあたり

1. in your penis?
2. in your testes?
3. around your scrotum?

どんな痛みですか.
□ What is the pain like?
□ Can you describe the pain for me?

1. 鈍い.
2. 鋭く,刺すような.
3. 焼けるような.
4. 圧迫されるような.
5. 引っ張られる〔ひきつる〕ような.

1. Dull ache?
2. Sharp and stabbing?
3. Burning?
4. Pressure-like?
5. Pulling〔Dragging〕sensation?

―痛みはほかの場所へ広がりますか〔移動しますか〕.
― Does it radiate〔move〕to another place?

―どこからどこですか.
― From where to where?

痛みがあるのは…ですか.
1. 勃起時
2. 射精時
3. 排尿時

- [ ] Does it occur...
    1. when you have erections?
    2. when you ejaculate?
    3. when you urinate?

痛みを…がありますか.
1. 軽くするもの［こと］
2. 悪化させるもの［こと］
—それは何ですか.

- [ ] Is there anything that makes it...
    1. better?
    2. worse?
— What is it?

初めて痛んだのはいつですか.

- [ ] When did you first get it?
- [ ] When did it start?

### 分泌物・精液

ペニス〔尿道口〕から分泌液が出ますか.

- [ ] Do you have any discharge from your penis〔urethral opening〕?

どんな分泌物ですか.

- [ ] What is the discharge like?
- [ ] Can you describe the discharge for me?

1. どろどろ［膿性］.
2. さらさら［漿液性］.
3. 血がにじんでいる.
—どんな色をしていますか.
1. 透明.
2. 白い.
3. 黄色い.
4. 赤っぽい.
5. その他.
—悪臭がしますか.

1. Thick like pus?
2. Thin?
3. Blood-tinged?
— What color is it?
1. Clear?
2. White?
3. Yellow?
4. Reddish?
5. Any other color?
— Does it have a bad smell?

精液はどんな色ですか.
1. 乳白色.
2. 黄色.
3. 血液がにじんでいる.

- [ ] What color is your semen?
    1. Milky?
    2. Yellow?
    3. Blood-tinged?

初めて気づいたのはいつですか.

- [ ] When did you first notice it?
- [ ] When did it start?

### 随伴症状

そのほか徴候や症状がありますか.

―それは何ですか.
1. 発熱.
2. かゆみ.
3. 皮膚の色の変化,たとえば,ペニスや陰嚢の赤み.
4. ペニスのただれ [潰瘍].
5. 潰瘍からの膿.
6. 鼠径部の腫れ.
7. 鼠径部,ペニス,陰嚢内のしこり.
8. ペニスや陰嚢のサイズの変化.
9. その他.

☐ Do you have any other signs or symptoms?
― What are they?
1. Fever?
2. Itching?
3. Change in the color of the skin, such as redness on your penis or scrotum?
4. Sores on your penis?
5. Pus from the sores?
6. Swelling in your groin?
7. Lump in your groin, penis, or scrotum?
8. Change in the size of your penis or scrotum?
9. Any other symptoms?

### 性機能

それではこれからあなたの性習慣についておうかがいします.
―個人的な質問になるかと思いますが,この情報はあなたの診療に役立てるためのものです.

―ここでお話になる内容は秘密厳守とさせていただきます.

性欲はありますか.

―最近,セックスに対して関心が薄れてきたと思いますか.

―性行為に対する嫌悪感がありますか.

☐ Now I'd like to ask about your sexual practices.
― I know these questions are very personal, but this information will help me take better care of you.
― Anything we discuss here will be completely confidential.

☐ Are you interested in sexual activity?
☐ Do you experience sexual desire?
― Do you think that you have been less interested in sexual activity recently?
― Do you have any dislike for sexual activity?

―自分の性器に対して劣等感を感じますか.
―自慰行為はしますか.

あなたは勃起力に問題がありますか.
1. ぜんぜん勃起しない.
2. 勃起が難しい.
3. 勃起が続かない.
4. 勃起が弱い.
―夜間睡眠時や朝目覚めたときなどに勃起することがありますか.

勃起不全のために薬を飲んでいますか.

―どんな薬ですか.

あなたは射精に問題がありますか.

1. ぜんぜん射精しない.
2. 射精が難しい.
    a. 射精が早すぎる.
    b. 射精に時間がかかる.
―射精量はどのくらいですか.
1. 普通.
2. 非常に少ない.

オルガスムに問題がありますか.

1. ぜんぜんない.
2. オルガスムに達するのが難しい.

性専門のカウンセラーに会って話をしたいですか.

— Do you have a sense of inferiority about your genitals?
— Do you masturbate?

☐ Do you have any difficulty with erection?
1. No erection?
2. Difficulty achieving it?
3. Difficulty maintaining it during sexual activity?
4. Weak erection?
— Do you have erections at other times, such as during sleep at night or upon awakening in the morning?

☐ Are you taking [using] any medications for erectile dysfunction [impotence]?
— What are they?

☐ Do you have any difficulty with ejaculation?
1. No ejaculation?
2. Difficulty ejaculating?
    a. Premature ejaculation?
    b. Delayed ejaculation?
— How much do you ejaculate?
1. Normal?
2. Too little?

☐ Do you have any difficulty with orgasm?
1. No orgasm?
2. Difficulty achieving it?

☐ Would you like to talk with a sexual counselor?

### 性生活

現在,性生活はありますか. □ Are you currently sexually active?

—性行為の相手は男性,女性,またはその両方ですか. — Are your partners men, women, or both?

—パートナーは2人以上いますか. — Do you have two partners or more?

—1か月に何人ですか. — How many different partners in a month?

—先月,パートナーは何人でしたか. — How many partners have you had in the past month?

—あなたは性生活に満足していますか. — Are you happy with your sex life?

—あなたのパートナーは性生活に満足していますか. — Is your partner happy with her [his] sex life?

—1番最近に性行為をしたのはいつですか. — When was the last time you had intercourse?

性感染症の予防を講じていますか. □ Do you take any precautionary measures to prevent having a sexually transmitted infection?

—どんな予防法を講じていますか. — What measures do you take?

☞「訊きにくい/尋ねにくい質問」(116ページ).

### 既往歴

これまでに性行為感染症にかかったことがありますか. □ Have you had any sexually transmitted infection?

—それは何でしたか. — What was the problem?
1. クラミジア感染症. 1. Chlamydia?
2. 淋菌感染症. 2. Gonorrhea?
3. トリコモナス感染症. 3. Trichomonas?
4. 性器ヘルペス. 4. Genital herpes?
5. 尖圭コンジローマ. 5. Genital warts [Condyloma acuminatum]?
6. 梅毒. 6. Syphilis?
7. HIV感染症〔エイズ〕. 7. HIV infection [AIDS]?
8. B型肝炎. 8. Hepatitis B?

—いつですか. — When (did you have it)?

| | |
|---|---|
| —どんな治療を受けましたか. | — How was it treated? |
| これまでに性行為感染症やエイズにかかっている人と性関係をもったことがありますか. | ☐ Have you ever had any sexual contact with anyone who had sexually transmitted infections or AIDS? |
| …の既往はありますか.<br>　1. 糖尿病<br>　2. 狭心症や心筋梗塞などの心臓の病気<br>　3. 高血圧か低血圧症<br>　4. 脳血管疾患<br>　5. 肝障害<br>　6. 網膜色素変性症 | ☐ Do you have a history of...<br>　1. diabetes?<br>　2. heart disease, such as angina pectoris or myocardial infarction?<br>　3. high blood pressure or low blood pressure?<br>　4. cerebrovascular disease?<br>　5. liver disorder?<br>　6. retinitis pigmentosa? |
| 尿生殖路〔脊髄〕を損傷したことがありますか. | ☐ Have you ever had an injury of the genitourinary tract〔the spinal cord〕? |
| —いつですか.<br>—どうしたのですか.<br>—その結果, どんな症状がありましたか.<br>—どんな治療を受けましたか. | — When did it occur?<br>— What happened?<br>— What symptoms did you develop as a result?<br>— How was your injury treated? |
| あなたは包茎手術をしていますか. | ☐ Are you circumcised? |
| これまでに…の手術を受けたことがありますか.<br>　1. 尿生殖路<br>　2. ヘルニア<br>　3. 骨盤内<br>　4. 脊髄<br>—いつですか.<br>—術後の合併症がありましたか.<br>—どんな合併症でしたか. | ☐ Have you ever had surgery...<br><br>　1. on your genitourinary tract?<br>　2. for a hernia?<br>　3. on your pelvis?<br>　4. on your spinal cord?<br>— When (did you have it)?<br>— Were there any complications after surgery?<br>— What complications did you have? |

常用している薬がありますか.

—それは何ですか.
1. 降圧薬.
2. 胃潰瘍治療薬.
3. 女性〔男性〕ホルモン薬.
4. 利尿薬.
5. 抗うつ薬.
6. ニトログリセリン.

☐ Are you taking any drugs or medications regularly?
— What are they?
1. Antihypertensives?
2. Medications for gastric ulcers?
3. Female〔Male〕hormones?
4. Diuretics?
5. Antidepressants?
6. Nitroglycerin?

---

**コラム**

## 訊きにくい／尋ねにくい質問

性生活など患者さんがオープンに話すことをためらう話題について訊ねる必要があると判断した場合には，事実関係を知るためにプロ意識をもって冷静に質問する．その際，プライバシーを確保し，患者さんが不愉快な思いをしないようにその気持ちに配慮して訊ねることが肝要である．

本題に入る前に，その質問が診察や治療に役立つ可能性について説明する．また，医療者側に守秘義務があることを伝える．例えば，"I know these questions are very personal, but they are important for diagnosis and treatment."（個人的な質問になるかと思いますが，診断や治療を行う上で重要なことがらになります．）や "Anything we discuss here will be completely confidential."（ここでお話になる内容は秘密厳守とさせていただきます．）などと前もって伝えれば患者さんは安心して話すことができる．

## 9　乳房・女性生殖器

☞「妊娠・分娩」(363 ページ).
☞「乳房の診察」(223 ページ).
☞「生殖器の診察」(226 ページ).

### 一般的な質問

乳房〔性器〕に何か問題がありますか.

- □ (Do you have) any problems with your breasts〔female organs〕?
- □ (Is there) anything wrong with your breasts〔female organs〕?

—どんな問題ですか.
— What kind of problems?

それはどのくらい続いていますか.
- □ How long have you had the problems?

—いつからですか.
— Since when?

このような問題は以前にもありましたか.
- □ Have you had these problems before?

☞「病歴をとるためのヒント」(22 ページ).

### 乳房変化

あなたは乳房の変化に気づきましたか.
- □ Have you noticed any changes in your breasts?

—どちらの乳房ですか. 右か左.
— Which breast? Right or left?

—どのような変化ですか.
— How has it changed?
  Can you describe it for me?

—…がありますか
— Do you have any...
  1. しこり
  2. 腫れ［盛り上がり］
  3. 皮膚の硬化
  4. へこみ［えくぼ］
  5. 乳首の陥没

  1. lumps?
  2. swelling?
  3. thickened skin?
  4. dimples?
  5. nipple(s) drawn into the breast?

—最初に気づいたのはいつですか.
— When did you first notice it〔them〕?

乳首から分泌物が出ていますか．

─分泌物は片方だけですか，それとも両方ですか．
─どちらの乳首ですか．右か左．
─どんな分泌物ですか．
─どんな色をしていますか．
　1．透明か白っぽい．
　2．乳白色．
　3．赤みがかった．
　4．緑がかった．
　5．茶色がかった．
─分泌物は…
　1．自然に出てきますか．
　2．押すと出るのですか．

乳房に発疹や湿疹が出ていますか．

─かゆいですか．

痛みがありますか．
　1．乳房に．
　2．乳首に．
　3．脇の下に．
─そこは…
　1．触ると痛みますか．
　2．焼け付くようですか．
　3．ひりひりしますか．
─痛みは…
　1．月経が始まる前にひどくなりますか．
　2．月経が始まると軽くなりますか．
─最近痛みはひどくなりましたか．

☐ Have you noticed any nipple discharge?
— Does it occur with only one nipple or both?
— Which nipple?  Right or left?
— What is it like?
— What is the color?
　1. Clear or whitish?
　2. Milky?
　3. Reddish?
　4. Greenish?
　5. Brownish?
— Does it come out...
　1. spontaneously?
　2. with squeezing or pressure?

☐ Is there any rash or eczema on your breast(s)?
— Are they 〔Is it〕 itchy?

☐ Do you have any pain...
　1. in your breast(s)?
　2. in your nipple(s)?
　3. under your arm(s)?
— Are they 〔Is it〕...
　1. tender?
　2. burning?
　3. feeling sore?
— Is the pain...
　1. worse just before you have menstrual periods?
　2. relieved after you start to have menstrual periods?
— Has it become more painful recently?

### 月経

今でも月経がありますか．

☐ Do you still have menstrual periods now?

| | |
|---|---|
| 最初の月経があったのは［初経年齢は］何歳のときですか． | ☐ How old were you when you started having periods? |
| 最後に月経があったのは［閉経年齢は］何歳のときですか． | ☐ How old were you when you had your last period? |
| あなたの…はいつでしたか．<br>　1．最近の月経［最終月経］<br>　2．その前の月経<br>―いつからいつでしたか． | ☐ When was...<br>　1．your last period?<br>　2．second to your last period?<br>— From when to when? |
| 月経と次の月経との間［月経周期］は通常何日ありますか． | ☐ How many days usually pass between periods?<br>☐ How often do your periods come? |
| ―月経は通常…ですか．<br>　1．規則的<br>　2．不規則<br>　3．25 日より短い<br>　4．38 日より長い | — Are your periods usually...<br>　1．regular?<br>　2．irregular?<br>　3．shorter than 25 days?<br>　4．longer than 38 days? |
| （月経期間は）何日くらい続きますか．<br>　1．3 日よりも短い．<br>　2．3〜7 日．<br>　3．7 日よりも長い． | ☐ How many days do they last?<br><br>　1．Shorter than 3 days?<br>　2．3 to 7 days?<br>　3．Longer than 7 days? |
| 出血量［経血量］はどうですか．<br>　1．少なめ．<br>　2．ふつう．<br>　3．多め．<br>―1 日に生理用ナプキン〔タンポン〕を何枚〔いくつ〕使いますか．<br>―最近，出血量に変化がありましたか．<br>　1．増えた．<br>　2．減った．<br>　3．同じ． | ☐ What is your usual flow?<br>　1．Light?<br>　2．Normal?<br>　3．Heavy?<br>— How many pads〔tampons〕do you use a day?<br>— Has your flow changed recently?<br><br>　1．Increased?<br>　2．Decreased?<br>　3．The same? |

―出血の中に血の塊が混じっていますか.
1. ごく少量.
2. ほどほど［中程度］.
3. 多量.

貧血があると言われたことがありますか.

月経中に痛みや不快感がありますか.

―どんな痛みですか.
1. 下腹部痛.
2. 腰痛.
3. 乳房痛.
4. 頭痛.

そのほかに徴候や症状がありますか.
―それは何ですか.
1. のぼせ.
2. 冷感.
3. むくみ.
4. 体重増加.
5. 食欲不振.
6. 吐き気.
7. 嘔吐.
8. 便通異常.
9. 抑うつ気分，情緒不安定などの気分のむら.

症状が起こるのはいつですか.
1. 月経の前.
2. 月経中.
―どのくらい長く続きますか.

— Have you noticed any clots in your flow?
1. A few?
2. Moderate number?
3. Many?

☐ Have you ever been told that you have anemia?

☐ Do you have any pain or discomfort during your periods?

— What kind of pain is it?
1. Cramps in the lower abdomen?
2. Low back pain?
3. Pain in your breasts?
4. Headache?

☐ Do you have any other signs or symptoms?
— What are they?
1. Hot flashes?
2. Chills?
3. Swelling?
4. Weight gain?
5. Loss of appetite?
6. Nausea?
7. Vomiting?
8. Problem with bowel movements?
9. Mood swings, such as depression or emotional instability?

☐ When does the symptom occur?
1. Before periods?
2. During periods?
— How long does it last?

―初めて症状を自覚したのはいつですか．
― When did you first notice it? When did it start?

―症状は徐々にひどくなっていますか．
― Is it getting worse?

鎮痛薬などの薬を飲みますか．
☐ Do you take any medications such as pain killers?

―仕事〔学校〕を休むか，就寝を余儀なくされますか．
― Do you have to be absent from work〔school〕, or go on bed rest?

毎朝，基礎体温を計っていますか．
☐ Do you take your（basal body）temperature every morning?

―記録を見せていただけますか．
― Can you show me the record?

### 不正出血

月経と次の月経の間に出血しますか．
☐ Do you ever bleed between your menstrual periods?

―その量はどのくらいですか．
― How much is it?
 1. ごく少量．
 2. 多量．
 1. A little bit ［A small amount］?
 2. A lot ［Abundant］?

―どのくらい長く続きますか．
― How long does it last?

―最初に気づいたのはいつですか．
― When did you first notice it? When did it start?

―最後に自覚したのはいつですか．
― When was the last time you noticed it?

性行為の後，腟から出血しますか．
☐ Do you ever have vaginal bleeding after intercourse?

出血傾向はありますか．
☐ Do you bleed easily?

閉経していますか．
☐ Have you undergone menopause?

―最後に月経があったのは［閉経年齢は］何歳のときですか．
― How old were you when you had your last period?

### 帯下(おりもの)

腟からおりもの[分泌物]が出ますか.
―どんな分泌物ですか.
1. 透明か白っぽい.
2. 灰色か緑色がかっている.
3. 黄色.
4. 褐色か暗赤色.
5. さらさら[漿液性].
6. どろどろ[膿性].
7. 血がにじんでいる.
8. チーズのような.
9. 泡のような.
―悪臭がしますか.

その量はどのくらいですか.
1. ごく少量.
2. 多量.

初めて気づいたのはいつですか.

そのほか徴候や症状がありますか.

―それは何ですか.
1. かゆみ.
2. 焼け付くような感じ.
3. 腫れ.
4. ただれ[潰瘍].
5. 発熱.

### 更年期症状

最近,月経の変化に気づきましたか.
―以前の月経と比べると,…ですか.

1. 期間が短い
2. 期間が長い

☐ Do you have any vaginal discharge?
— What is it like?
1. Clear or whitish?
2. Gray or greenish?
3. Yellow?
4. Dark brown or dark red?
5. Thin?
6. Thick like pus?
7. Blood-tinged?
8. Cheesy?
9. Frothy?
— Does it have a bad smell?

☐ How much is it?
1. A little bit [A small amount]?
2. A lot [Abundant]?

☐ When did you first notice it?
☐ When did it start?

☐ Do you have any other signs or symptoms?
— What are they?
1. Itching?
2. Burning sensation?
3. Swelling?
4. Sores?
5. Fever?

☐ Have you recently noticed any change in your periods?
— Compared with your previous periods, are your periods...
1. shorter?
2. longer?

3. 不規則
  4. 出血量が少ない
  5. 出血量が多い

そのほかに徴候や症状がありますか.
― それは何ですか.
  1. のぼせ［ほてり］.
  2. 発汗.
  3. 動悸.
  4. 腟の乾燥.
  5. 性交時の痛みや不快感.
  6. 不眠.
  7. 疲労感.
  8. 気分のむら，例えば…
     a. 落ち込み［うつ状態になる］.
     b. 不安.
     c. いらいら.
  9. その他，頭痛，肩こり，腰痛，冷え，息切れ，しびれ，めまいなど.

  3. irregular?
  4. lighter in their flow?
  5. heavier in their flow?

☐ Do you have any other signs or symptoms?
― What are they?
  1. Hot flashes?
  2. Sweating?
  3. Palpitations?
  4. Vaginal dryness?
  5. Pain or discomfort during intercourse?
  6. Insomnia?
  7. Fatigue?
  8. Mood swings, such as...
     a. depression?
     b. nervousness?
     c. irritability?
  9. Others, such as headache, stiff neck, low back pain, chills, shortness of breath, numbness, or dizziness?

### 性生活

それではこれからあなたの性習慣についておうかがいします.
― 個人的な質問になるかと思いますが，この情報はあなたの診療に役立てるためのものです.

― ここでお話になる内容は秘密厳守とさせていただきます.

現在，性生活はありますか.

― 性行為の相手は男性，女性，またはその両方ですか.

☐ Now I'd like to ask about your sexual practices.
― I know these questions are very personal, but this information will help me take better care of you.

― Anything we discuss here will be completely confidential.

☐ Are you currently sexually active?

― Are your partners men, women, or both?

| | |
|---|---|
| ―パートナーは 2 人以上いますか. | — Do you have two partners or more? |
| ―1 か月に何人ですか. | — How many different partners in a month? |
| ―先月, パートナーは何人でしたか. | — How many partners have you had in the past month? |
| ―あなたは性生活に満足していますか. | — Are you happy with your sex life? |
| ―あなたのパートナーは性生活に満足していますか. | — Is your partner happy with his [her] sex life? |
| ―1 番最近に性行為をしたのはいつですか. | — When was the last time you had intercourse? |
| 性感染症の予防を講じていますか. | ☐ Do you take any precautionary measures to prevent having a sexually transmitted infection? |
| ―どんな予防法を講じていますか. | — What measures do you take? |

避妊していますか.　☐ Do you practice birth control?
―何を使っていますか.　— What do you use?

1. コンドーム.
2. ピル〔経口避妊薬〕.
3. 子宮内避妊具.
4. ペッサリー〔頸管キャップ〕.
5. 避妊用フォーム〔フィルム／クリーム／ゼリー〕.
6. ホルモン避妊インプラント〔パッチ／注射〕.
7. 基礎体温.
8. その他.

1. Condoms?
2. Birth control pills?
3. Intrauterine device [IUD]?
4. Diaphragm [Cervical cap]?
5. Contraceptive foam [film/cream/jelly]?
6. Hormonal implant [patch/injection]?
7. Basal body temperature?
8. Something else?

| | |
|---|---|
| 性生活のことで問題がありますか. | ☐ Do you have any problem with your sex life? |
| ―どんな問題ですか. | — What is it? |
| ―初めて気づいたのはいつですか. | — When did you first notice it? When did it start? |
| ―性交中に痛みや不快感がありますか. | — Do you feel any pain or discomfort during intercourse? |
| ―性交後出血しますか. | — Do you bleed after intercourse? |

あなたの性行為の相手の性器に異常がありますか.

1. ペニス〔腟〕からの分泌物.
2. 性器のただれ［潰瘍］.

☐ Does your sexual partner have any problems with his〔her〕genitals?
1. Discharge from his penis〔her vagina〕?
2. Genital sores?

### 既往歴・家族歴

これまでに性行為感染症にかかったことがありますか.
―それは何でしたか.
1. クラミジア感染症.
2. 淋菌感染症.
3. トリコモナス感染症.
4. 性器ヘルペス.
5. 尖圭コンジローマ.
6. 梅毒.
7. HIV 感染症〔エイズ〕.
8. B 型肝炎.
9. パピローマウイルス感染症.
―いつですか.
―どんな治療を受けましたか.

☐ Have you had any sexually transmitted infection?
— What was the problem?
1. Chlamydia?
2. Gonorrhea?
3. Trichomonas?
4. Genital herpes?
5. Genital warts〔Condyloma acuminatum〕?
6. Syphilis?
7. HIV infection〔AIDS〕?
8. Hepatitis B?
9. Papillomavirus infection?
— When (did you have it)?
— How was it treated?

以前…を受けたことがありますか.
1. 乳房診察
2. マンモグラフィ検査
3. 乳房超音波検査
4. 子宮頸がん検診［パップスメア検査］
―この前受けたのはいつですか.
―その結果は…でしたか.
1. 正常
2. 異常

☐ Have you ever had...
1. a breast examination?
2. a mammogram?
3. a breast ultrasound?
4. a Pap smear?
— When was your last test?
— Were the results...
1. normal?
2. abnormal?

乳房の自己触診をやっていますか.
―いつやりますか. どのくらいの頻度ですか.

☐ Do you do self breast exams?
— When do you do them? How often?

| | |
|---|---|
| 妊娠したことがありますか． | ☐ Have you ever been pregnant? |
| ―妊娠回数と分娩回数を教えて下さい． | — Please tell me how many times you were pregnant and how many babies [deliveries] you had. |
| ―1番下のお子さんは何歳ですか． | — How old is your last child? |
| 現在も授乳していますか． | ☐ Are you breast-feeding now? |
| ご家族に乳がんの人がいますか． | ☐ Has anyone in your immediate family had breast cancer? |
| ―どなたですか． | — Who is it? |
| ―何歳でしたか． | — How old was she when she had it? |
| ご家族に婦人科の病気にかかった人がいますか． | ☐ Has anyone in your immediate family had any gynecologic problem? |
| ―誰ですか． | — Who is it? |
| ―何の異常でしたか． | — What was the problem? |

## 10 代謝・内分泌

### 一般的な質問

ホルモンに何か問題がありますか．
- □ (Do you have) any problems with your hormones?
- □ (Is there) anything wrong with your hormones?

―どんな問題ですか．
― What kind of problems?

それはどのくらい続いていますか．
- □ How long have you had the problems?

―いつからですか．
― Since when?

このような問題は以前にもありましたか．
- □ Have you had these problems before?

☞「病歴をとるためのヒント」(22 ページ)．

### 体重変化

☞「単位の換算表」(216 ページ)．

体重はどのくらいありますか．
- □ How much do you weigh now?
- □ What's your weight?

―昨年，体重はどのくらいありましたか．
― How much did you weigh last year?

―最高の体重はいくらですか．
― What's the most you've weighed?

―最低の体重はいくらですか．
― What's the least you've weighed?

最近，体重に変化がありましたか．
- □ Has your weight changed recently?
  1. 増えましたか．
  2. 減りましたか．
  1. Have you gained weight?
  2. Have you lost weight?

―1 週間〔月／年〕で何キロ〔ポンド〕増え〔減り〕ましたか．
― How many kilos〔pounds〕did you gain〔lose〕within a week〔month/year〕?

―説明のつかない体重増加〔減少〕ですか．
― Is it an unexplained weight gain〔loss〕?

| | |
|---|---|
| 体重増加のほかに徴候や症状がありますか. | ☐ Do you have any other signs or symptoms, accompanied by your weight gain? |
| ―それは何ですか. | — What are they? |

1. にきび.
2. 多毛.
3. 高血圧.
4. 皮膚のかさかさ.
5. 便秘.
6. 寒がり.
7. 声がれ.

1. Pimples?
2. Excessive hair growth?
3. High blood pressure?
4. Increased dryness or roughness of your skin?
5. Constipation?
6. Feeling the cold more than you used to?
7. Hoarseness?

| | |
|---|---|
| 体重減少のほかに徴候や症状がありますか. | ☐ Do you have any other signs or symptoms, accompanied by your weight loss? |
| ―それは何ですか. | — What are they? |

1. 吐き気.
2. 嘔吐.
3. 下痢.
4. 食欲不振.
5. 過食.
6. 口渇.
7. 多飲.
8. 多尿.
9. 動悸.
10. 発汗.
11. 震え.
   ―手や指が震えますか.
12. 頭痛.
13. 高血圧.
14. 皮膚や口腔粘膜の色素沈着.

1. Nausea?
2. Vomiting?
3. Diarrhea?
4. Loss of appetite?
5. Excessive eating?
6. Dry mouth?
7. Excessive thirst?
8. Increased urination?
9. Palpitations?
10. Sweating?
11. Trembling?
    — Do your hands or fingers tremble or shake?
12. Headache?
13. High blood pressure?
14. Darkening of your skin or your oral mucous membrane?

| | |
|---|---|
| 食欲はどうですか. | ☐ How is your appetite? Has it... |

1. 増えましたか.
2. 減りましたか.
3. これまでと同じですか.

1. increased?
2. decreased?
3. stayed about the same?

|  |  |
|---|---|
| バランスの良い食事を規則的にとっていますか. | ☐ Do you eat well-balanced meals at regular times? |
| ―暴飲暴食していますか. | ― Do you eat and drink too much? |
| ―不規則な食生活ですか. | ― Do you eat at irregular times? |
| ―以前より食べる量が多いのに体重が増えないのですか. | ― Do you eat more and not gain weight? |
| ふだん運動をしていますか. | ☐ Do you usually do any exercise? |
| ―どんな運動ですか. | ― What do you do? |

☞「食習慣」,「運動」(202, 207 ページ).

### 口渇・多飲・多尿

|  |  |
|---|---|
| 異常なほど喉が渇きますか. | ☐ Do you feel unusually thirsty? |
| ―初めて気づいたのはいつですか. | ― When did you first notice the problem? |
| ―その状態はどのくらい続いていますか. | ― How long have you felt this way? |
| 1日にどの〔何リットル〕くらいの水分を飲んでいますか. | ☐ How much liquid〔How many liters of liquid〕do you drink each day? |
| 以前より汗をたくさんかきますか. | ☐ Do you perspire more than you used to? |
| 排尿は1日に何回ありますか. | ☐ How often [How many times] do you urinate a day? |
| ―以前より回数が多い〔少ない〕ですか. | ― Do you urinate more〔less〕often than you used to? |
| ―以前より尿の量は多い〔少ない〕ですか. | ― Do you pass more〔less〕urine than you used to? |
| ―夜間, トイレに何回起きますか. | ― How many times do you wake up to go to the bathroom during the night? |
| 口の渇きのほかに徴候や症状がありますか. | ☐ Do you have any other signs or symptoms, accompanied by your dry mouth? |
| ―それは何ですか. | ― What are they? |

chapter 3 現病歴（代謝・内分泌）

| | |
|---|---|
| 1. 発熱. | 1. Fever? |
| 2. 嘔吐. | 2. Vomiting? |
| 3. 下痢. | 3. Diarrhea? |
| 4. 体重減少. | 4. Weight loss? |
| 5. 目がごろごろする〔涙が少ない〕. | 5. Feeling something gritty in your eyes〔Dry eyes〕? |

### 前頸部腫瘤

| | |
|---|---|
| 首のしこり［腫れ］に気がつきましたか. | ☐ Have you noticed a lump in your neck? |
| —初めてしこりに気づいたのはいつですか. | — When did you first notice the lump? |
| しこりは… | ☐ Is it... |
| 1. 大きくなっていますか. | 1. growing [getting bigger]? |
| 2. ひいてきていますか. | 2. decreasing [getting smaller]? |
| 3. 変化なしですか. | 3. the same? |
| 前頸部腫瘤のほかに徴候や症状がありますか. | ☐ Do you have any other signs or symptoms, accompanied by your lump? |
| —それは何ですか. | — What are they? |
| 1. 発熱. | 1. Fever? |
| 2. 痛み. | 2. Pain? |
| 3. 動悸. | 3. Palpitations? |
| 4. 発汗. | 4. Sweating? |
| 5. 手の震え. | 5. Trembling hands? |
| 6. 体重減少. | 6. Weight loss? |
| 7. 皮膚のかさかさ. | 7. Increased dryness or roughness of your skin? |
| 8. むくみ. | 8. Swelling [Edema]? |
| 9. 便秘. | 9. Constipation? |
| 10. 寒がり. | 10. Feeling the cold more than you used to? |
| 11. 声がれ. | 11. Hoarseness? |

### その他

最近，頭痛がしますか．
☐ Do you have or have you recently had a headache?

―吐き気や嘔吐がありますか．
― Do you feel like vomiting or have you vomited?

最近，視力に問題がありますか．
☐ Have you had any visual problems recently?

1. 視野が狭くなった．
2. ものがかすんで見える．
3. ものが二重に見える．

1. Is your visual field getting narrowed?
2. Are you having blurred vision?
3. Are you having double vision?

顔つき〔容貌〕が変化しましたか．
☐ Have you noticed any change in your facial features?

―指輪がきつくなりましたか．
― Do your rings feel tight?

―靴がきつくてサイズを大きくしましたか．
― Do your shoes feel tight, so now do you wear bigger size shoes?

月経が変化しましたか．
☐ Have you noticed any change in your menstrual periods?

―月経がなくなりましたか．
― Have your periods stopped?

性欲が変化しましたか．
☐ Have you noticed any change in your desire for sexual relations?

1. 性欲がなくなった〔ほとんどなくなった〕．
2. インポテンツになった．

1. Do you have no 〔little〕 interest in sex?
2. Do you have difficulty achieving and maintaining an erection?

乳房が小さくなりましたか．
☐ Have your breasts become smaller?

陰毛や脇毛が薄くなりましたか．
☐ Has your pubic hair or the hair of your armpits become thin?

最近,皮膚に変化がありましたか.

―皮膚の色が…
1. 薄くなった.
2. 黒ずんだ.

疲れやすいですか.

出産後にもかかわらず乳汁がみられないのですか.
―妊娠や出産がないのに乳汁が出ますか.

(男性で)乳房が大きくなりましたか.

☐ Have you noticed any change in your skin?
— Has your skin become...
1. paler?
2. darker?

☐ Do you get tired easily?

☐ Do you have no flow of milk even after you had a baby?
— Do you have a flow of milk even though you are not pregnant or you did not have a baby?

☐ Have you noticed development of your breasts?

### 既往歴・家族歴

これまでに…と診断されたことがありますか.
1. 糖尿病
2. 甲状腺の病気
3. 高血圧
4. 腎結石
5. 尿路結石
6. その他
―診断されたのはいつですか.
―どんな治療を受けましたか.

最近,出産しましたか.

常用している薬がありますか.

―それは何ですか.
1. 降圧薬.
2. 利尿薬.
3. 抗コリン薬.
4. 抗ヒスタミン薬.
5. 向精神薬.

☐ Have you ever been diagnosed that you have...
1. diabetes?
2. thyroid disease?
3. high blood pressure?
4. kidney stones?
5. urinary stones?
6. any other disorders?
— When was it diagnosed?
— How was it treated?

☐ Have you recently had a baby?

☐ Are you taking any drugs or medications regularly?
— What are they?
1. Antihypertensives?
2. Diuretics?
3. Anticholinergic drugs?
4. Antihistamines?
5. Psychotropic drugs?

| | |
|---|---|
| 6. 抗うつ薬. | 6. Antidepressants? |
| 7. 制酸薬. | 7. Gastric antiacids? |
| 8. 経口避妊薬. | 8. Birth control pills? |
| 9. ステロイド薬. | 9. Steroids? |

ご家族に肥満, やせの人がいますか. — ☐ Is anyone else in your immediate family overweight or underweight?

ご家族に…の病気にかかっている人がいますか. — ☐ Does anyone in your immediate family have illnesses of...

1. 下垂体
2. 膵臓
3. 副甲状腺
4. 甲状腺
5. 副腎
6. その他

1. the pituitary gland?
2. the pancreas?
3. the accessory [para-] thyroid gland?
4. the thyroid gland?
5. the adrenal gland?
6. any other organs?

---

### 名句・ことわざ

**The best doctors in the world are Dr. Diet, Dr. Quiet, and Dr. Merryman.**

この世の名医とは「食事」医,「安静」医, それに「快活」医なり

『ガリバー旅行記』で有名な英国の風刺作家スウィフト (Jonathan Swift, 1667-1745, *Polite Conversation*) の名言.

## 11 血液

### 一般的な質問

血液に問題があると言われたことがありますか.

—どんな問題ですか.

それはどのくらい続いていますか.

—いつからですか.

このような問題は以前にもありましたか.

☞「病歴をとるためのヒント」(22 ページ).

☐ Have you ever been told that you have problems with your blood?
— What kind of problems?

☐ How long have you had the problems?
— Since when?

☐ Have you had these problems before?

### 貧血

人から「顔色が悪い」と言われたことがありますか.
—いつもより…ですか.

1. 青白い
2. 黄色い

ほかに徴候や症状はありますか.

—それは何ですか.
1. 倦怠感.
2. 動悸.
3. 息切れ.
4. 立ちくらみ.
5. 頭痛.
6. 舌痛.
7. 嚥下障害.

最近, 便の色が変わりましたか.

☐ Has anyone told you that you look pale?
— Has your color become ... than your normal skin?
 1. paler
 2. more yellowish

☐ Do you have any other signs or symptoms?
— What are they?
 1. Fatigue?
 2. Palpitations?
 3. Shortness of breath?
 4. Feeling dizzy when you stand up?
 5. Headache?
 6. Pain in the tongue?
 7. Difficulty swallowing?

☐ Have you noticed any change in the color of your stools?

―どんな便でしたか.

1. 血が混じっていた.
2. タール様.

月経に変化がありましたか.

―月経はいつもより…
1. 周期が短いですか.
2. 期間が長いですか.
3. 血の量が多いですか.

これまでに何か大きな病気をしましたか.
―…の既往がありますか.
1. 痔
2. 胃手術
3. 婦人科疾患

血液検査で貧血と言われたことがありますか.

―いつですか.
―どんな治療を受けましたか. どのくらいの期間ですか.

…は受けましたか.
1. 胃検診
2. 大腸検診
3. 婦人科検診

最近飲んでいる薬がありますか.

―それは何ですか.

— What were they like?
Can you describe them for me?
Was [Were] there...
1. any blood mixed in with your stools?
2. any tarry stools?

☐ Have you noticed any change in your menstrual periods?

— Are they...
1. shorter than usual?
2. longer than usual?
3. heavier than usual?

☐ Have you had any serious illnesses?
— Have you ever had...
1. hemorrhoids?
2. stomach surgery?
3. women's [gynecological] disease?

☐ As a result of the blood test, have you ever been told that you are anemic?

— When was it?
— How were you treated? How long?

☐ Did you have...
1. a stomach checkup?
2. a colon checkup?
3. a gynecologic checkup?

☐ Have you taken or are you taking any drugs or medications?

— What are they?

chapter 3 現病歴（血液）

### 出血傾向

出血しやすいですか．

☐ Do you bleed easily?

最近，異常に出血しましたか．

☐ Have you noticed any unusual bleeding recently?

—出血の場所はどこですか．
1. 鼻．
   a. いつも決まった側から．
   b. 両側から．
2. 口．
3. 歯茎［歯肉］．
4. その他．

— Where is the bleeding?
1. Your nose?
   a. Always from the same side?
   b. From both sides?
2. Your mouth?
3. Your gums?
4. Any other part of your body?

出血したあと血が止まらないことがありましたか．例えば，

1. 傷口から．
2. 抜歯をしたあと．
3. 月経時．
4. 手術後．
5. 出産後．

—その時に輸血をしましたか．

☐ Have you had an experience of bleeding that wouldn't stop? For example,
1. from a cut?
2. after having your tooth pulled?
3. at the time of your menstrual periods?
4. after surgery?
5. after having a baby?

— Then, did you have a blood transfusion?

皮下出血を起こしやすいですか．
—場所はどこですか．
—気がつかない間にあざができていることはありますか．

☐ Do you bruise easily?
— Where are the bruises?
— Do you ever have bruises［skin discoloration］for no obvious reason?

初めて気づいたのはいつですか．

☐ When did you first notice it?
☐ When did it start?

—出血傾向は生まれつきですか．

— Were you born with the bleeding tendency?

| | |
|---|---|
| 最近,吐いたことがありますか. | ☐ Have you vomited recently? |
| ―どんな色でしたか. | ― What color was the vomit? |
|   1. 真っ赤. |   1. Bright red? |
|   2. 茶色. |   2. Brown? |
|   3. 黒. |   3. Black? |
|   4. その他. |   4. Any other color? |
| ―吐いた物に血が混じっていましたか. | ― Have you noticed any blood in the vomit? |
| 咳をしたとき血が出たことがありますか. | ☐ Have you coughed up blood? |
| 最近,尿の色が変わりましたか. | ☐ Have you noticed any change in the color of your urine? |
| ―どんな色でしたか. | ― What color was it? |
|   1. ピンクがかった. |   1. Pinkish? |
|   2. 真っ赤. |   2. Bright red? |
|   3. 茶褐色. |   3. Dark brown? |
|   4. その他. |   4. Any other color? |
| ―尿に血が混じっていましたか. | ― Have you noticed any blood in the urine? |
| 便に血が混じっていることがありますか. | ☐ Have you noticed any blood in your stools? |
| ―どんな色でしたか. | ― What color were they? |
|   1. 真っ赤. |   1. Bright red? |
|   2. 黒ずんだ色. |   2. Dark? |
|   3. 血がにじんだ. |   3. Blood tinged? |
|   4. その他. |   4. Any other color? |
| 黒い,タール様の便が出たことがありますか. | ☐ Have you had any black, tarry stools? |
| 常用している薬がありますか. | ☐ Are you taking any drugs or medications regularly? |
| ―それは何ですか. | ― What are they? |
|   1. ステロイド. |   1. Steroids? |
|   2. 鎮痛解熱薬. |   2. Pain killers and medications for fever [Analgesic-antipyretic drugs]? |

| | |
|---|---|
| 3. 制酸薬. | 3. Gastric antacids? |
| 4. 抗血小板薬. | 4. Antiplatelets? |
| 5. 抗凝固薬. | 5. Anticoagulants? |
| —薬草［漢方薬］を飲んでいますか. | — Are you taking any herbal medications? |
| 最近, 大きな病気をしましたか. | ☐ Have you recently had any serious illnesses? |
| —それは何ですか. | — What are they? |
| ご家族のどなたかに出血傾向のある人がいますか. | ☐ Is there anyone else in your immediate family who has a bleeding tendency? |

---

### 名句・ことわざ

**頭寒足熱**

〔英訳〕**A cool head and warm feet live long.**

英語には, "A cool mouth and warm feet live long."（口を冷やし足を温めると長生きできる）や "Keep your mouth wet, feet dry."（口は濡らして足は乾かしておけ）という類似のことわざがある.

## 12 筋・骨格

☞「骨格の診察」(227 ページ).

### 一般的な質問

骨, 関節, 筋肉に何か問題がありますか.
- ☐ (Do you have) any problems with your bones, joints, or muscles?
- ☐ (Is there) anything wrong with your bones, joints, or muscles?

―どんな問題ですか.
― What kind of problems?

それはどのくらい続いていますか.
- ☐ How long have you had the problems?

―いつからですか.
― Since when?

このような問題は以前にもありましたか.
- ☐ Have you had these problems before?

☞「病歴をとるためのヒント」(22 ページ).

### 痛み

☞「痛みの表現」(31 ページ).

#### 症状の特徴

筋肉, 関節, または骨のどこかが痛みますか.
- ☐ Are you having pain in any of your muscles, joints, or bones?

どこが痛みますか.
- ☐ Where is the pain?
- ☐ Where does it hurt [ache]?

1. 首.
2. 肩.
3. 肘.
4. 手首.
5. 指.
6. 背骨.
7. 腰.
8. 股関節.
9. 膝.
10. 足首.

1. Neck?
2. Shoulders?
3. Elbows?
4. Wrists?
5. Fingers?
6. Spine?
7. Lower back?
8. Hip joints?
9. Knees?
10. Ankles?

11. その他.
— 両方ですか，それとも片方ですか．
— 右ですか，左ですか．
— 痛む所を指でさして下さい．

痛みは他の場所へ広がりますか〔移動しますか〕．
— どこからどこへですか．
— 1つの関節に限局していますか，複数の関節に及んでいますか．

どんなふうに痛みますか．

1. 軽い．
2. 激しい．
3. 鈍い．
4. 鋭い［ナイフで刺すような］．
5. ずきずきする．
6. 焼け付くような．
7. 圧迫されるような．
8. こわばった感じ．
9. その他．

いつ痛むのですか．

1. 早朝．
2. 日中．
3. 夜間．
4. 睡眠中．
5. 1日中．

時期によって痛みがひどくなりますか．
1. 寒いとき．
2. 雨が降るとき．
3. じめじめしたとき．

11. Any other part of your body?
— Do you have it on both sides or only one side?
— Right or left?
— Please point to the place (where you have the pain).

☐ Does the pain radiate [move] to another place?
— From where to where?
— Is it confined to one joint, or does it affect more joints?

☐ What is the pain like?
☐ Can you describe the pain for me?
  1. Mild?
  2. Severe?
  3. Dull ache?
  4. Sharp [Stabbing-like a knife]?
  5. Throbbing?
  6. Burning?
  7. Pressure-like?
  8. Stiff?
  9. Any other kind of pain?

☐ When do you have the pain?
☐ When does it hurt?
  1. Early in the morning?
  2. During the day?
  3. At night?
  4. During sleep?
  5. All day long?

☐ Does the pain bother you during certain times of the year?
  1. When it is cold?
  2. When it rains?
  3. When it is damp?

どんな動作をすると痛みますか〔痛みがひどくなりますか〕.

1. 首を曲げる.
2. 腕を上にあげる.
3. 手を使う.
4. 手足を曲げたり,伸ばしたりする.
5. 体を曲げる〔かがむ〕.
6. ひざまずく.
7. 椅子から立ち上がる.
8. 歩く.
9. 階段を上る.
10. 運動する.
11. その他.

☐ What kind of movements bring on the pain〔make the pain worse〕?
1. When you turn your head?
2. When you raise your arms?
3. When you use your hands?
4. When you bend or stretch your hands, arms, or legs?
5. When you bend over?
6. When you kneel?
7. When you get up from a chair?
8. When you walk?
9. When you climb stairs?
10. When you exercise?
11. Any other movement?

**時間経過**

痛むようになったのは…ですか.
1. つい最近
2. かなり前
   a. 数週間.
   b. 数か月.
   c. 数年.

☐ Did you have the pain...
1. just recently?
2. some time ago?
   a. Over weeks?
   b. Over months?
   c. Over years?

初めて痛みに気づいたのはいつですか.突然起こりましたか.
―その時の状況を教えて下さい.
1. 転んだ.
2. 何かにぶつかった.
3. ボールを投げた.
4. 手を引っ張られた.
5. 突き指をした.
6. 寝違えた.
7. 骨折した.
8. その他.

☐ When did you first notice the pain? Did it come on suddenly?
— Please tell me what happened?
1. Did you fall?
2. Did you bump into something?
3. Did you throw a ball?
4. Did you get pulled on the hand?
5. Did your finger get sprained?
6. Did you develop a crick in your sleep?
7. Did you have a fracture?
8. Something else?

| 痛みは徐々に数か月〔数年〕にかけて起こりましたか. | ☐ Did the pain come on gradually over months〔years〕? |

どのくらいの頻度で痛みますか.
- How often do you have the pain?
  1. 絶えず.
  2. 頻繁に.
  3. 時々.
  1. Constantly?
  2. Frequently?
  3. Occasionally [Once in a while]?

### 運動制限

体のどこかが動かしにくいですか.
☐ Do you have difficulty moving any part of your body?

―どこですか.
― Where?

痛むので動かせないのですか.
☐ Does the pain keep you from moving?

腕〔足〕に力が入らない感じがありますか.
☐ Do your arms〔legs〕feel weak?
☐ Do you have no strength in your arms〔legs〕?

―片方ですか, 両方ですか.
― In one or both arms〔legs〕?

足元がふらつきますか.
☐ Do you feel unsteady [shaky] on your feet?

### こわばり・突っ張り

どこかこわばって〔突っ張って〕いるところがありますか.
☐ Do you have stiffness anywhere?

―どこですか.
― Where?

―その場所を指でさして下さい.
― Please point to the place (where you have the stiffness).

こわばるのはいつですか.
☐ When do you have the stiffness?
1. 早朝.
2. 日中.
3. 夜間.
4. 睡眠中.

1. Early in the morning?
2. During the day?
3. At night?
4. During sleep?

5. 1日中.
―朝のこわばりは1時間以上続きますか.

こわばり始めたのはいつですか.
1. つい最近.
2. かなり前.
    a. 数週間.
    b. 数か月.
    c. 数年.

関節を動かすときにきしるような音を聞いたり感じたりすることがありますか.

### 腫れ

腫れているところがありますか.
―どこですか.
―その場所を指でさして下さい.

どんなふうな腫れですか.
―ほてって[熱をもって]いますか.
―何もしなくても痛みますか.
―そこを押すと痛みますか.
―動かすと痛みますか.

腫れに初めて気づいたのはいつですか.

腫れをとるのに何かしましたか.

1. 温めましたか.
2. 冷やしましたか.

---

5. All day long?
— Does morning stiffness last more than an hour?

☐ When did the stiffness start?
1. Just recently?
2. Some time ago?
    a. Over weeks?
    b. Over months?
    c. Over years?

☐ Do you sometimes hear a grating sound or feel a grating sensation when you move your joint(s)?

☐ Have you noticed any swelling?
— Where?
— Please point to the place (where you have the swelling).

☐ What is the swelling like?
— Does the overlying skin feel hot?
— Is it painful even when resting?
— Is the area tender?
— Is it painful with some movements?

☐ When did you first notice the swelling?

☐ Did you try anything to reduce the swelling?
1. Did you apply heat?
2. Did you apply ice?

### 随伴症状

ほかに徴候や症状がありますか.

― それは何ですか.
1. 発熱.
2. 発疹.
3. しびれ感, または感覚の消失.
4. 手足の冷感.
5. 筋肉の脱力感.
6. その他.

☐ Do you have any other signs or symptoms?
― What are they?
1. Fever?
2. Rash?
3. Numbness or loss of sensation?
4. Cold feeling of your hands and feet?
5. Muscle weakness?
6. Any other symptoms?

### 生活歴・既往歴・家族歴

最近, 体重が増えましたか.

― 何キロ〔ポンド〕増えましたか. どのくらいの期間ですか.

☞「単位の換算表」(216 ページ).

☐ Have you recently gained weight?
― How many kilos〔pounds〕did you gain? Within how long?

仕事でいつも同じ姿勢だったり, 重いものを持ったりしますか.

☐ Do you always assume the same posture, or do you lift heavy objects during work?

何かスポーツをしていますか.

☐ Do you play any sports?

靴は足にフィットしていますか.

☐ Do your shoes fit well?

あなたはどちらの手を多く使いますか.
1. 右手.
2. 左手.
3. 両手を同じくらい.

☐ Which hand do you use most?
1. The right?
2. The left?
3. Both the same?

お酒を飲みますか.
― 平均して 1 日にどれくらいの量を飲みますか.

☐ Do you drink alcohol?
― How much do you drink a day on the average?

| | |
|---|---|
| あなたは…と言われたことがありますか.<br>　1. 関節炎<br>　2. 骨粗鬆症<br>　3. 痛風<br>　4. 膠原病 | ☐ Have you ever been told that you have...<br>　1. arthritis?<br>　2. osteoporosis?<br>　3. gout?<br>　4. collagen disease? |
| これまでに骨折したことがありますか. | ☐ Have you ever broken any of your bones? |
| これまでに…に損傷を受けたことがありますか.<br>　1. 筋肉<br>　2. 関節<br>　3. 靭帯<br>　4. 腱<br>―いつですか.<br>―どうしたのですか.<br>―どういう治療を受けましたか.<br>―それ以来,その部分に何か問題がありますか. | ☐ Have you ever injured your...<br>　1. muscle?<br>　2. joint?<br>　3. ligament?<br>　4. tendon?<br>— When did it occur?<br>— What happened?<br>— How was it treated?<br>— Have you had any problem in that area since then? |
| 骨,関節,筋肉の手術を受けたことがありますか.<br>―いつですか.<br>―それ以来,その部分に何か問題がありますか. | ☐ Have you ever had any surgery involving bones, joints, or muscles?<br>— When?<br>— Have you had any problem in that area since then? |
| 歩くとき補助具を使っていますか.<br>―何を使いますか.<br>　1. ステッキ.<br>　2. 松葉杖.<br>　3. 特別な靴.<br>　4. 歩行器. | ☐ Are you using any assistive devices when you walk?<br>— What do you use?<br>　1. Cane?<br>　2. Crutches?<br>　3. Special shoes?<br>　4. Walker? |
| ステロイドを内服していますか〔いましたか〕. | ☐ Are you 〔Have you been〕 taking oral steroid medications? |

chapter 3　現病歴(筋・骨格)

―どのくらいの量をどのくらいの期間内服していますか〔していましたか〕.

ご家族のどなたかが…にかかったことがありますか.
1. 関節リウマチ
2. 骨粗鬆症
3. 結核
4. その他

— How much and how long?

☐ Has anyone in your immediate family had...
1. rheumatoid arthritis?
2. osteoporosis?
3. tuberculosis?
4. any other disorders?

## 13 神経

☞「神経の診察」(229 ページ).

### 一般的な質問

具合の悪いところをお聞かせ下さい.
― どんな問題ですか.
1. 意識を失った.
2. 痙攣する〔した〕.
3. 上手く話せない.
4. 手足に力が入らない.
5. 立てない,歩けない.
6. 感覚がおかしい.
7. 手足が勝手に動く.
8. その他.

☐ Please tell me your problems.
― What kind of problems?
1. Have you lost consciousness?
2. Do you have〔Have you had〕convulsions or spasms?
3. Do you have difficulty speaking?
4. Do your hands, arms, or legs feel weak?
5. Do you have difficulty standing or walking?
6. Do you have any problems with sensations?
7. Do you make any unconscious and unintentional movements of your hands, arms, or legs?
8. Any other problems?

(付き添いの人に) 認知症の症状がありますか.

☐ Does he〔she〕have any symptom of dementia?

それはどのくらい続いていますか.
― いつからですか.

☐ How long have you had the problems?
― Since when?

このような問題は以前にもありましたか.

☐ Have you had these problems before?

☞「病歴をとるためのヒント」(22 ページ).

### 意識障害・失神

あなたは意識を失いましたか．
―それはどのような状況でしたか．

1. 強い不安や痛みを経験したとき．
2. 急に立ち上がったときや，急に体を起こしたとき．
3. 排尿時．
4. 発作的に咳込んだとき．
5. その他．

―どのくらいの間，意識を失っていましたか．
―意識が回復した後，麻痺の症状がありましたか．

☐ Did you lose consciousness?
― In what situations did it happen?

1. When you experienced strong anxiety or severe pain?
2. When you stood up suddenly? When you rose from a lying or bending position?
3. When you passed urine?
4. When you had a coughing spell?
5. In any other situations?

― How long were you unconscious?
― Have you noticed paralysis in any part of your body after you recovered consciousness?

### 痙攣

痙攣を起こし〔起こしたことがあり〕ますか．

痙攣は…ですか．
1. 全身
2. 体の一部
―体の一部から全身へと広がる痙攣ですか．

どのような痙攣ですか．

―筋肉が一時的に強直するような痙攣ですか．

☐ Do you have〔Have you had〕convulsions [seizures]?

☐ Do the convulsions appear...
1. all over the body?
2. in one part of the body?
― Do the convulsions radiate from one part to the whole body?

☐ What are the convulsions like?
☐ Can you describe the convulsions for me?
― Does your body become rigid for a time due to strong muscular contractions?

―筋肉が強直と弛緩を交互に繰り返す痙攣ですか.
― Do the muscles contract and relax by turns [alternately]?

―手足を投げ出すような痙攣ですか.
― Do you make violent flinging and jerky arm and leg movements?

―一部の筋肉が瞬間的に不規則に収縮するような痙攣ですか.
― Does a muscle or group of muscles twitch or have sudden involuntary jerks?

―痛みを伴った突然の足の筋収縮[こむらがえり]ですか.
― Do you have a sudden, painful muscle cramp in your leg?

―筋肉がぴくぴく動く[ひきつる]感じですか.
― Does any of your muscles twitch?

―手や指が震える感じですか.
― Do your hands or fingers tremble or shake?

―痙攣は毎回,どのくらい続きますか.
― How long do the convulsions last each time?
1. 2, 3 秒.
2. 2, 3 分.
3. もっと長く.
1. For a few seconds?
2. For a few minutes?
3. Longer?

痙攣時に意識を失いますか.
☐ With the convulsions do you lose consciousness?

―痙攣後はどのくらい長く…
― After a convulsion, how long are you...
1. 意識を失っていますか.
2. 意識が混乱しますか.
1. unconscious?
2. confused?

初めて起こったのはいつですか.
☐ When did you have your first convulsion?

―最近[最後]に起こったのはいつですか.
― When did you have your last convulsion?

―どのくらいの頻度で起こりますか.
― How often do you have convulsions?
1. 頻繁に起こる.
2. さほど頻繁ではない.
3. めったに起こらない.
1. Often [Frequently]?
2. Not so often [Infrequently]?
3. Rarely?

痙攣のために薬を飲んでいますか.
☐ Are you taking any medications for the convulsions?

―どんな種類の薬ですか.
― What kind?

―どのくらい長く飲んでいますか．いつから？
― For how long have you been taking them? Since when?

―規則的に飲んでいますか．
― Are you taking them regularly?

―痙攣は…
1. 改善していますか．
2. ひどくなっていますか．
3. 変わりませんか．

― Have your convulsions...
1. improved?
2. gotten worse?
3. stayed the same?

### 認知障害

(付き添いの人への質問)

#### ▶ 記憶・思考・判断の障害

最近，忘れっぽくなっていますか．
☐ Has he〔she〕been forgetting things recently?

記憶力に変化が起こりましたか．
☐ Have you noticed any changes in his〔her〕ability to remember things?

―忘れるのは…ですか．
1. 最近の出来事
2. 昔の出来事

― Does he〔she〕lose memory...
1. for recent events?
2. for past events?

―同じことを何度も訊くことがありますか．
― Does he〔she〕repeat the same questions many times?

―忘れっぽいことを自覚していますか．
― Is he〔she〕aware of being forgetful of things?

迷子になることがありますか．
☐ Does he〔she〕ever get lost?

よく知っている物の意味がわからなくなることはありますか．例えば，自動車と電車の共通点，相違点はわかりますか．
☐ Does he〔she〕ever get confused about the meaning of familiar things? Can he〔she〕tell the similarity or difference between automobiles and trains?

物事や状況に対する判断がおかしいと思うことはありますか．例えば，台所が火事になったらどうするかわかりますか．
☐ Does he〔she〕make a poor judgment about things or situations? Does he〔she〕know what to do if the kitchen is on fire?

### ▶ 失語

言葉を話したり，聞いたり，読んだり，書いたりするのに問題がありますか．
— どんな問題ですか．

1. あまり話をしなくなった．
2. 明瞭に〔流暢に〕話せない．
3. 思っている言葉が見つからない，使えない．
4. 言い間違えが多い．
5. 話し方が回りくどい．
6. 復唱できない．
7. 訊かれたことが理解できない．
8. 読んだことが理解できない．
9. 書けない．

☐ Does he 〔she〕 have any problem with speaking, listening, reading, or writing?
— What kind of problem is it? Does he 〔she〕...

1. talk less than before?
2. have difficulty speaking clearly 〔fluently〕?
3. have difficulty finding or using the words he 〔she〕 is thinking?
4. often use wrong words?
5. talk in a roundabout way?
6. have difficulty repeating what others say?
7. have difficulty understanding what he 〔she〕 has been asked?
8. have difficulty understanding what he 〔she〕 has read?
9. have difficulty writing?

### ▶ 失認

見えている空間の左側に存在するものに気づかなかったり，無視することはありますか．

☐ When he 〔she〕 is looking ahead, does he 〔she〕 fail to recognize or ignore something that is on his 〔her〕 left?

見えている物が理解できないことがありますか．

☐ Does he 〔she〕 see objects but still fail to recognize them?

知り合いの人の顔が見分けられないことはありますか．

☐ Can he 〔she〕 not consciously recognize familiar faces?

自分の障害や病気を否認することがありますか．

☐ Does he 〔she〕 deny his 〔her〕 problem or disease?

### ▶ 失行

| | |
|---|---|
| 洋服を上手に着られなくなりましたか. | ☐ Does he〔she〕have difficulty getting dressed by himself〔herself〕? |
| 使い慣れた物の操作ができなくなりましたか. | ☐ Does he〔she〕have difficulty handling familiar things he〔she〕used to do before? |
| ―テレビのリモコンが操作できませんか. | ― Can he〔she〕not turn on or off the TV with the remote control? |
| パズルをしたり, 図形を描いたりできなくなりましたか. | ☐ Does he〔she〕have difficulty working on a puzzle or making a drawing? |

### 脳神経障害

| | |
|---|---|
| 最近, 嗅覚が変化しましたか. | ☐ Have you recently had any changes in your sense of smell? |

☞「嗅覚」(65 ページ).

| | |
|---|---|
| 最近, 視力や視野が変化しましたか. | ☐ Have you recently had any changes in your vision? |

☞「眼」(54 ページ).

| | |
|---|---|
| 顔の感覚がおかしいと感じますか. | ☐ Have you noticed something wrong with your facial sensations? |
| 食べ物を噛みにくいですか. | ☐ Do you have difficulty chewing? |
| 口笛を吹きにくいですか. | ☐ Do you have difficulty whistling? |
| 涙や唾液が出にくいと感じますか. | ☐ Do you feel that tears or saliva won't flow easily? |
| 最近, 味覚が変化しましたか. | ☐ Have you recently had any changes in your sense of taste? |

☞「味覚」(73 ページ).

| 物音ががんがん響きますか. | ☐ Do you hear a banging [roaring] sound in your ear(s)? |

最近,聴力が変化しましたか. ☐ Have you had any changes in your hearing?

☞「聴力」(60 ページ).

めまいがしますか. ☐ Do you feel dizzy or lightheaded?

☞「めまい」(43 ページ).

物を飲み込みにくいですか. ☐ Do you have difficulty swallowing?

食事中によくむせますか. ☐ Do you often choke while eating?

声は変わりましたか.鼻声になったり,嗄れた声になったりしましたか. ☐ Have you had any changes in your voice? Nasal or hoarse?

### 運動障害

#### ▶ 錐体路系症状

筋力に何か問題がありますか. ☐ Do you have any problems with your muscle strength?

どこの場所ですか.どの筋肉ですか. ☐ Where? Which muscles?
  1. 体.
  2. 手や腕.
  3. 足.

  1. Of your body?
  2. Of your hands and [or] arms?★
  3. Of your feet and [or] legs?★

---

★ arm は肩から手首まで,hand は手首より先,leg はももの付け根から足首まで,foot は足首から先を指す.なお,arm は上肢全体,leg は下肢全体を表す言葉として用いられることもある.

chapter 3 現病歴(神経)

| | |
|---|---|
| どんな問題ですか. | ☐ What kind of problem is it? |
| 1. 脱力感がある［力が入らない］. | 1. Do you feel weakness in your muscles? |
| 2. よく転倒する［つまずいて転ぶ］. | 2. Do you often have falls [tumble down]? |
| 3. よく物を落とす. | 3. Do you often drop things? |
| 4. 上手く歩けない. | 4. Do you have difficulty walking? |
| 5. 足を引きずって歩く. | 5. Do you shuffle? |
| 6. その他. | 6. Any other problems? |

### ▶ 錐体外路系症状

| | |
|---|---|
| 自分の意思によらずに, 勝手に筋肉が動いてしまうことはありますか. | ☐ Do your muscles ever move unintentionally and unconsciously? |
| どこの場所ですか. どの筋肉ですか. | ☐ Where? Which muscles? |
| 1. 顔面, 瞼, 舌. | 1. Of your face, eyelids, or tongue? |
| 2. 首, 体幹. | 2. Of your neck or torso? |
| 3. 手や腕. | 3. Of your hands and〔or〕arms? |
| 4. 足. | 4. Of your feet and〔or〕legs? |
| どのような動きですか. | ☐ What kind of movement is it? |
| 1. 規則的［リズミック］ですか. 不規則的ですか. | 1. Regular [rhythmic] or irregular? |
| 2. 発作的ですか. 持続的ですか. | 2. Convulsive or continuous? |
| 3. 速いですか. ゆっくりですか. | 3. Fast or slow? |
| 4. 細かいですか. 粗いですか. | 4. Fine or gross? |
| 5. 体をくねらせる感じですか. | 5. Writhing? |
| 6. その他. | 6. Any other movement? |
| 何か誘因はありますか. | ☐ What triggers such movement? |

| | |
|---|---|
| どういうときに出現しますか. | In what situations does it appear? |
| 1. 決まった姿勢をとるときですか. | 1. When adopting the same posture? |
|    a. 立っているとき. |    a. Standing? |
|    b. 座っているとき. |    b. Sitting? |
|    c. 手をあげるとき. |    c. Raising your hand(s)? |
|    d. じっとしているとき. |    d. Posture at rest? |
| 2. 何かをしようとするときですか. | 2. When trying to do some tasks? |
| 3. 精神的にプレッシャーを感じるときですか. | 3. When feeling emotional pressure? |
| 4. その他. | 4. In any other situations? |

### ▶ 小脳系症状

| | |
|---|---|
| 立っている時, ふらつきますか. | When you are standing still, do you feel unsteady? |
| バランスを保つのが難しいですか. | Do you find it difficult to balance yourself? |
| 歩きにくいですか. | Do you have difficulty walking? |
| —どんな問題ですか. | — What kind of difficulty is it? |
| 1. よろける. | 1. Do you stagger? |
| 2. バランスをくずす. | 2. Do you lose your balance? |
| 3. よちよち歩く. | 3. Do you waddle? |
| 字が下手になったと感じますか. | Do you feel that your handwriting has become poorer? |
| 手先が不器用になったと感じますか. | Do you feel that you have become more clumsy with your hands? |
| —それはどういう時ですか. | — In what situations do you feel that way? |

|  |  |
|---|---|
| ろれつが回らない，またはしゃべりにくいと感じるときがありますか． | Do you ever feel that your speech is slurred or that you have difficulty speaking? |

### 感覚障害

|  |  |
|---|---|
| 感覚に何か問題がありますか． | ☐ Do you have any problems with your sensations? |
| どんな問題ですか． | ☐ What kind of problems are they? |
| —…が鈍っていますか． | — Are your...dull [less sharp/less acute]? |
| —…が過敏ですか．<br>　1. 触った感覚<br>　2. 痛みの感覚<br>　3. 温度の感覚<br>　4. 振動の感覚 | — Are your ... sharp?<br>　1. touch sensations<br>　2. pain sensations<br>　3. heat and cold sensations<br>　4. sensations of vibration |
| しびれ感がありますか．<br>—どこの場所ですか．<br>　1. 体．<br>　2. 手や腕．<br>　3. 足．<br>—その場所を指でさして下さい． | ☐ Do you have numbness?<br>— Where?<br>　1. Your body?<br>　2. Your hands and〔or〕arms?<br>　3. Your feet and〔or〕legs?<br>— Please point to the place (where you have the numbness). |
| 本来とは異なった感覚として感じられることがありますか． | ☐ Do you ever have sensations that are not natural [normal]? |
| 刺激がなくてもしびれてピリピリする感じがしますか． | ☐ Do you have a feeling of pins and needles even without any stimulus? |
| ひりひり感がありますか． | ☐ Do you have tingling sensations? |
| 刺されるような鋭い自発痛や焼け付くような自発痛がありますか． | ☐ Do you have any spontaneous stinging or burning pain? |

### 自律神経障害

立ちくらみをしやすいですか．
☐ Do you often get dizzy on standing up?

排尿をコントロールするのが難しいですか．
☐ Do you have difficulty controlling your bladder?

排便をコントロールするのが難しいですか．
☐ Do you have difficulty controlling your bowel movements?

汗が出にくいですか．
☐ Do you sweat very little?
☐ Do you sweat less?

涙や唾液が少ないですか．
☐ Do you have little amount of tears or saliva?

まぶしいですか．
☐ Are you sensitive to light?

### 随伴症状

そのほかに徴候や症状がありますか．
―それは何ですか．
1. 発熱．
2. 頭痛．
3. 嘔吐．
4. 意識障害．
5. めまい．
6. 痙攣．
7. しびれ．

☐ Do you have any other signs or symptoms?
— What are they?
1. Fever?
2. Headache?
3. Vomiting?
4. Disturbance of consciousness?
5. Dizziness?
6. Convulsions [Seizures]?
7. Numbness?

（付き添いの人への質問）

最近，気持ちの変化がありますか．

1. 無気力．

☐ Have you recently noticed any change in his〔her〕mood?
1. Lethargic [Having no energy, and feeling lazy and tired all the time]?

2. 無関心.

3. 頑固.
4. 怒りやすい.
5. 疑い深い.

2. Apathetic [Losing interest in things he 〔she〕 usually enjoys]?
3. Obstinate?
4. Irritable?
5. Suspicious?

### 既往歴・家族歴

これまでに…と診断されたことがありますか.
1. 頭部外傷
2. 首や背中の外傷
3. 脳血管疾患
4. 脳炎
5. 髄膜炎
6. 脊椎の病気
7. 不整脈やその他の心疾患
8. 高血圧
9. 糖尿病
10. 出生時の異常
11. その他

—その診断を受けたのはいつですか.
—どういう治療を受けましたか.

ご家族のどなたかに同じような症状の人はいますか.

☐ Have you ever been diagnosed with...
1. a head injury?
2. a neck or back injury?
3. cerebrovascular disease?
4. encephalitis?
5. meningitis?
6. a spinal disorder?
7. irregular pulse or other heart problems?
8. high blood pressure?
9. diabetes?
10. a problem at birth?
11. any other disorders?

— When was it diagnosed?
— How was it treated?

☐ Does anyone in your immediate family have a similar symptom?

## 14 皮膚

### 一般的な質問

皮膚〔ほくろ／頭髪・体毛／爪〕に何か問題がありますか.
- [ ] (Do you have) any problems with your skin〔moles/hair/nails〕?
- [ ] (Is there) anything wrong with your skin〔moles/hair/nails〕?

―どんな問題ですか.
― What kind of problems?

それはどのくらい続いていますか.
- [ ] How long have you had the problems?

―いつからですか.
― Since when?

このような問題は以前にもありましたか.
- [ ] Have you had these problems before?

☞「病歴をとるためのヒント」(22 ページ).

### 発疹

**症状の特徴**

皮膚にどんな問題がありますか.
- [ ] What kind of skin problems do you have?

発疹がありますか.
- [ ] Do you have rashes?

どんな発疹ですか.
　1. 赤い発疹.
　2. 水疱状の発疹.
　3. 蕁麻疹のような発疹.
　4. 潰瘍のような発疹.
　5. その他.
- [ ] What kind of rash is it?
  1. Red rash?
  2. Blistery rash?
  3. Rash like hives?
  4. Rash like ulcers?
  5. Any other kind of rash?

発疹の場所はどこですか.

　1. 頭皮.
　2. 顔.
　3. 口唇.
　4. 首.
- [ ] Where on your body do you have rashes?
  1. Scalp?
  2. Face?
  3. Lips?
  4. Neck?

| | |
|---|---|
| 5. 胸. | 5. Chest? |
| 6. 背中. | 6. Back? |
| 7. 手〔腕〕. | 7. Hand(s)〔Arm(s)〕? |
| 8. 足. | 8. Leg(s)〔Foot/Feet〕? |
| 9. 性器. | 9. Genital area? |
| 10. 他の場所. | 10. Any other body areas? |
| 11. 体全体. | 11. All over your body? |

—どこから始まりましたか. — Where did they start?
—その場所を指でさして下さい. — Please point to the place.
—ほかの部位に広がっていますか. — Have they spread to other areas?
—どこからどこへ. — From where to where?

☐ かゆみがありますか. ☐ Do you feel itchy?
—どの程度のかゆみですか. — How bad is the itching?
　1. ひどくかゆい. 　1. Intensely itchy?
　2. 軽度にかゆい. 　2. Mildly itchy?
—かゆみの頻度はどのくらいですか. — How often do you feel itchy?
　1. いつも. 　1. All the time [Constantly]?
　2. 時々. 　2. Occasionally?
—かゆみはとれたり, かゆくなったりしますか. — Does the itching clear up and then come back?

☐ (炎症による)痛みがありますか. ☐ Do you have sores?

☐ 皮膚の色が変化しましたか. ☐ Has your skin changed its color?
—どう変わりましたか. — How has it changed?
　1. 黒ずんだ. 　1. Darker?
　2. 赤みを帯びた. 　2. Reddish?
　3. 黄色っぽくなった. 　3. Yellowish?

☐ 他に皮膚の問題がありますか. ☐ Do you have any other skin problems?

—潰瘍がありますか. — Do you have ulcers?
—乾燥, ざらざら感がありますか. — Is your skin dry or rough?
—表皮のはがれがありますか. — Is your skin flaky?
—脂っぽさがありますか. — Is your skin oily?
—外傷〔切り傷／擦り傷／やけど〕がありましたか. — Did you have injuries〔cuts/scrapes/burns〕?
—あざがありますか. — Do you have bruises?

―その他.

症状を…がありますか.

1. 悪化させるもの
2. 軽くするもの

―それは何ですか.

1. 水,お湯〔お風呂またはシャワー〕.
2. 寒さ,暑さ.
3. 日光.
4. 薬品.
5. ストレス.
6. 運動.
7. 月経.
8. その他.

**時間経過**

その問題に初めて気づいたのはいつですか.

―どんな起こり方をしましたか.

1. (有害なものに接触してから) 突然.
2. 徐々に.

症状は…
1. 改善していますか.
2. 悪化していますか
3. 変わりませんか.

肌触りは以前とくらべてどうですか.
1. なめらかですか.
2. ざらざらしていますか.
3. 厚く硬くなっていますか.

— Any other problems?

☐ Does anything make the problem...
  1. worse?
  2. better?
— What is it?
  1. Water or hot water〔Bath or shower〕?
  2. Cold or heat?
  3. Sunshine?
  4. Some medications?
  5. Stress?
  6. Exercise?
  7. Menstruation?
  8. Any other causes?

☐ When did you first notice the problem?
— How has the problem developed?
  1. Suddenly (after exposure to something harmful)?
  2. Gradually?

☐ Has the symptom been...
  1. improving?
  2. getting worse?
  3. staying the same?

☐ How has your skin been in texture?
  1. Finer?
  2. Rougher?
  3. More thickening and tightening?

**随伴症状**

発疹のほかに徴候や症状がありますか.

- ☐ Do you have any other signs or symptoms?

それは何ですか.
―発熱はありますか.
―発熱が先行していますか.

―発熱と同時に発疹が出ましたか.

―風邪症状の先行はありましたか.

―呼吸困難はありますか.

―関節症状はありますか.

―出血傾向はありますか〔あざができやすいですか〕.

- ☐ What are they?
- — Do you have a fever?
- — Did you have a fever before the rash developed?
- — Did the fever and the rash develop at the same time?
- — Did you have cold symptoms before the rash developed?
- — Do you have breathing difficulties?
- — Do you have any joint problems?
- — Do you bleed easily〔Do you bruise easily〕?

**その他**

今の皮膚の状態は何かに関係があると思いますか. 例えば,
1. ふだんと違う銘柄の化粧品, 石鹸, 洗剤.
2. 染料や化学物質.
3. 抗生物質や鎮痛解熱薬などの薬品.
4. 食品.
5. 虫刺され.
6. つたうるしなどの植物.
7. 暑さ〔寒さ〕.
8. 日光.
9. ストレス.
10. 麻疹, 風疹, 水痘, 手足口病, 疥癬など感染性の発疹疾患.

- ☐ Does your skin problem seem related to anything, such as...
  1. a different brand of cosmetics, soap, or detergent?
  2. a dye or a chemical?
  3. a medication such as an antibiotic, or a pain reliever and a fever reducer?
  4. foods?
  5. an insect bite?
  6. a plant like poison ivy?
  7. heat〔cold〕?
  8. sunlight?
  9. stress?
  10. infectious eruptive disease, such as measles, rubella〔German measles〕, chickenpox, hand-foot-and-mouth disease, or scabies?

| | |
|---|---|
| 11. 感染性の発疹疾患にかかっている患者との接触. | 11. being exposed to someone with infectious eruptive disease? |
| 12. 怪我. | 12. an injury? |
| 13. その他. | 13. any other causes? |

発疹を改善させるために何を使っていますか. ☐ What have you been using on it to relieve your problem?
—それは何ですか.市販薬,それとも医師からの処方薬ですか. — What is it? Is it an over-the-counter drug or a prescribed drug?

1. クリーム. 1. Creams?
2. ローション. 2. Lotions?
3. 軟膏. 3. Ointments?
4. 湿布. 4. Compresses?
5. 薬の服用. 5. Medications?
6. その他. 6. Any other drugs?

—効果はありますか. — Does it help?

同じ症状は以前にもありましたか. ☐ Have you ever had the same symptom before?

—それはいつですか. — When was it?
—思い当たる誘因はありましたか. — Was there any cause that you could identify?

—その時医師の診察を受けましたか.何と診断されましたか. — Did you consult a doctor? How was it diagnosed?
—どんな治療を受けましたか. — How was it treated?

家でペットを飼っていますか. ☐ Do you have pets in your house?

どんな種類の石鹸,クリーム,ローション,シャンプーを使っていますか. ☐ What type of soap, cream, lotion, or shampoo do you use?
—化粧品や香水を使っていますか. — Do you use cosmetics or perfumes?

—毎日ですか. — Do you use them every day?

これまでにアレルギー反応を起こしたことがありますか.何にですか. ☐ Have you ever had any allergic reactions? To what?

☞「アレルギー」(195 ページ).

| | |
|---|---|
| 麻疹, 風疹, 水痘など感染性の発疹性疾患にかかったことがありますか. | ☐ Have you ever had infectious eruptive disease, such as measles, rubella [German measles], or chickenpox? |
| ―何歳のときですか | ― How old were you, then? |
| ―麻疹, 風疹, 水痘の予防接種は受けましたか. | ― Did you have vaccinations for measles, rubella [German measles], and chickenpox? |
| ご家族に同じ症状の人はいますか. | ☐ Does anyone else in your family have similar symptoms? |

### ほくろ

| | |
|---|---|
| ほくろがありますか. | ☐ Do you have any moles? |
| ―どこですか. | ― Where? |
| 最近, ほくろのサイズ, 形や色などに変化が起こりましたか. | ☐ Have you noticed any change in the size, shape or color of your moles? |
| ―どんな変化ですか. | ― What kind of change is it? |
| ―…に気づきましたか. | ― Have you noticed... |
| 1. 縁の形が不規則なこと | 1. an irregular edge? |
| 2. 色に濃淡の差が目立つこと | 2. an uneven color? |
| 3. サイズの増大 | 3. growing in size? |
| 4. 盛り上がり | 4. a raised appearance [a raised lump]? |
| 5. 出血 | 5. bleeding? |
| 6. 分泌物 | 6. discharge? |
| 7. 痛み | 7. pain? |
| 8. かゆみ | 8. itching? |

### 頭髪・体毛

| | |
|---|---|
| 頭髪や体毛に変化がありますか. | ☐ Have you noticed any change in your hair? |
| ―どこですか. | ― Where? |
| ―毛の量は… | ― Has it been getting... |
| 1. 薄くなっていますか. | 1. thinner? |
| 2. 濃くなっていますか. | 2. thicker? |

| 最近，ひどく脱毛しましたか． | ☐ Have you recently noticed any excessive hair loss? |
|---|---|

1. 全体にわたる脱毛．
2. むらのある脱毛．
— どこですか．
— いつ気づきましたか．
— 範囲は広がっていますか．

1. Overall [Extensive] hair loss?
2. Patchy hair loss?
— Where?
— When did you first notice it?
— Has it increased in size?

何か脱毛の誘因として考えられるものはありますか．例えば…

☐ What do you think is causing your hair loss? For example, ...

1. 生まれつき．
2. 毛髪をぬく癖がある．
3. 頭皮の感染．
4. 頭皮の怪我．
5. ポニーテールなどでいつも髪を引っ張っている．
6. 長期にわたって寝たきりだった．
7. 最近，化学物質に触れた．
8. 化学療法を受けた．
9. 放射線治療を受けた．
10. 最近，大きな手術を受けた．
11. 最近，出産した．
12. 最近，ストレスが多い．
13. 甲状腺の病気がある．
14. 糖尿病，エリテマトーデスなどの全身的な病気がある．

1. was it present at birth?
2. do you have a habit of pulling your hair?
3. have you had a scalp infection?
4. have you had an injury to your scalp?
5. does your hairstyle pull on your hair like a ponytail?
6. have you been confined to bed for a long time?
7. have you recently been exposed to any chemicals?
8. have you had chemotherapy?
9. have you had radiation therapy?
10. have you recently had any major surgery?
11. have you recently had a baby?
12. have you been under stress these days?
13. do you have thyroid disease?
14. do you have systemic disease, such as diabetes or lupus?

これまでに何か治療薬を試したことがありますか．
— 今も使用していますか．

☐ Have you ever tried any medication for your hair loss?
— Are you using it now?

1. 市販の育毛剤.
2. 医師の処方薬.

— 効果はありましたか.

髪はどのくらいの頻度で洗いますか.
1. 毎日.
2. 1日おき.
3. 週に2回.
4. もっと少ない回数.

— どんなシャンプーを使っていますか.

髪を染めていますか.

脱毛剤を使っていますか.

かつらを使っていますか.

ご家族で脱毛症の人はいますか.

— 誰ですか.

### 爪

爪の状態に変化がありましたか.

— どういう変化ですか.

1. 湾曲した.
2. 肥厚した.
3. くぼみやへこみができた.
4. はがれた.
5. すぐ割れる.
6. すぐ亀裂が入る.

色が変化しましたか. どんな色にですか.

---

1. Over-the-counter hair restorer?
2. Prescribed drug?

— Did it help?

☐ How often do you wash your hair?
1. Every day?
2. Every other day?
3. Twice a week?
4. Less often?

— What type of shampoo do you use?

☐ Do you dye your hair?

☐ Do you use a depilatory?

☐ Do you wear a wig?

☐ Is there anyone else in your immediate family affected by hair loss?

— Who is it?

### Nails

☐ Have you noticed any change in your nails?

— What kind of change is it? How have they become?
1. Curved?
2. Thickened?
3. Pitted or dimpled?
4. Loosened?
5. Easily broken?
6. Easily split?

☐ Have your nails changed color? How?

1. 黒.
2. 褐色.
3. 青みがかった色.
4. その他.

爪の周囲の皮膚はどうですか.

1. 腫れている.
2. 赤くなって, 痛む.

これまでに何か治療薬を試したことがありますか.
―今も使用していますか.
1. 市販薬.
2. 医師の処方薬.
3. 飲み薬.
4. 塗り薬.
―効果はありましたか.

1. Black?
2. Brown?
3. Bluish?
4. Any other color?

☐ How is the skin around your nails?
1. Swollen?
2. Red, and painful?

☐ Have you ever tried any medication for your problem?
— Are you using it now?
1. Over-the-counter drug?
2. Prescribed drug?
3. Internal medication?
4. Ointment?
— Did it help?

## 15 精神・心理

### 一般的な質問

それでは，あなたのことについておうかがいいたします．
☐ Now I'd like to ask you a few questions about yourself.

ご自分のことについて話して下さい。
☐ Tell me about yourself.

☞「病歴をとるためのヒント」(22 ページ)．

### 睡眠障害

睡眠に何か問題がありますか．
☐ Do you have any problems sleeping?

―どんな問題ですか．
— What kind of problems?
 1. 寝つきが悪い．
 1. Difficulty falling asleep?
 2. 早朝目が覚めてその後なかなか眠れない．
 2. Waking up early in the morning and not being able to get back to sleep?
 3. 夜中に目が覚める．
 3. Waking up in the middle of the night?
 4. 熟睡した感じがしない．
 4. Feeling unable to have a sound sleep?
 5. 眠りが浅いような気がする．
 5. Feeling like you sleep poorly?
 6. ふだんより眠りすぎる．
 6. Sleeping more than usual?
―いつ頃からですか．
— When did you first notice the problem?

実際の睡眠時間を教えて下さい．
☐ Please tell me how many hours you sleep a day?
 1. 何時に床につきますか．
 1. What time do you go to bed?
 2. 眠りにつくまでにどのくらいの時間がかかりますか．
 2. How long does it take to fall asleep?
 3. 何時に起床しますか．
 3. What time do you get up in the morning?

不眠が日常生活〔仕事／学業〕に悪影響を及ぼしていると思いますか．
☐ Does sleeplessness affect your everyday life〔work/schoolwork〕?

1. 居眠りが多い.
2. 物事に集中できない.
3. ミスが多い.

不眠の原因に心当たりはありますか.

1. 職場からの帰宅時間が不規則で生活のリズムが乱れがち.
2. 最近, ストレスが多い.
3. 病気のために身体的苦痛がある.
4. 昼寝をしている.
5. カフェインを含むコーヒー, お茶, コーラなどの飲み物を飲む.
6. お酒を飲む.
7. その他.

眠れないときには, どのように対処していますか.
1. あきらめて起きている.
2. 睡眠薬を飲む.
3. お酒を飲む.
4. その他.

### ストレス

最近, いつもより多くストレスを受けていますか.

1. Do you often nod off to sleep?
2. Do you have difficulty concentrating?
3. Do you often make careless mistakes?

☐ What do you think is causing your sleeplessness?
☐ Is there any cause you can identify?
1. Is the rhythm of your life often disturbed because of the irregular time when you return home from work?
2. Have you recently been under much stress?
3. Have you been physically suffering from an illness?
4. Do you often take naps?
5. Do you take drinks containing caffeine, such as coffee, tea, or cola?
6. Do you drink alcohol?
7. Any other causes?

☐ How do you cope with sleeplessness?
1. Giving up sleeping and staying awake?
2. Taking sleeping drugs?
3. Drinking alcohol?
4. Any other coping strategies?

☐ Have you been under more stress recently?

chapter 3 現病歴（精神・心理）

| | |
|---|---|
| ストレスがたまっていますか. | ☐ Do you have too much stress?<br>☐ Do you recognize stress in your life? |
| どんなことがストレスになりますか.<br>1. 自分の健康状態.<br>2. 家族の病気.<br>3. 配偶者の死.<br>4. 結婚生活.<br>5. 別居.<br>6. 離婚.<br>7. 経済問題.<br>8. 仕事.<br>9. 学業.<br>10. 人間関係.<br>11. その他. | ☐ What causes you to feel stress?<br>1. Your own health problems?<br>2. Illness in your family?<br>3. Your husband's〔wife's〕death?<br>4. Marriage?<br>5. Separation?<br>6. Divorce?<br>7. Financial problems?<br>8. Work?<br>9. School work?<br>10. Personal relations?<br>11. Any other causes? |
| ストレス状況でどんな症状を起こしますか.<br>1. 頭痛.<br>2. 口の渇き.<br>3. 吐き気.<br>4. 下痢や便秘.<br>5. 肩こり.<br>6. 腰痛.<br>7. 動悸.<br>8. 疲労. | ☐ What happens to you when you're in a stressful situation?<br>1. Headache?<br>2. Dry mouth?<br>3. Nausea?<br>4. Diarrhea and〔or〕constipation?<br>5. Stiff shoulders?<br>6. Low back pain?<br>7. Palpitations?<br>8. Fatigue? |
| どうやってストレスを解消しますか.<br>1. 運動.<br>2. 喫煙.<br>3. 飲酒.<br>4. 甘い物を食べる.<br>5. コーヒー,お茶,ソフトドリンクを飲む. | ☐ What do you do to get rid of〔cope with〕stress?<br>1. Exercising?<br>2. Smoking?<br>3. Drinking alcohol?<br>4. Eating sweets?<br>5. Drinking coffee, tea, or soft drinks? |

### 不安・恐怖

**症状の特徴**

| | |
|---|---|
| あなたは心配性のほうですか. | ☐ Do you tend to be an anxious or nervous person?<br>☐ Do you worry often? |
| あなたは几帳面な性格のほうですか. | ☐ Do you tend to be precise in everything you do?<br>☐ Do you have a meticulous [compulsive] personality? |
| ずっと不安な気持ちがしているのですか. | ☐ Do you feel anxious or nervous most of the time? |
| 漫然とした不安感ですか. | ☐ Do you feel anxious or nervous without an apparent cause? |
| 不安になるとどんな症状が出ますか. | ☐ When you feel anxious or nervous, what symptoms do you have? Do you... |

1. 落ち着きがなくなる.
2. 疲れやすくなる.
3. 集中できなくなる.
4. 怒りっぽくなる.
5. 首や肩が凝る.
6. 眠れなくなる.
7. 動悸がはげしくなる.
8. 冷や汗が出る.
9. 体や手足が震える.
10. 息切れがする.
11. 息が苦しくなる〔窒息するような感じがする〕.
12. 胸が痛む.
13. 吐き気がする.
14. めまいがする,頭がふらつく.
15. しびれる感じがする.

1. feel restless?
2. get tired easily?
3. have difficulty concentrating?
4. get irritable?
5. have a stiff neck or stiff shoulders?
6. have difficulty sleeping?
7. feel your heart beating fast [pounding]?
8. have a cold sweat?
9. tremble or shake?
10. get short of breath?
11. feel you can hardly breathe [feel you're choking]?
12. have chest pain?
13. feel like vomiting?
14. get dizzy or lightheaded?
15. get numb?

| | |
|---|---|
| 16. 突然顔がほてる，悪寒がする． | 16. have sudden hot flashes or chills? |
| 17. 尿が近くなる． | 17. urinate more frequently? |
| 18. 自分が自分でない感じがする． | 18. feel that you are not yourself? |
| 19. 自分を制御できなくなるのでは，取り乱してしまうのでは，狂ってしまうのではないかという恐怖を覚える． | 19. fear that you won't be able to control yourself, lose your self-control, or go out of your mind? |
| 20. 死ぬのではないかという恐怖を覚える． | 20. fear that you may be dying? |
| 21. その他． | 21. have anything else? |

突然，発作的に不安な気持ちにかられるのですか．

☐ Do your feelings of anxiety come on suddenly or without warning?
☐ Do they come as panic attacks?

不安にかられるのはどんな状況のときですか．例えば，…

☐ In what situations do you feel anxious or nervous? Do you feel this way when you're...

1. 人に会う，パーティに出る．
2. バスや電車に乗る．
3. 高い場所や混んだ場所にいる．
4. 旅行にでかける．
5. 家にひとりきりでいる．
6. そばに動物や昆虫がいる．

1. meeting people or going to parties?
2. taking buses or trains?
3. in high places or crowded places?
4. traveling away from home?
5. staying home alone?
6. around animals or insects?

もっと頻繁に発作が起きるのではないかという不安がありますか．

☐ Do you fear your panic attacks will occur more frequently?

ある一定の動作，例えば，手を洗う，火の元や鍵を確認するなどを繰り返さないと気がすまないことがありますか．

☐ Do you feel you must repeat certain actions, such as washing your hands, checking and rechecking that the stove is off, or that the door is locked?

重い病気にかかっているのではと思いますか.
—医師から異常がないと言われてもやっぱり気になりますか.

- [ ] Do you feel you have a serious illness?
— When reassured by your doctor that nothing is wrong, do you still worry about your health?

あなたが感じている不安や心配,恐怖が日常生活〔仕事／学業〕に悪影響を及ぼしていると思いますか.

- [ ] Do your anxiety, worry, or fear affect your everyday life〔work/schoolwork〕?

### 時間経過

このような状態はどのくらい続いていますか.
1. 2, 3 日.
2. 1 週間.
3. 2, 3 週間.
4. 5, 6 か月.
5. 5, 6 年.

- [ ] How long have you felt this way?
   1. A few days?
   2. A week?
   3. A few weeks?
   4. Several months?
   5. Several years?

症状は…
1. 徐々に悪化していますか.
2. 変化がありませんか.
3. 反復していますか. 日によって調子のよいときと悪いときがありますか.

- [ ] Has the symptom been...
   1. getting worse?
   2. staying the same?
   3. recurrent? Do you have ups and downs in your mood, feeling good one day and feeling anxious the next?

( 抑うつ状態 )

### 症状の特徴

最近, ご気分はどうですか.

- [ ] How has your mood been recently?
- [ ] How have your spirits been recently?
   Do you feel...

1. 気分が減入っている.
2. 悲しい, むなしい.
3. 涙もろい.
4. いらいらする［怒りっぽい］.
5. 気力がわかない.

   1. depressed?
   2. sad or empty?
   3. tearful?
   4. irritable?
   5. a lack of energy?

6. いつも疲れている.
7. 仕事へ行ったり, 友人と会ったりするのが億劫である.

ふだんやっていることに興味がわかないことがありますか. 例えば, …
1. 買い物.
2. 家事.
3. 身だしなみ.
4. 友人との付き合い.
5. テレビを見る, 新聞を読む.
6. 趣味.
7. 性行為.
8. その他.

こんなふうに感じることがありますか. 例えば, …
1. 事がうまくいかないのは自分のせいだと気がとがめる.
2. 自分に自信がもてない.
3. 自分は生きている価値がない.
4. 将来が絶望的だ.

集中できないとか, いろいろ迷って決断できないことがありますか.

気分が落ち込むのはいつですか.
1. 朝.
2. 夕方.
3. 1日中.

気分が落ち込んだために生活に影響が出ましたか.

気分がひどく落ち込んだとき, 死んだほうがましだと思ったことがありますか.

- 6. tired all the time?
- 7. reluctant to go to work or meet your friends?

☐ Have you lost interest in your usual activities, such as...
1. shopping?
2. housework?
3. self-care?
4. meeting friends?
5. watching TV or reading newspapers?
6. enjoying your hobbies?
7. sex?
8. any other activities?

☐ Do you ever feel this way, such as feeling...
1. guilty about everything that goes wrong?
2. insecure about yourself?
3. worthless?
4. hopeless about your future?

☐ Do you have difficulty concentrating or making decisions?

☐ When do you feel depressed?
1. In the morning?
2. In the late afternoon?
3. All day long?

☐ Has your depression affected your life?

☐ With all the depression you've been under, have you ever thought that you'd be better off dead?

| | |
|---|---|
| 自殺を計画したり，試みたりしたことがありますか． | ☐ Have you planned or attempted to kill yourself [suicide]? |
| (付き添いの人への質問)<br>ひどく落ち込んでいますか． | ☐ Is he [she] very depressed? |
| 自分は生きている価値がないと言いますか． | ☐ Does he [she] say that he [she] is too worthless to live? |
| 自殺について話すことがありますか． | ☐ Does he [she] talk about killing himself [herself] or suicide? |
| 自分を傷つけようとしたことがありますか． | ☐ Has he [she] ever tried to harm himself [herself] in some way? |

## 時間経過

| | |
|---|---|
| このような状態はどのくらい続いていますか．<br>1. 2, 3 日．<br>2. 1 週間．<br>3. 2, 3 週間．<br>4. 5, 6 か月．<br>5. 5, 6 年． | ☐ How long have you felt this way?<br>1. A few days?<br>2. A week?<br>3. A few weeks?<br>4. Several months?<br>5. Several years? |
| 何かきっかけはありましたか．例えば，失恋，離婚，金銭問題，近親者の死，仕事上のミス，リストラなど． | ☐ Was there any trigger for your symptom, such as disappointment in love, divorce, money worries, the death of someone you have loved, errors at work, or loss of your job? |

## 随伴症状

| | |
|---|---|
| 最近，体重に変化がありましたか．<br><br>1. 体重が減った．<br>2. 体重が増えた． | ☐ Has your weight changed recently?<br>1. Have you lost weight?<br>2. Have you gained weight? |
| 食欲はどうですか．<br>1. 食欲がほとんどない． | ☐ How about your appetite?<br>1. Do you have almost no appetite? |

| | |
|---|---|
| 2. どんどん食べてしまう. | 2. Are you eating more and more? |

| | |
|---|---|
| 睡眠はどうですか. 何か問題がありますか. | ☐ How about your sleeping patterns? Do you have any problems sleeping? |
| 1. 寝つきが悪い | 1. Difficulty falling asleep? |
| 2. 早朝目が覚めてその後なかなか眠れない. | 2. Waking up early in the morning and not being able to get back to sleep? |
| 3. 熟睡した感じがない. | 3. Feeling unable to have a sound sleep? |
| 4. ふだんより眠りすぎる. | 4. Sleeping more than usual? |

### 躁状態

| | |
|---|---|
| 最近, ご気分はどうですか. | ☐ How has your mood been recently? |
| | ☐ How have your spirits been recently? Do you feel... |
| 1. すごく幸せな気分. | 1. very happy? |
| 2. いつもよりエネルギッシュだ. | 2. more energetic than usual? |
| 3. いらいらする [怒りっぽい]. | 3. irritable? |
| このような状態はどのくらい続いていますか. | ☐ How long have you felt this way? |
| 1. 2, 3 日. | 1. A few days? |
| 2. 1 週間. | 2. A week? |
| 3. 2, 3 週間. | 3. A few weeks? |
| 4. 5, 6 か月. | 4. Several months? |
| 5. 5, 6 年. | 5. Several years? |
| このような気分の高揚は周期的に起こりますか. | ☐ Does this heightened mood occur periodically? |
| 高揚感の他にどのような徴候がありますか [どのような気分ですか]. 例えば, … | ☐ In addition to the heightened mood, do you have any other signs, such as... |
| 1. 自分は何でもできる感じがする. | 1. feeling that there's nothing that you can't do? |

2. 睡眠時間はふだんより短くてもたりる．例えば，2,3時間．

3. いつもより口数が多い，声が大きい，早口で話す．
4. 考えが次々に湧き出して追いつかないほどだ．

5. することが次々に出てくるが時間がたりない．

6. 気が散って，落ち着かない．
7. 物事に集中できない，いろいろ迷って決断できない．
8. ふだんより精力的に活動している．
9. 仕事〔学業〕を頑張っている．
10. 性欲が強い．
11. お金を気前よく使う．

(付き添いの人への質問)
過度なほど幸せそうな様子ですか．

2. feeling less need for sleep? For example, sleeping a few hours at night?
3. talking more than usual, louder, and more rapidly?
4. feeling you have so many thoughts that it's hard to keep track of them all?
5. feeling that you have more and more to do and less and less time in which to do it?
6. feeling distracted or restless?
7. having difficulty concentrating or making decisions?
8. finding yourself taking on more activities than usual?
9. working harder?
10. having more sexual drive?
11. spending money lavishly?

☐ Does he〔she〕appear excessively happy?

### アルコール依存

**飲酒歴・飲酒量**

お酒を時々飲みますか．

☐ Do you have a drink now and then?

楽しみというより習慣になっていますか．
—仕事上，必要に迫られて飲酒することがありますか．

☐ Is your drinking more a habit than a pleasure?
— Do you drink out of necessity because of your job expectations?

最後にお酒を口にしたのはいつですか．

☐ When was the last time you drank?

| | |
|---|---|
| 飲酒量はどのくらいですか. | ☐ How much do you drink? |
| 　1. 気分がリラックスするほど. | 　1. Enough to make you feel relaxed? |
| 　2. 酔っ払うほど. | 　2. Enough to get drunk? |
| 　3. 酔いつぶれて意識がなくなるほど. | 　3. Enough to pass out? |
| いつも適量以上飲んでいますか. | ☐ Do you regularly drink more than a moderate amount of alcohol? |
| 適量で止めようと思っても，ついつい飲み続けてしまうのですか. | ☐ Even when you want to stop after a moderate amount, do you keep drinking more? |
| 周囲の人から酒豪だと言われていますか. | ☐ Have you been told by people around you that you are a heavy drinker? |
| ―どんな種類のお酒を1日にどのくらい〔何リットル〕飲みますか. | ― What do you usually drink? How much〔How many liters〕do you drink a day? |
| ―いつごろから飲酒量が増えてきたのですか. | ― When did you start drinking large amounts of alcohol? |
| ―アルコール消費量が徐々に増えて今の量になったのですか. | ― Has your alcohol consumption increased steadily over a period of time to the present level? |
| ―午前中に飲むことがありますか. | ― Do you ever drink before noon? |
| 何かきっかけはありましたか．例えば，仕事内容や職場の人間関係におけるストレス，仕事上のミス，リストラ，金銭問題，失恋，離婚，近親者の死など. | ☐ Was there any trigger for it, such as stress from your duties or unhappy relationship at work, errors at work, loss of your job, money worries, disappointment in love, divorce, or the death of someone you have loved? |

**飲酒による身体障害・社会障害**

| | |
|---|---|
| 朝，よく二日酔いになりますか. | ☐ Do you often have hangovers in the morning? |

―二日酔いを治すために，翌朝からまた飲酒したことはありますか．

飲んだ翌朝，前夜のことを切れ切れにしか思い出せないといった経験がありますか．

これまでに…と診断されたことがありますか．
1. 糖尿病
2. 膵炎
3. 肝障害
4. 胃・十二指腸潰瘍

―いつ診断されましたか．
―どのような治療を受けていますか．

飲むのを止めるとどんな症状が出ますか．

1. 体や手足が震える．
2. 汗がひどく出る．
3. 不安になる，イライラする．
4. 眠れなくなる．
5. 吐き気がする，吐く．
6. その他．

飲酒のため問題がありましたか．例えば，…
1. 仕事でトラブルを起こした．
2. 失職した．
3. 妻〔夫／友人／同僚〕と口論した．
4. 飲酒運転〔飲酒行為〕で逮捕された．
5. 入院した．

― Have you drunk again to recover from hangovers the next morning after drinking?

☐ The next morning after drinking, do you have experiences like remembering only snatches of the night before?

☐ Have you ever been told that you have...
1. diabetes?
2. pancreatitis?
3. liver disorder?
4. gastric and duodenal ulcer?

― When was it diagnosed?
― How have you been treated?

☐ When you stop drinking, what symptoms do you have? Do you...
1. tremble or shake?
2. sweat excessively?
3. feel nervous or irritable?
4. have difficulty sleeping?
5. have nausea or vomiting?
6. have anything else?

☐ Because of your drinking, have you ever...
1. gotten into trouble at work?
2. lost your job?
3. argued with your wife 〔husband/friends/co-workers〕?
4. been arrested for drunk driving 〔drunk behavior〕?
5. been hospitalized?

| | |
|---|---|
| 6. その他. | 6. had any other problem? |

**飲酒の制御**

| | |
|---|---|
| お酒を飲むことに気がとがめますか. | ☐ Do you feel guilty about drinking? |
| ご自分はアルコールに依存していると思いますか. | ☐ Do you feel you have a drinking problem?<br>☐ Do you feel you are dependent on alcohol? |
| 断酒しようとしたことがありますか.<br>—それはいつですか.<br>—上手くいきましたか. | ☐ Have you ever tried to stop drinking?<br>— When was it?<br>— Did it work well? |
| 断酒したいですか. | ☐ Do you want to stop drinking? |

### 摂食障害

| | |
|---|---|
| 体重の減量やダイエットに強い思い込みがありますか. | ☐ Do you have intense interest in weight loss and diets? |
| 格好よくするには痩せなくてはと思いますか. | ☐ Do you feel you must be thin to look OK? |
| 今の体型はまだ太りすぎだと感じますか.<br>—太るのは怖いですか.<br>—もっと痩せたいですか. | ☐ Do you see yourself still overweight?<br>— Are you afraid of gaining weight?<br>— Do you want to be thinner? |
| 体重の変動が激しいですか. | ☐ Does your weight fluctuate dramatically? |
| ダイエット〔減量〕を始めたのはいつですか.<br>—ダイエット〔減量〕前の体重はいくらでしたか. | ☐ When did you first try to diet 〔lose weight〕?<br>— What weight were you before you started to diet〔lose weight〕? |

| | |
|---|---|
| —今の体重はいくらですか． | — What weight are you now? |
| —これまでの最高体重はいくらありましたか． | — What has been your heaviest weight? |

食べることにこだわりがありますか． ☐ Do you take eating seriously?

食べることに気がとがめますか． ☐ Do you feel guilty about eating?

食事を避けたり，食べ物を隠したりすることがありますか． ☐ Do you ever avoid meals or hide food?

空腹のあまり大量に食べることがありますか． ☐ Do you ever eat [binge on] large amounts of food in a frenzy of hunger?

食べ始めると止まらなくなることはありますか． ☐ Once you start eating, do you ever find it difficult to stop?

食べたあと無理に吐くことがありますか． ☐ Do you ever induce vomiting after eating?

やせ薬，下剤，浣腸，利尿剤を使いますか． ☐ Do you use diet pills, laxatives, enemas, or diuretics?

月経が止まったり，不規則になったりしていますか． ☐ Have your menstrual periods stopped or become irregular?

平均的な1日の食事内容を教えて下さい． ☐ Please tell me what you eat on a typical day.

### 妄想

他の人の考えが入ってくる，自分の考えが他の人に筒抜けになると感じますか． ☐ Do you feel other people can put thoughts or ideas into your head, or take them out of your head?

| | |
|---|---|
| 誰かがあなたに嫌がらせをしたり，危害を加えようとしたりしていると感じますか． | ☐ Do you feel that someone is harassing you or trying to harm you? |
| 見たり聞いたりした人や物が，あなただけに特別なメッセージを出していると感じますか．例えば，テレビの出演者とか． | ☐ Do you feel that someone or a thing you see or hear has a special message just for you? For example, people on TV? |
| 自分の考えや行動を外部の人や物にコントロールされていると感じますか． | ☐ Do you feel someone or something is controlling your thoughts or actions from afar? |
| 自分は特別な人間だ，他の人にはない能力をもっていると感じますか． | ☐ Do you feel that you are a special person or that you have special abilities no one else has? |

こういう状態はどのくらい続いていますか．
1. 2, 3 日．
2. 1 週間．
3. 2, 3 週間．
4. 5, 6 か月．
5. 5, 6 年．

☐ How long have you felt this way?
1. A few days?
2. A week?
3. A few weeks?
4. Several months?
5. Several years?

### 幻覚・性格変化

| | |
|---|---|
| 周りに誰もいないのに，人の声が聞こえたことがありますか．その声は何と言いましたか． | ☐ Have you ever heard voices where there was nobody around? What did the voices say? |
| 自分の頭の中に浮かんだ考えが声になって聞こえてくることはありますか． | ☐ Do you ever hear thoughts that pop into your head? |
| 他の人には見えない物が見えることがありますか． | ☐ Do you ever see things other people can't see? |

| | |
|---|---|
| 皮膚の上を虫が這い回ったり，電気が走ったりする感触はありますか． | ☐ Do you feel as if insects are crawling over or as if electricity flows through your body? |
| 他の人が気づかないにおいを感じることがありますか． | ☐ Do you ever smell things other people wouldn't notice? |
| こういう状態はどのくらい続いていますか．<br>1. 2, 3 日．<br>2. 1 週間．<br>3. 2, 3 週間．<br>4. 5, 6 か月．<br>5. 5, 6 年． | ☐ How long have you felt this way?<br>1. A few days?<br>2. A week?<br>3. A few weeks?<br>4. Several months?<br>5. Several years? |
| （付き添いの人への質問）<br>非現実的な経験について話したことがありますか． | ☐ Has he〔she〕ever talked about unrealistic experiences he〔she〕had? |
| ―現実には存在しない物が見えたり，声や音が聞こえたりしますか． | ― Does he〔she〕see imaginary things, or hear imaginary voices or noises? |
| いつもとは違う行動をしますか． | ☐ Does he〔she〕act differently from the way he〔she〕usually does? |
| ―どんな奇妙な行動ですか．<br><br>1. ぶつぶつ独り言を言う．<br><br>2. 独り笑いをする．<br><br>3. 目が据わっている．<br>4. 話のつじつまが合わない．<br><br>5. 話しかけても反応がない．<br><br>6. 異常な動作をする． | ― What does he〔she〕do that is strange?<br>1. Muttering to himself〔herself〕?<br>2. Chuckling to himself〔herself〕?<br>3. His〔Her〕eyes fixed?<br>4. His〔Her〕words making no sense?<br>5. Not responding when you talk to him〔her〕?<br>6. Making unusual movements? |

| | |
|---|---|
| 7. 理由もなく攻撃的になったり，暴力をふるったりする． | 7. Becoming aggressive or violent without any apparent reason? |

表情が乏しくなったり，口数が減ったりしていますか．

☐ Does he [she] have poor facial expressions or speak less than usual?

部屋に閉じこもって，何もしないでいることが多いですか．

☐ Does he [she] stay in his [her] room most of the time without doing anything?

初めて変化に気づいたのはいつですか．

☐ When did you first notice the change in him [her]?

### 職歴・学歴・既往歴・家族歴

現在の仕事はどのような職種ですか．

☐ What type of work do you do?

どのような仕事内容ですか．

☐ What are your duties and responsibilities?

—いつから，現在の仕事に就いていますか．
—残業は多いですか．
—仕事内容や職場の人間関係でストレスを感じますか．

— How long have you had this job?

— Do you often work overtime?
— Do you feel stress from your duties or unhappy relationships at work?

最終学歴を教えて下さい．

☐ Please tell me how much schooling you've had.
☐ Please tell me about your last level of school.

学校での成績はどうでしたか．

☐ How well did you do at school?
☐ How was your school record?

1. 優秀．
2. 良いほう．
3. 普通．
4. 悪いほう．

1. Excellent?
2. Good?
3. Average?
4. Poor?

| | |
|---|---|
| それでは，これまでの健康状態についてうかがいましょう． | ☐ OK, let's talk about your past health. |
| これまでに健康面で大きな問題がありましたか．それは何でしたか． | ☐ Have you ever had any serious health problems? What was it? |
| これまでに感情面あるいは精神面での問題がありましたか．それは何でしたか． | ☐ Have you ever had any emotional or psychiatric problems? What was it? |
| ご家族のことをお聞かせ下さい． | ☐ Now I'd like to know a little about your family.<br>☐ Tell me about your family. |
| ご家族のどなたかに感情面あるいは精神面での問題をおもちの人がいますか．それは何ですか． | ☐ Has anyone in your immediate family had any emotional or psychiatric problems? What is it? |
| ご家族のなかに，同じ症状をもつ人がほかにいますか． | ☐ Does anyone else in your immediate family have this same problem? |
| ご家族に遺伝性と思われる病気がありますか． | ☐ Is there any disease that seems to run in your family? |

---

### 名句・ことわざ

#### A sound mind in a sound body.
#### 健全な身体に宿る健全な精神

古代ローマの諷刺詩人ユウェナリス Juvenal（55 ? - 130 ? *Satires*）の名言．原典は "You should pray for a sound mind in a sound body." で，「あなた方は，健全な身体に健全な精神が宿るように祈るべきだ」という意味．人間は健全な身体と健全な精神の両方を合わせ持てるよう神に祈るべきだと説いている．

## ➔ 健診異常

| | |
|---|---|
| 健診を受けたのですね.何と言われましたか. | ☐ I understand you had a general physical checkup. What have you been told about your problem? |
| ―いつ,どこで受けた健診ですか. | ― When did you have the checkup? And where? |
| ―結果報告書があれば見せて下さい. | ― Did you bring the results? Can I see them? |
| 症状はありますか. | ☐ Have you had any symptoms? |
| 昨年の健診は受けましたか. | ☐ Did you have a general physical checkup last year? |
| 精密検査を勧められたのは今回が初めてですか. | ☐ Is it the first time a thorough examination was recommended? |
| ―初めて異常を指摘されたのですか. | ― Is it the first time you were told about your problem? |
| これまでに同様の指摘をされたことがありますか. | ☐ Have you ever been told by a doctor that you have the same problem? |
| ―他の医療機関で精密検査を受けたことがありますか. | ― Have you ever had a thorough examination for your problem in another clinic or hospital? |
| ―いつ,どこでですか. | ― When did you have it? And where? |
| ―どのような検査を受けましたか. | ― What kind of tests did you have? |
| ―結果は正常〔異常〕でしたか. | ― Were the results normal〔abnormal〕? |
| ―結果についてどのような説明を受けましたか. | ― What did your doctor tell you about the results? |
| ―どんな治療を受けましたか. | ― How were you treated? |

# 既往歴

## ⊃ これまでの健康状態

| | |
|---|---|
| それでは，これまでの健康状態についてうかがいましょう． | ☐ OK, let's talk about your past health. |
| これまで健康状態はどうでしたか． | ☐ How has your health been up until now? |
| 1. 大変よい． | 1. Excellent? |
| 2. よい． | 2. Good? |
| 3. まあまあ． | 3. Fair? |
| 4. 悪い． | 4. Poor? |

## ⊃ かかりつけの医師

| | |
|---|---|
| かかりつけの医師がいますか． | ☐ Do you have your own doctor? |
| | ☐ Do you have a regular doctor? |
| ―その医師のお名前〔住所／電話〕を教えて下さい． | ― What's his 〔her〕 name 〔address/telephone number〕? |
| 最後に診察を受けたのはいつですか． | ☐ When was the last time you went to his 〔her〕 office? |
| ―診察の理由は何でしたか． | ― What was the visit for? |
| ―検査を何かしましたか． | ― Did your doctor run any test for you? |
| ―異常があると言われましたか． | ― Were you told that you have a problem? |
| ―どんな治療を受けましたか． | ― How was it treated? |

## ⊃ 既往症

| | |
|---|---|
| それでは，これまでにかかった病気についてお聞きします． | ☐ Now I'd like to ask you about any illnesses [any medical problems] you've had in the past. |
| 大きな病気にかかったことがありますか． | ☐ Have you ever had any serious illnesses? |
| ―何の病気でしたか． | ― What were they? |

|  |  |
|---|---|
| ―その時何歳でしたか． | — How old were you then? |
| ―どんな治療を受けましたか． | — How were they treated? |
| …にかかったことがありますか． | ☐ Have you ever had＿＿? |

☞「主要な病気」（189 ページ）．

|  |  |
|---|---|
| 他に何か病気にかかったことがありますか． | ☐ Have you had any other illnesses? |
| これまでにかかったその他の病気について全部話して下さい． | ☐ Please tell me about all the other illnesses you have had. |
| あなたに何か遺伝性の病気がありますか． | ☐ Do you have any hereditary [genetic] diseases? |

---

### 名句・ことわざ

**Habit is a second nature.**

**習慣は第二の天性である**

古代ローマの政治家で雄弁家として有名なキケロ（Marcus Tullius Cicero, 106- 43 B.C., *De Finibus Bonarum et Malorum*）の名言．フランスの哲学者・物理学者パスカル（Blaise Pascal, 1623-1662, *Pansées*）はこの言葉を引用して，習慣という第二の天性のために，人間に本来備わっている第一の天性が壊されることがなければよいのだがと警告している．

# 用語・表現ファイル

## 病名　その1　主要な病気

### 1. 感染症

1. 麻疹
2. 風疹 [三日ばしか]
3. 流行性耳下腺炎
4. 水痘
5. ヘルペス
6. HIV 感染症
7. エイズ
8. 溶血性連鎖球菌感染症
9. しょう紅熱
10. リウマチ熱
11. 百日咳
12. 淋菌感染症
13. 梅毒
14. 性行為感染症
15. マラリア

1. measles
2. rubella [German measles]
3. mumps
4. chickenpox
5. herpes
6. HIV infection
7. AIDS
8. hemolytic streptococcal infection
9. scarlet fever
10. rheumatic fever
11. whooping cough [pertussis]
12. gonorrhea
13. syphilis
14. sexually transmitted infection
15. malaria

### 2. 生活習慣病

1. 肥満
2. 糖尿病
3. 脂質異常症
4. 高コレステロール血症
5. 高中性脂肪血症
6. 高尿酸血症 [痛風]
7. 高血圧
8. 低血圧
9. 動脈硬化

1. obesity
2. diabetes (mellitus)
3. dyslipidemia
4. high blood cholesterol
5. high blood triglycerides ★
6. hyperuricemia [gout]
7. high blood pressure
8. low blood pressure
9. arteriosclerosis

### 3. 悪性腫瘍

がん

cancer

## 用語・表現ファイル（つづき）

### 4. 呼吸器疾患

1. 気管支炎
2. 肺炎
3. 結核
4. 喘息
5. 慢性閉塞性肺疾患
6. 過換気症候群
7. 睡眠時無呼吸症候群

1. bronchitis
2. pneumonia
3. tuberculosis
4. asthma
5. COPD [chronic obstructive pulmonary disease]
6. hyperventilation syndrome
7. sleep apnea syndrome

### 5. 心血管疾患

1. 心筋梗塞
2. 不整脈
3. 静脈瘤
4. 血栓性静脈炎
5. 動脈瘤
6. 川崎病

1. heart attack [myocardial infarction]
2. irregular pulse [arrhythmia]
3. varicose veins ★
4. thrombophlebitis
5. aneurysm
6. Kawasaki disease

### 6. 消化器疾患

1. 胃潰瘍
2. 痔
3. 肝炎
   —B 型肝炎
   —C 型肝炎
4. 胆石

1. gastric ulcer
2. hemorrhoids ★
3. hepatitis
   —hepatitis B
   —hepatitis C
4. gallstone(s)

### 7. 腎泌尿器疾患

1. 腎炎
2. 腎結石〔尿路結石〕
3. 前立腺肥大

1. nephritis
2. kidney stone(s)〔urinary calculus〕
3. enlargement of the prostate gland [benign prostatic hypertrophy]

## 用語・表現ファイル（つづき）

### 8. 血液疾患, 免疫異常

1. （鉄欠乏性）貧血
2. 出血傾向

<br>

1. (iron deficiency) anemia
2. bleeding tendency

### 9. 脳神経疾患

1. 脳梗塞
2. 脳出血
3. 痙攣
4. てんかん

<br>

1. stroke [cerebrovascular accident]
2. brain [intracerebral] hemorrhage
3. convulsions ★
4. epilepsy

### 10. 精神疾患

1. 精神遅滞
2. 精神的な問題
3. うつ病
4. 神経症
5. アルコール〔薬物〕依存症
6. 心的外傷後ストレス障害

<br>

1. mental retardation
2. psychiatric problem
3. depression
4. neurosis
5. alcohol [drug] dependence
6. PTSD [post-traumatic stress disorder]

### 11. アレルギー疾患

1. アトピー性皮膚炎
2. 花粉症

<br>

1. eczema [atopic dermatitis]
2. hay fever [pollen allergy]

### 12. 眼疾患

1. 白内障
2. 緑内障
3. 近視
4. 遠視
5. 乱視

<br>

1. cataract
2. glaucoma
3. near-sightedness [myopia]
4. far-sightedness [hyperopia]
5. distorted vision [astigmatism]

☞「小児に多い病気」(395 ページ).

---

★ 通例, 複数形で用いる.

## ● 事故・怪我

| | |
|---|---|
| 大きな事故や怪我をしたことがありますか. | ☐ Have you ever had any serious accidents or injuries? |
| 骨折したことがありますか. | ☐ Have you ever broken bones? |
| これまでに…傷を受けたことがありますか.<br>1. 頭に<br>2. 背中に<br>3. 神経に<br>4. その他の部位に | ☐ Have you ever had an injury...<br>1. to your head?<br>2. to your back?<br>3. to your nerve?<br>4. to other areas? |
| どうしたのですか [何が起こったのですか].<br>―転倒したのですか.<br>―交通事故にあったのですか. | ☐ What happened to you?<br>― Did you fall?<br>― Did you get involved in a traffic accident? |
| いつのことですか.<br>―何歳のときですか. | ☐ When was it?<br>― How old were you? |
| 医師に診てもらいましたか. | ☐ Did you see a doctor? |
| どんな治療を受けましたか. | ☐ What type of treatments did you get?<br>☐ How were you treated? |
| 入院しましたか. | ☐ Were you hospitalized? |

## ● 入院

| | |
|---|---|
| 入院したことがありますか. | ☐ Have you ever been admitted to the hospital?<br>☐ Have you ever been hospitalized? |
| 入院の理由は何でしたか. | ☐ Why were you admitted to the hospital? |

|  |  |
|---|---|
|  | ☐ What were you hospitalized for? |
| 何の治療を受けたのですか. | ☐ What were you treated for? |
| それはいつでしたか. | ☐ When was it? |
| 入院期間はどのくらいでしたか. | ☐ How long were you there?<br>☐ How long did you stay in the hospital? |
| どこの病院でしたか. | ☐ Which hospital was it?<br>☐ What was the name of the hospital? |
| 住所はどこですか. | ☐ What is the address? |

## ● 手術

| | |
|---|---|
| 手術を受けたことがありますか. | ☐ Have you ever had surgery before? |
| 何の手術でしたか. | ☐ What surgery did you have? |

…の手術を受けましたか.
　1. 扁桃
　2. 虫垂
　3. 大腸
　4. 痔
　5. 胆嚢
　6. 乳房
　7. 子宮
　8. 卵巣
　9. 前立腺
　10. 鼠径ヘルニア
　11. 白内障

☐ Did they operate…
　1. on your tonsil(s)?
　2. on your appendix?
　3. on your large intestine?
　4. on your hemorrhoids?
　5. on your gallbladder?
　6. on your breast(s)?
　7. on your uterus?
　8. on your ovary〔ovaries〕?
　9. on your prostate?
　10. for an inguinal hernia?
　11. for cataract(s)?

| | |
|---|---|
| それはいつでしたか. | ☐ When was it? |
| どこの病院でしたか. | ☐ Which hospital was it? |

## 🔹 血液型・輸血歴

| | |
|---|---|
| ご自分の血液型を知っていますか. | ☐ Do you know your blood type? |
| —何ですか. | — What is it? |
| — Rh 血液型は陽性〔陰性〕ですか. | — Is it Rh positive〔negative〕? |

輸血を受けたことがありますか. ☐ Have you ever had a blood transfusion?

—いつですか. — When was it?
—輸血が必要となった理由はなんですか. — What was it for? Why did you have the transfusion?
—輸血後体調に変化がありましたか. — Did you have any problems after the transfusion?

## 🔹 補完代替医療

補完代替医療を受けたことがありますか. ☐ Have you ever used any complementary and alternative treatment [therapy]?

—それは何ですか. — What was it?
1. 鍼灸. 　1. Acupuncture and/or moxibustion?
2. マッサージ. 　2. Massage therapy?
3. ヨガ. 　3. Yoga?
4. 太極拳. 　4. Tai chi?
5. カイロプラクティック. 　5. Chiropractic?
6. その他. 　6. Other?

## 🔹 薬歴

薬を何か常用していますか.
☐ Do you take any drugs or medications regularly?
☐ Are you taking any drugs or medications regularly?

何という薬ですか. ☐ What medications (are you now taking)?

—なぜ飲んでいるのですか. — Why are you taking them?

| | |
|---|---|
| ―飲み始めてどのくらいになりますか. | ― How long have you been taking them? |
| ―医師の処方による薬ですか. | ― Are they prescribed by your doctor? |
| ―市販の薬ですか. | ― Are they bought "over-the-counter"? |
| その薬を持ってきましたか. | ☐ Did you bring them with you? |
| ―見せて下さい. | ― May I see them? |
| ―お薬手帳があれば見せて下さい. | ― If you have your personal medication record, please show it to me. |
| これまでに薬の副作用はありましたか. | ☐ Have you ever had any side effects after taking medications? |
| ―どんな症状でしたか. | ― What happened to you? |
| 　1. 湿疹が出る. | 　1. Having a rash? |
| 　2. 気分が悪くなる. | 　2. Feeling sick? |
| ―どの薬ですか. | ― Which medications are they? |
| 飲んではいけない薬がありますか. | ☐ Are there any medications that you shouldn't take? |
| 薬草〔漢方薬〕か栄養補助食品〔サプリメント〕を使用していますか. | ☐ Do you use any herbs or nutritional supplements? |

## ● アレルギー

| | |
|---|---|
| アレルギーがありますか. | ☐ Are you allergic to anything? |
| | ☐ Do you have any allergies? |
| ―どんなアレルギーがありますか. | ― What type〔types〕of allergies do you have? |
| ―症状は…出ますか. | ― Does it occur... |
| | 　Does it bother you... |
| 　1. しょっちゅう | 　1. all the time? |
| 　2. ある特定の時期に | 　2. at just certain times of the year? |
| これまでに喘息〔花粉症〕になったことがありますか. | ☐ Have you ever had asthma〔hay fever〕? |

…にアレルギーがありますか.
1. 食べ物
    a. 卵
    b. 乳製品
    c. 小麦
    d. そば

    e. ナッツ
    f. 大豆
    g. 魚介類
    h. 果物
2. 昆虫
    a. ハチ
    b. ダニ
3. 動植物
    a. 犬
    b. 猫
    c. 鳥
    d. つたうるし
    e. 春〔初夏／秋〕の花粉

4. 医薬品
    a. 抗生物質
        ペニシリン
        サルファ剤
    b. 鎮痛解熱薬

        アスピリン
        イブプロフェン
    c. 造影剤〔ヨウ素〕
    d. 麻酔薬
5  化粧品
6  その他のアレルゲン
    a. ほこり
    b. ウール
    c. かび

どんなアレルギー反応を起こしますか.

☐ Are you allergic to...
1. foods?
    a. eggs?
    b. milk products?
    c. wheat?
    d. soba [buckwheat noodles]?
    e. nuts [peanuts]?
    f. soy beans?
    g. fish and shellfish?
    h. fruit?
2. insects?
    a. hornets [wasps/bees]?
    b. mites?
3. animals and plants?
    a. dogs?
    b. cats?
    c. birds?
    d. poison ivy?
    e. pollen in the spring [the early summer/the fall]?
4. medications?
    a. antibiotics?
        penicillin?
        sulfa drugs?
    b. analgesic-antipyretic drugs?
        aspirin?
        ibuprofen?
    c. contrast medium [iodine]?
    d. anesthetics?
5. cosmetics?
6. other allergens?
    a. dust?
    b. wool?
    c. mold?

☐ What happens to you when you have an allergic reaction? Do you get...

| | |
|---|---|
| 1. 発疹. | 1. a rash? |
| 2. 蕁麻疹. | 2. hives? |
| 3. かゆみ. | 3. itching? |
| 4. 腫れ. | 4. swelling? |
| 5. 鼻水. | 5. a runny nose? |
| 6. 涙. | 6. watery eyes? |
| 7. 目のかゆみ. | 7. itchy eyes? |
| 8. 息切れ. | 8. shortness of breath? |
| 9. 呼吸困難. | 9. difficulty breathing? |
| 10. 頭痛. | 10. a headache? |
| 11. 腹痛. | 11. an abdominal pain? |
| 12. アナフィラキシーショック. | 12. an anaphylactic shock? |

| | |
|---|---|
| 他にお話になりたいことがありますか. | ☐ Is there anything else you would like to tell me? |

## ❷ 妊娠・授乳

☞「妊娠歴」「分娩歴」(364 ページ).

| | |
|---|---|
| 妊娠の可能性がありますか. | ☐ Is there any possibility of getting pregnant?<br>☐ Could you be pregnant? |
| 妊娠の疑いがありますか. | ☐ Do you feel that you may have gotten pregnant? |
| 現在,妊娠していますか. | ☐ (To your knowledge, ) are you now pregnant? |
| —妊娠何週目ですか. | — How many weeks pregnant are you? |
| —予定日はいつですか. | — When is your baby due? |
| 妊娠したことがありますか. | ☐ Have you ever been pregnant? |
| —これまでに何回妊娠しましたか. | — How many times have you been pregnant? |
| —これまでに何回出産しましたか. | — How many babies have you had?<br>How many deliveries have you experienced? |

| 現在，授乳中ですか． | ☐ Are you now breast-feeding? |

## ➲ 予防接種

☞「予防接種」(400ページ)．

| これまでにどんな予防接種を受けましたか． | ☐ What vaccinations [shots] have you had? |

| あなたは…の予防接種を受けましたか． | ☐ Have you had vaccinations for... |

1. ジフテリア
2. 百日咳
3. 破傷風
4. ポリオ
5. 風疹
6. 麻疹
7. BCG
8. 日本脳炎
9. 水痘
10. 流行性耳下腺炎
11. インフルエンザ
12. 肺炎球菌
13. A型肝炎
14. B型肝炎
15. 腸チフス
16. コレラ
17. 黄熱
18. ペスト
19. 狂犬病

1. diphtheria?
2. whooping cough [pertussis]?
3. tetanus?
4. polio?
5. rubella [German measles]?
6. measles?
7. BCG?
8. Japanese encephalitis?
9. chickenpox?
10. mumps?
11. influenza [flu]?
12. pneumococcus?
13. hepatitis A?
14. hepatitis B?
15. typhoid?
16. cholera?
17. yellow fever?
18. the plague?
19. rabies?

―いつ受けましたか． — When did you have it [them]?
―最後に受けた予防注射はいつでしたか． — When was your last shot?
―予防接種後に具合が悪くなったことはありますか． — Have you had any problems after the shot?

## ➲ 健診・人間ドック

| この前健診を受けたのはいつですか． | ☐ When did you last have a general physical checkup? |

| | |
|---|---|
| ―何か異常所見はありましたか. | — Did they find anything wrong with you? |
| ―精密検査を受けましたか. | — Did you get a thorough examination? |
| ―どのような指導を受けましたか. | — What recommendation did you have from your doctor? |
| ―どのような治療を受けましたか. | — What type of treatment did you get? |

最後に撮った胸部X線写真はいつでしたか.
― どこで撮りましたか.
― 結果は正常〔異常〕でしたか.

☐ When was your last chest X-ray?
— Where was it taken?
— Were the results normal〔abnormal〕?

乳房X線写真を撮ったことがありますか.
― いつですか.
― 結果は正常〔異常〕でしたか.

☐ Have you ever had a mammogram?
— When?
— Were the results normal〔abnormal〕?

子宮頸がん検診〔パップスメア検査〕を受けたことがありますか.
― いつですか.
― 結果は正常〔異常〕でしたか.

☐ Have you ever had a Pap smear?
— When?
— Were the results normal〔abnormal〕?

☞「検査項目」(292 ページ).

## ● 海外渡航歴

これまでに日本の国外へ出てどこかへ旅行しましたか.
― いつですか.
― どこの国ですか．どのくらいの期間滞在しましたか.
― 渡航理由は何ですか．旅行ですか．仕事ですか.

☐ Have you ever traveled anywhere out of Japan?
— When?
— Which country〔countries〕? How long did you stay there?
— What was the purpose of the trip? A pleasure trip or a business trip?

# 家族歴

## ➡ 家族構成

| | |
|---|---|
| ご家族のことをうかがいます. | ☐ Now I'd like to know a little about your immediate family.<br>☐ Tell me about your immediate family. |
| ご両親はご健在ですか.<br>―お父さん〔お母さん〕はご健在ですか.<br>―今何歳ですか.<br>―亡くなられたとき何歳でしたか.<br>―亡くなられた原因は何でしたか. | ☐ Are your parents still living?<br>― Is your father〔mother〕living?<br>― How old is he〔she〕?<br>― How old was he〔she〕when he〔she〕died?<br>― What did he〔she〕die of? What was the cause of death? |
| お子さんはいますか.<br>―お子さんは全部で何人ですか. | ☐ Do you have any children?<br>― How many children do you have? |
| きょうだいはいますか.<br>―きょうだいは何人ですか. | ☐ Do you have brothers or sisters?<br>― How many brothers and sisters do you have? |

## ➡ 家族の病気

| | |
|---|---|
| ご家族のどなたかに健康上の問題か障害がありますか. | ☐ Does anyone in your immediate family have any health problems or disability? |
| ご家族の中に,あなたと同じ症状だった人はいますか. | ☐ Has anyone else in your immediate family had this same problem? |
| ご家族に遺伝性の病気の人はいますか. | ☐ Is there any disease that seems to run in your immediate family? |

| | |
|---|---|
| ご主人に何か遺伝性の病気がありますか. | ☐ Does your husband have any hereditary [genetic] diseases? |
| 血縁のある方で…にかかっているかかかった人がいますか. | ☐ Do you know of any blood relative that has or had... |

- 血縁のある方で…にかかっているかかかった人がいますか.
  1. がん
  ―どこの臓器ですか？
  2. 脳卒中
  3. 心筋梗塞
  4. 高血圧
  5. 糖尿病
  6. 花粉症
  7. アトピー性皮膚炎
  8. 喘息
  9. 結核
  10. 腎臓病
  11. 関節炎
  12. 甲状腺腫
  13. てんかん
  14. 白血病
  15. 神経症
  16. 自殺
- ご関係を教えて下さい.

☞「主要な病気」(189 ページ).

- Do you know of any blood relative that has or had...
  1. cancer?
  —What organ?
  2. stroke?
  3. heart attack [myocardial infarction]?
  4. high blood pressure?
  5. diabetes?
  6. hay fever?
  7. (atopic) eczema?
  8. asthma?
  9. tuberculosis?
  10. kidney disease?
  11. arthritis?
  12. goiter?
  13. epilepsy?
  14. leukemia?
  15. nervous breakdown?
  16. suicide?
- Tell me the relationship.

## 生活習慣・活動

生活習慣についておうかがいします. □ I'd like to ask you some questions about your routines.

### ➔ 睡眠

☞「精神・心理」(168 ページ).

夜はよく眠れますか. □ Do you sleep well at night?

夜はたいてい何時間眠りますか. □ How many hours do you usually sleep at night?

何時に寝ますか？ □ What time do you go to bed?

睡眠薬を飲んでいますか. □ Are you using sleeping pills to help you sleep?

### ➔ 食習慣

食習慣についてお話し下さい. □ Please tell me about your eating habits.

食欲はいかがですか. □ How is your appetite?
―このところ食欲はどうでしたか. ― How has your appetite been?

食事は規則的にしていますか. □ Do you eat at regular times?
―食事は 1 日何回食べますか. ― How many times a day do you eat?

―食事を抜くことがありますか. ― Do you skip one or more meals during the day?

―昼間あるいは夜寝る前に間食しますか. ― Do you eat between meals or before going to bed?

食事は外食が多いですか. □ Do you eat out mostly?
―家で食べますか. ― Do you eat at home?
―自分で調理しますか. ― Do you cook for yourself?
―誰が食事を調理しますか. ― Who prepares the meals?

ふだんの日に何を食べているかを教えて下さい.

□ Tell me what you eat on a typical day.

ふだん何を食べていますか.
1. パン.
2. お米のご飯.
3. めん類.
4. 牛肉・豚肉.
5. 鶏肉.
6. 魚.
7. 乳製品.
8. 青野菜.
9. 黄色野菜.
10. 豆類.
11. 果物.
12. 菓子類.

□ What do you usually eat?
1. Bread?
2. Rice?
3. Noodles?
4. Beef or pork?
5. Chicken?
6. Fish?
7. Milk products?
8. Green vegetables?
9. Yellow vegetables?
10. Beans?
11. Fruit?
12. Sweets?

食べ物はふつう…が多いですか.
1. 揚げもの
2. 炒めもの
3. 生もの
4. 煮たり,焼いたりしたもの
5. 電子レンジもの
6. 塩辛いもの
7. 香辛料のきいたもの
8. 甘いもの

□ Is the food usually...
1. deep-fried?
2. pan-fried?
3. raw?
4. boiled or broiled?
5. microwaved?
6. salty?
7. spicy?
8. sweet?

食べ物はどんなものがお好きですか.

□ What kind of foods do you like?

食べないものがありますか.
―何ですか.
―その理由は…ですか.
1. 好きではないから
2. 気持ちが悪くなるから
3. アレルギーがあるから
4. 宗教に反するから
5. 食べたことがないから

□ Is there anything you won't eat?
— What is it?
— Because...
1. you don't like it?
2. it makes you feel bad?
3. you are allergic to it?
4. it is against your religion?
5. you haven't eaten it before?

菜食主義者ですか.

□ Are you a vegetarian?

| | |
|---|---|
| ダイエットをしていますか. | ☐ Are you on a diet? |
| 飲み物はふだん何を飲みますか. | ☐ What do you usually drink? |
| 1. コーヒー. | 1. Coffee? |
| 2. 紅茶. | 2. Black tea? |
| 3. 緑茶. | 3. Green tea? |
| 4. ジュース. | 4. Fruit juice? |
| 5. 清涼飲料水. | 5. Soft drinks? |
| ― 1 日に何杯飲みますか. | ― How many cups〔glasses〕do you drink each day? |
| ―甘味料を使いますか. | ― Do you use sweeteners〔sugar substitutes〕? |
| 1 日に水分をどのくらいとりますか. | ☐ How much liquid do you drink during the day? |

## ● 便通

☞「便通異常」(96 ページ).

| | |
|---|---|
| 便通は規則的にありますか. | ☐ Do you have regular bowel movements? |
| ―毎日ありますか, 1 日おきですか. | ― Every day or every other day? |
| ―何日おきにありますか. | ― How many days apart do you have them? |
| ―頻度はどのくらいですか. | ― How often do you have them? |
| 便秘がちですか. | ☐ Do you tend to have constipation? |
| 下痢がちですか. | ☐ Do you tend to have diarrhea? |
| ― 1 日に何回便通がありますか. | ― How many times do you move your bowels? |
| ―昨日は何回下痢しましたか. | ― How many times did you have diarrhea yesterday? |
| 1. 1, 2 回. | 1. Once or twice? |
| 2. 3 回以上. | 2. Three times or more? |
| 3. なし. | 3. No movement? |

| | |
|---|---|
| 下痢と便秘を交互に繰り返しますか. | ☐ Do you have diarrhea alternating with constipation? |

## ➡ 喫煙・飲酒・麻薬

### 喫煙

| | |
|---|---|
| タバコを吸いますか. | ☐ Do you smoke? |
| ―タバコを吸ったことがありますか. | ― Have you ever smoked? |
| ―タバコは1日何本吸いますか〔ましたか〕. | ― How many cigarettes do〔did〕you smoke a day? |
| ―吸い始めたのは何歳のときですか. | ― How old were you when you started? |
| いつから禁煙していますか. | ☐ When did you stop smoking? <br> ☐ Since when have you stopped smoking? |
| ―最後に吸ってからどのくらい経ちますか. | ― About how long has it been since you last smoked? |
| ―吸うのをやめようとしたことがありますか. | ― Have you ever tried to stop? |
| ―吸うのをやめたいですか. | ― Would you like to stop? |
| ご家族や仕事場でタバコを吸う人がいますか. | ☐ Does anyone in your family or workplace smoke? |

### 飲酒

☞「アルコール依存」(177ページ).

| | |
|---|---|
| お酒を飲みますか. | ☐ Do you drink alcohol? |
| ふだん何を飲みますか. <br> 　1. ビール. <br> 　2. ワイン. <br> 　3. ウイスキー. <br> 　4. 日本酒. | ☐ What do you usually drink? <br> 　1. Beer? <br> 　2. Wine? <br> 　3. Whiskey? <br> 　4. Sake? |

|  |  |
|---|---|
| どのくらいの頻度で飲みますか. | How often do you drink? |
| 1. 毎日. | 1. Every day? |
| 2. 週3回. | 2. Three times a week? |
| 3. 週末. | 3. On weekends? |

平均して,毎日〔1週間に〕どのくらいの量を飲みますか.
- How much do you drink a day 〔a week〕, on the average?
  1. グラス1杯〔3杯〕. / One glass〔3 glasses〕?
  2. ボトル1本〔2本〕. / One bottle〔2 bottles〕?

どういうとき飲みますか. / When do you drink?
Do you drink when you are...
1. 1人のとき. / alone?
2. 悲しいとき. / sad?
3. 憂うつなとき. / depressed?
4. 楽しいとき. / happy?
5. 付き合いのときのみ. / in a social situation only?

ご自分はアルコールに依存していると思いますか. / Do you feel you have a drinking problem?

援助をお望みですか. / Would you like help?

### 麻薬

快楽用の麻薬を使ったことがありますか. / Have you ever used any recreational drugs?
—どんな麻薬を使いましたか. / — What kind of drugs did you use?

—それは何でしたか. / — What was it?
1. マリファナ. / Marijuana [Pot]?
2. コカイン. / Cocaine?
3. ヘロイン. / Heroin?
4. LSD 幻覚剤. / LSD [Lysergic acid diethylamide]?

—どのくらいの頻度で使いましたか. / — How often did you use it?
—どのくらいの期間使いましたか. / — How long did you use it?

―だれかと注射針を共有したことがありますか.
1. 肝炎の人.
2. エイズの人.

— Have you ever shared needles with someone?
1. Someone with hepatitis?
2. Someone with AIDS?

## 趣味・運動

### 趣味

どんな趣味をおもちですか.

☐ What hobbies do you have?
☐ What are your hobbies?

リラックスしたいときには何をしますか.
1. スポーツ.
2. 読書.
3. 映画.
4. 音楽.
5. 絵画.
6. 写真.
7. 旅行.
8. 庭仕事.

☐ What do you do for relaxation?
Do you enjoy...
1. sports?
2. reading?
3. movies?
4. music?
5. painting?
6. photography?
7. traveling?
8. gardening?

何かクラブに所属していますか.

☐ Do you belong to any club?

### 運動

何かスポーツをしますか.
―どんなスポーツをしますか.

☐ Do you play any sports?
— What sports do you play?

何か運動をしていますか.
―どんな運動をしていますか.

1. 散歩.
2. 水泳.
3. ジョギング.
4. テニス.
5. ゴルフ.
6. 美容体操.

☐ Do you do any exercises?
— What type of exercises do you do? Do you enjoy...
1. walking?
2. swimming?
3. jogging?
4. playing tennis?
5. golfing?
6. calisthenics?

— 1週何回くらいしますか．— How many times per week do you exercise?

— 1回につきどのくらい（長く）運動しますか．— How long do you spend exercising each time?

お仕事中どのくらい体を動かしますか．— How much physical labor does your work require?

## ● ペット

ペットを飼っていますか．— Do you have any pets?
— どんなペットですか．— What kind of pets do you have?
1. 犬．
2. 猫．
3. 鳥．
4. ハムスター．

1. Dogs?
2. Cats?
3. Birds?
4. Hamsters?

---

**名句・ことわざ**

**風邪は万病のもと**

〔英訳〕**A cold can lead to all kinds of diseases.**

英語には "A May cold is a thirty-day cold."（5月に風邪を引くと治るのに30日かかる）という類似のことわざがある．

## 問診の最後に

| | |
|---|---|
| 私からの質問はこれで終わりです. | ☐ OK, I think that's about all the questions I have for now. |
| 何かご質問はありますか. | ☐ Do you have any questions? |
| それでは,診察をしましょう. | ☐ Now, let's do your physical exam. |

---

### 名句・ことわざ

**Art is long, life is short.**
**医術の修得には時間が長くかかるが、人生は短い**

近代医学の祖とされる古代ギリシャの医師ヒポクラテス (Hippocrates, 460 ? - 377 B.C., *Aphorisms*) の箴言. W. H. S. Jones (Loeb Classical Library) の翻訳では, "Life is short, the art long, opportunity fleeting, experiment★ treacherous, judgment difficult."（人生は短く, 術の道は長く, 機会は一瞬にして消え去り, 経験には危険が潜み, 判断は難しい) となっている.〔★かつては experience（経験）の意味で用いられていた。〕

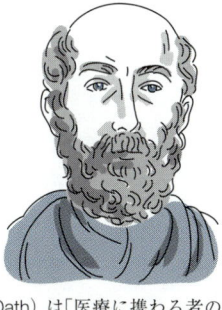

有名なヒポクラテスの誓い (the Hippocratic Oath) は「医療に携わる者の職業倫理についての誓い」で, 欧米では医学部の卒業式などのときに唱えて, 医療の現場に旅立つ前にこの誓いの言葉を心に刻むという.「治療の機会に見聞きしたことや, 治療と関係なくても他人の私生活についての漏らすべきでないことは, 他言してはならないとの信念をもって, 沈黙を守ります….」(小川政恭訳) という誓いは医療従事者すべてに当てはまる. 看護師にはこの誓いをもとに作られた看護師の誓い (the Nursing Oath, the Nightingale Oath) がある.

## 問診のီ変化

他に何か質問はございますか？   OK, I think that's about all the questions I have for now.

他にご質問は？ありますか   Do you have any questions?

では、診察をしましょう   Now, let's do your physical exam.

chapter **4**

# 身体の診察

## Physical Examination

**診察前** 212
**身体計測・バイタルサイン** 212
**系統別診察** 217
 頭頸部(頭頸・眼・耳鼻咽喉)の診察 217
 胸背部・乳房の診察 222
 腹部(消化器・鼠径)の診察 224
 直腸診・生殖器の診察 225
 骨格(上肢・下肢・脊柱)の診察 227
 神経の診察 229
**診察の終了** 234

## 診察前

眼鏡，入れ歯，装飾品はすべてとって下さい．
☐ Please remove your glasses, dentures and all of your jewelry.

服は…脱いで下さい．
1. 上半身を
2. 下半身を
3. ぜんぶ

☐ Please take off your clothes...
1. from the waist up.
2. from the waist down.
3. completely.

このガウンを着て下さい．
―前を〔後ろを〕開けて着て下さい．

☐ Please put on this gown.
― Please put it on with the opening in the front〔back〕.

診察中にご気分が悪くなったら言って下さい．
☐ Please let me know if you feel sick during the examination.

## 身体計測・バイタルサイン

### ➔ 身体計測

身長と体重を測りましょう．
☐ I'm going to [Let me] measure your height and weight.

―靴を脱いで，この台の上に乗って下さい．
― Please take off your shoes and stand on this scale.

―身長は 178 cm，体重は 74 kg です．
― You're 178 centimeters in height, and 74 kilos in weight.

## ◯ バイタルサイン

熱［体温］を測りましょう. 　　　　　　☐ I'm going to [Let me] take your temperature.

—体温計をピーッと鳴るまでわきの下にはさんで下さい. 　　　— Please keep this thermometer under your arm until it beeps.

—この体温計を額にかざします. 　　　— I'm going to [Let me] place this thermometer just in front of your forehead.

—熱は摂氏 37.5℃です. 　　　— Your temperature is thirty-seven point five degrees Celsius.

☞外国の患者さんには華氏で言ってもよい.「単位の換算表」(216 ページ).

血圧を測りましょう. 　　　　　　☐ I'm going to [Let me] take your blood pressure.

—右手を出して下さい. 　　　— Please hold out your right hand.
—腕をまくって下さい. 　　　— Roll up your sleeve.
—腕にこのカフ［腕帯］を巻きましょう. 　　　— Let me put this cuff on your arm.

（機械の場合）
—白いカフの中に手を入れて下さい. 　　　— Please put your arm inside this white cuff.
—腕の力を抜いて下さい. 　　　— Relax your arm.
—血圧は上が 138, 下が 85 です. 　　　— Your blood pressure is 138 over 85.

脈を測りましょう. 　　　　　　☐ I'm going to [Let me] take your pulse.

—右手を出して下さい. 　　　— Please hold out your right hand.
—脈は 1 分間に 80 です. 　　　— Your pulse is 80 a minute.

酸素濃度を測りましょう. 　　　　　　☐ I'm going to [Let me] measure your oxygen level.

—このパルスオキシメーターに指を入れて下さい. 　　　— Please insert your finger into this pulse oximeter.
—数値は 98 です. 　　　— Your reading is 98.

## 用語・表現ファイル
## 数字の読み方

**1. 電話番号，診察券，クレジットカードなど，長い数字が続くもの**

　　──→数を1字ずつ棒読みにする．
　　（例）　03−3451−6208　　　　zero-three, three-four-five-one,
　　　　　　　　　　　　　　　　　　six-two-zero-eight ★1

**2. 時刻**

　　──→数をそのままの順序で言う．
　　（例）　いま…です．　　8:00　It's eight o'clock.
　　　　　　　　　　　　　　　　　It's eight a.m.
　　　　　　　　　　　　9:15　It's nine fifteen.
　　　　　　　　　　　　　　　　　It's a quarter after [past] nine.
　　　　　　　　　　　　9:30　It's nine thirty.
　　　　　　　　　　　　　　　　　It's half past nine.
　　　　　　　　　　　　　　　　　It's half nine.
　　　　　　　　　　　　9:45　It's nine forty-five.
　　　　　　　　　　　　　　　　　It's a quarter of [to] ten.
　　　　　　　　　　　　3:10　It's three ten.
　　　　　　　　　　　　　　　　　It's ten after [past] three.
　　　　　　　　　　　　3:55　It's three fifty-five.
　　　　　　　　　　　　　　　　　It's five of [to] four.

**3. 日付**

　　（例）　5月12日　　　　　　　May (the) twelfth ★2

**4. 西暦年号**

　　（例）　1965年　　　　　　　nineteen sixty-five
　　　　　2000年　　　　　　　two thousand
　　　　　2005年　　　　　　　two thousand and five
　　　　　2013年　　　　　　　two thousand and thirteen

## 用語・表現ファイル（つづき）

### 5. 病室番号

⟶ 100 の位で分けて言うか，あるいは 1 字ずつ言う．

（例）外科病棟 321 号室　　　Room three twenty-one [three-two-one], the Surgical Floor

### 6. 温度

（例）38.2 ℃　　　　　thirty-eight point two degrees Celsius [centigrade]

　　96.5 °F　　　　　ninety-six point five degrees Fahrenheit

### 7. 検査値，計測値，薬量

⟶ 整数は普通の読み方，小数点以下は数を 1 つずつ棒読みにする．

（例）中性脂肪値 224　　　two hundred (and) twenty four

　　血糖値 130 mg/dl　　　one hundred (and) thirty milligrams per deciliter

　　尿酸値 5.6　　　　　　five point six

　　総ビリルビン値 0.8　　point eight ★3

　　身長 183 cm　　　　　one hundred (and) eighty-three centimeters

　　体重 78 kg　　　　　　seventy-eight kilos

　　薬 0.25 mg　　　　　　point-two-five milligrams ★4

### 8. 救急車

⟶ 数を 1 字ずつ棒読みにする．

（例）119　　　　　　　　one-one-nine

### 9. その他大きい数字の読み方

⟶ hundred や thousand のあとに名詞形がくるときには hundreds, thousands と "s" をつけた複数形にしない．

（例）350 人の入院患者　　three hundred (and) fifty inpatients

## 用語・表現ファイル(つづき)

| | |
|---|---|
| 10,000 人の症例 | ten thousand cases |
| 人口 100,000 人 | a [one] hundred thousand population, a population of one hundred thousand |

[*1] 0 は,[zíerou] あるいは [óu] という.
[*2] 英国では "the twelfth of May" という.
[*3] 0 を読まない.または zero point eight ともいう.
[*4] 0 を読まない.または zero point-two-five milligrams ともいう.

## 用語・表現ファイル
### 単位の換算表(概算)

| 体重 | | 身長 | | | 体温 | |
|---|---|---|---|---|---|---|
| キログラム | ポンド | センチメートル | インチ | フィート/インチ | 摂氏 | 華氏 |
| kg | lb | cm | in | ft/in [*1] | ℃ | °F |
| 80 | 176 | 180 | 71 | 5'11" [*2] | 40 | 104.0 |
| 70 | 154 | 170 | 67 | 5'7" | 39 | 102.2 |
| 60 | 132 | 160 | 63 | 5'3" | 38 | 100.4 |
| 50 | 110 | 150 | 59 | 4'11" | 37 | 98.6 |
| 40 | 88 | 140 | 55 | 4'7" | 36 | 96.8 |

◎重さ　ポンド　lb＝(kg)×2.2
　　　　キログラム　kg＝(lb)×0.45
◎長さ　インチ　in＝(cm)×0.4
　　　　センチメートル　cm＝(in)×2.54
◎温度　華氏　°F＝(℃×1.8)＋32
　　　　摂氏　℃＝(°F−32)×5/9

[*1] フィート　1 foot＝12 inches
[*2] 5'11" は 5 ft 11 in (five feet eleven inches) と読む.

# 系統別診察

## ● 頭頸部（頭頸・眼・耳鼻咽喉）の診察

### 頭頸

| | |
|---|---|
| 頭を診察しましょう． | ☐ I'm going to [Let me] examine your head. |
| 痛む所〔しこり〕を指でさして下さい． | ☐ Please point to where the pain is [where you have the lump]. |
| 首を診察しましょう． | ☐ I'm going to [Let me] examine your neck. |
| 真っ直ぐ前を見て下さい． | ☐ Please look straight ahead. |
| 痛む場所があれば教えて下さい． | ☐ If you have any pain, let me know where. |
| 唾をゆっくり飲み込んで下さい． | ☐ Please swallow some saliva slowly. |
| ―もう一度やって下さい． | ― Again. |

### 眼

| | |
|---|---|
| 目を診察しましょう． | ☐ I'm going to [Let me] examine your eyes. |
| コンタクトレンズは外して下さい． | ☐ Please take out [remove] your contact lenses. |
| コンタクトレンズは外さなくても結構です． | ☐ It's OK to wear your contact lenses.<br>☐ You don't have to take out [remove] your contact lenses. |
| どうぞこれを読んで下さい． | ☐ Please read this. |
| 頭を動かさないで下さい． | ☐ Please don't move your head. |

| 目を開けて真っ直ぐ前を見て下さい． | ☐ Please keep your eyes open and look straight ahead. |

右〔左〕目を手で隠して下さい． ☐ Please cover your right〔left〕 eye with your hand.

—私の指がはっきり見えますか． — Can you see my finger(s) clearly?

—指が何本見えますか． — How many fingers am I holding up?

—頭を動かさずに目で追って下さい． — Follow it〔them〕without moving your head.

—私の指が動いたら教えて下さい． — Let me know when my finger moves〔my fingers move〕.

どうぞ…(を) 見て下さい． ☐ Please look...
1. 上
2. 下
3. 右
4. 左
5. ずっと上まで
6. ずっと下まで
7. 真っ直ぐ
8. ここ

1. up.
2. down.
3. to the right.
4. to the left.
5. all the way up.
6. all the way down.
7. straight.
8. here.

目にペンライトの光が入りますが，真っ直ぐ前を見て下さい． ☐ I'm going to shine this penlight into your eye(s), so please look straight ahead.

—まぶしいですよ． — It may be a little bright. You might see some glare.

(これで) 目に触りますよ． ☐ I'll touch your eye(s)（with this）.

結膜をみせて下さい． ☐ Let me look at your conjunctiva.

うわまぶたを裏返します． ☐ I'm going to flip your upper eyelid(s).

散瞳するために点眼薬を入れます． ☐ I'm going to put eye drops in your eye(s) to dilate your pupil(s).

| | |
|---|---|
| あごと額をこの台の上に載せて下さい． | ☐ Please put your chin and forehead on this support. |
| ―目を開けて〔閉じて〕下さい． | — Open 〔close〕 your eyes. |
| ―目を動かさないで下さい． | — Don't move your eyes. |
| ―光が見えますか． | — Do you see a light? |
| ―その光をずっと見ていて下さい． | — Please continue looking at it. |
| ―ちょっとの間，まばたきしないで下さい． | — Don't blink for just a second. |
| ―まばたきをしてもいいですよ． | — Now, you can blink. |
| ―目を大きく開けたままで，黒い点を追いかけて下さい． | — Keep your eyes open wide, and follow the black spot. |
| こちらを見てここにピントを合わせて下さい． | ☐ Please look this way and focus here. |

### 耳鼻咽喉

| | |
|---|---|
| …を診察しましょう． | ☐ I'm going to [Let me] examine your... |
| 1．耳 | 1. ears. |
| 2．鼻 | 2. nose. |
| 3．口 | 3. mouth. |
| 4．のど | 4. throat. |

#### ▶ 耳

| | |
|---|---|
| 私の声が聞こえますか． | ☐ Can you hear me speaking? |
| ―私は今，何と言いましたか． | — What did I say? |
| (指をこすり合わせて) 聞こえますか． | ☐ Do you hear anything? |
| ―左右差はありますか． | — Do you hear the same in both ears? |
| ―どちらが聞こえにくいですか． | — Which ear has more difficulty in hearing? |
| 音叉をあてます． | ☐ I'm going to place this tuning fork on you. |
| (音叉を耳に近づけて) …教えて下さい． | ☐ Please tell me when... |

| | |
|---|---|
| 1. これ [この音] が聞こえなくなったら | 1. you can't hear this any more. |
| 2. これ [この音] が聞こえたら | 2. you can hear this. |

耳の中を診察しましょう. □ I'm going to [Let me] examine the inside of your ear(s).

---

### ▶ 鼻

鼻の中を診察しましょう. □ I'm going to [Let me] examine the inside of your nose.

(副鼻腔を叩きながら) 痛みますか. □ Does it hurt?

頭を後ろに傾けて下さい. □ Please lean your head backward.

鼻で息をして下さい. □ Breathe through your nose.

目を閉じて下さい.
―片方の鼻を押さえて下さい.
―何かにおいがしますか.
―何のにおいですか.
―このにおいは…ですか.
 1. ミント
 2. 香水
 3. タバコ

□ Please close your eyes.
— Pinch one side of your nose.
— Do you smell something?
— What do you smell?
— Does this smell like...
 1. mint?
 2. perfume?
 3. tobacco?

---

### ▶ 咽喉

入れ歯をしていたらはずして下さい. □ If you wear dentures, please remove them.

口の中を診察しましょう. □ I'm going to [Let me] examine the inside of your mouth.

まず舌を見せて下さい. □ Let me see your tongue first.

口を (もっと) 大きく開けて下さい.
―「アー」と言って下さい.

□ Please open your mouth wider.
— Say "ah."

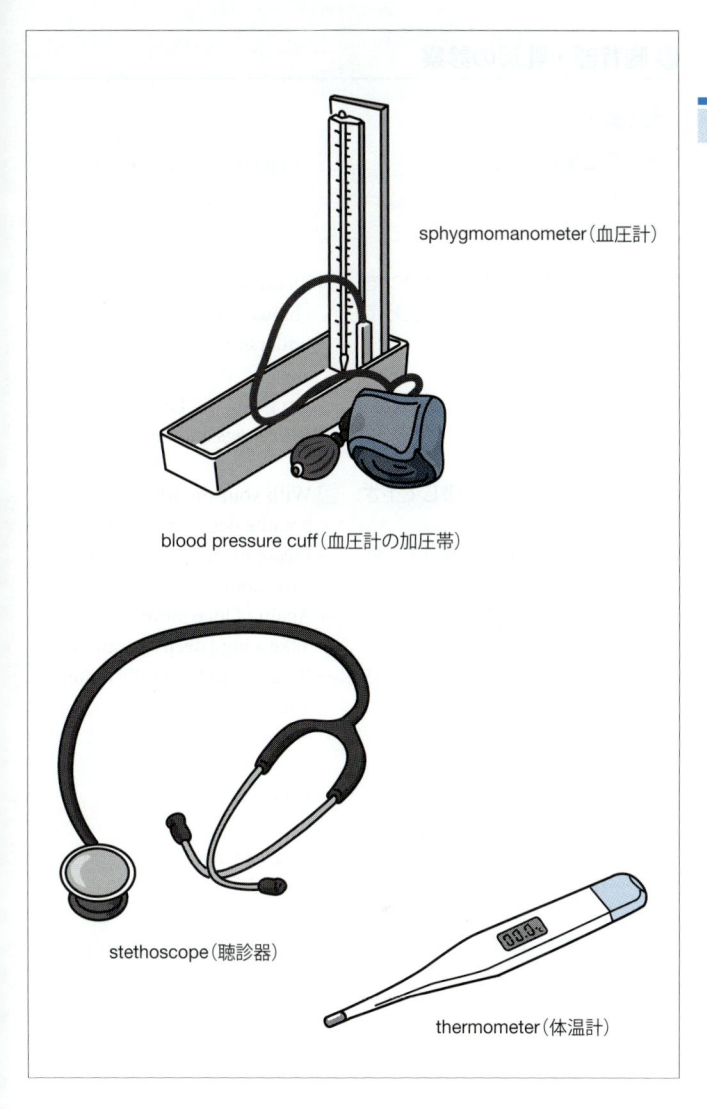

- sphygmomanometer（血圧計）
- blood pressure cuff（血圧計の加圧帯）
- stethoscope（聴診器）
- thermometer（体温計）

## 胸背部・乳房の診察

### 胸背部

| | |
|---|---|
| …を診察しましょう.<br>　1. 肺<br>　2. 心臓 | ☐ I'm going to [Let me] examine...<br>　1. your lungs.<br>　2. your heart. |
| ワイシャツ〔ブラウス〕のボタンをはずして下着のシャツを引き上げて下さい. | ☐ Please unbutton your shirt [blouse] and pull up your undershirt. |
| 胸の音を聴きましょう. | ☐ I'm going to [Let me] listen to your lungs and heart. |
| 口を開けてゆっくり深呼吸して下さい.<br>―息を吸って,吐いて,吸って,吐いて.<br>―もう一度やって下さい.<br>―大きく息を吸って下さい.<br>―できるだけ勢いよく吐いて下さい.<br>―けっこうです.楽にして下さい. | ☐ With your mouth open, please breathe deeply and slowly.<br>― Please breathe in, breathe out, ...in, ...out.<br>― Again [Once more].<br>― Take a big [deep] breath in.<br>― Breathe out forcefully as hard and fast as you can.<br>― Good [OK], please relax. |
| 背中を診ましょう. | ☐ Let me see your back. |
| 後ろを向いて下さい.<br>―「イー」と言ってみて下さい. | ☐ Please turn around.<br>― Say "e." |
| 背中を押します〔叩きます〕. | ☐ I'm going to press〔tap〕your back. |
| ―ここを押す〔叩く〕と痛みますか. | ― Does it hurt when I press〔tap〕here? |
| ―痛いところがあったら言って下さい. | ― Let me know if you have any pain. |

### 乳房

| | |
|---|---|
| 乳房の診察をしましょう． | ☐ I'm going to [Let me] examine your breasts. |
| 服は上半身脱いで下さい． | ☐ Please take off your clothes from the waist up. |
| 手を横にして真っ直ぐに座って下さい． | ☐ Please sit up with your hands at your side. |
| —痛む所〔しこり〕を指でさして下さい． | — Please point to where the pain is 〔where you have the lump〕. |
| —腕を前に出して下さい． | — Hold your arms out straight. |
| —手をあげて頭の上に載せて下さい． | — Lift up your hands and put them on your head. |
| —手を降ろして下さい． | — Lower your hands. |
| —体を前かがみにして下さい． | — Lean forward. |
| —手〔腕〕をこんなふうにあげて下さい． | — Put your hands 〔arms〕 up like this. |
| 診察台の上に，仰向けに寝て下さい． | ☐ Please lie down on your back on the examination table. |
| —乳房を触診します． | — I'm going to palpate your breasts. |
| —乳頭をつまんで，分泌物がないかチェックします． | — I'm going to pinch [squeeze] your nipple(s) to make sure there's no discharge coming out of it 〔them〕. |
| 腋窩〔脇の下〕を触診しましょう． | ☐ I'm going to [Let me] palpate your armpit(s). |
| —軽く両腕をあげて下さい． | — Please put up both your arms gently. |
| —降ろしてけっこうですよ． | — Now, you can lower them. |

## 🢂 腹部（消化器・鼠径）の診察

### 消化器

お腹を診察〔触診〕しましょう．
- I'm going to [Let me] examine 〔palpate〕your abdomen.

診察台の上に，仰向けに寝て下さい．
- Please lie down on your back on the examination table.

ズボン〔スカート〕を下げて，お腹を見せて下さい．
- Please lower your pants〔skirt〕and show me your abdomen.

両膝を立てて，お腹の力を抜いて下さい．
- Please pull [bring] your knees up, and relax your abdomen.

痛いところやしこりがあったら言って下さい．
—指でさして教えて下さい．
—ここを押すと痛みますか．
—手を急に離すと痛みますか．
- Let me know if you have any pain or lump.
— Please point to the place.
— Does it hurt when I press here?
— Does it hurt when I release my hand suddenly?

—大きく息を吸って下さい．
—お腹をふくらませて下さい．
—お腹をひっこめて下さい．
— Take a big breath in.
— Push out [Inflate] your stomach.
— Suck in your stomach.

今度は…に寝て下さい．
　1．右向き
　2．左向き
- Please lie on your...
  1. right side.
  2. left side.

### 鼠径

鼠径部を触診しましょう.

☐ I'm going to [Let me] palpate the groin.★

痛みがあれば教えて下さい.

☐ Let me know if you have any pain.

## ● 直腸診・生殖器の診察

### 直腸診

直腸診をしましょう.

☐ I'm going to [Let me] examine your rectum.

下着を脱いで下さい.

☐ Please remove your underwear.

左向きに寝て下さい.
—膝を曲げて胸のほうにつけて下さい.

☐ Please lie on your left side.
— Bend your knees and bring them toward your chest.

それでは,肛門に指を入れます.

—体の力を抜いて下さい.
—口で息をして,楽にしていて下さい.
—ここを押すと痛みますか.

☐ Now, I'm going to insert my finger into the anus.
— Relax your muscles.
— Breathe through your mouth and relax.
— Does it hurt when I press here?

けっこうです.楽にして下さい.

☐ Good [OK], please relax.

---

★ the inguinal region ともいう.

### 生殖器

| | |
|---|---|
| 骨盤〔腟,（子宮）頸部,子宮〕の診察をしましょう. | ☐ I'm going to [Let me] do a pelvic exam 〔examine your vagina, cervix and uterus〕. |
| 下着を脱いで下さい. | ☐ Please remove your underwear. |
| 診察台にあがって下さい. | ☐ Please go up onto the examination table. |
| ―診察台が動きます. | ― The table will move you. |
| ―足をこのあぶみに入れて下さい. | ― Put your feet into these stirrups. |
| ―台の端にもっと体をずらして下さい. | ― Pull yourself all the way down to the end of the table. |
| ―足をもう少し開いて下さい. | ― Open your legs a little more. |
| それでは内診します. | ☐ Now, I'm doing the (gynecologic) exam. |
| ―体の力を抜いて下さい. | ― Relax your muscles. |
| ―口で息をして,楽にしていて下さい. | ― Breathe through your mouth and relax. |
| ―ここを押すと痛みますか. | ― Does it hurt when I press here? |
| ―次に,器具を入れますよ.少し冷たいかもしれません. | ― Next, I'm inserting an instrument. It may be a little cold. |
| ―けっこうです.楽にして下さい. | ― Good [OK], please relax. |
| 後で少し出血するかもしれませんが,心配はありません. | ☐ You may notice slight bleeding later, but please don't worry. |

## ● 骨格（上肢・下肢・脊柱）の診察

### 上肢

右腕〔左腕〕をあげて下さい．
―もっとあげて下さい．
―今度は，反対のほうをあげて下さい．
―手や腕で動かしにくいところがあったら言って下さい．

- Raise your right 〔left〕 arm.
— Raise it more.
— Now, the other, please.
— Let me know if you have any difficulty moving your hands or arms.

力を抜いて下さい．私が右腕〔左腕〕を動かしてみましょう．
―痛いところがあったら言って下さい．

- Please relax and let me move your right 〔left〕 arm.
— Let me know if you have any pain.

ここを押すと痛みますか．

- Does it hurt when I press here?

### 下肢

足を見せて下さい．

- Let me look at your leg(s).

靴下〔ストッキング〕を脱いで下さい．

- Please take off your socks 〔stockings〕.

診察台の上に寝て下さい．

―仰向けに．
―うつ伏せ［腹ばい］に．

- Please lie down on the examination table.
— Lie on your back.
— Lie on your stomach.

右足〔左足〕をあげて下さい．
―もっとあげて下さい．
―今度は，反対のほうをあげて下さい．
―動かしにくいところがあったら言って下さい．

- Raise your right 〔left〕 leg.
— Raise it more.
— Now, the other, please.
— Let me know if you have any difficulty moving your legs.

| | |
|---|---|
| 力を抜いて下さい．私が右足〔左足〕を動かしてみましょう． | ☐ Please relax and let me move your right 〔left〕 leg. |
| ―痛いところがあったら言って下さい． | ― Let me know if you have any pain. |
| ここを押すと痛みますか． | ☐ Does it hurt when I press here? |

### 脊柱

| | |
|---|---|
| 背中を診ましょう． | ☐ I'm going to 〔Let me〕 look at your back. |
| 後ろを向いて下さい． | ☐ Please turn around. |
| 身をかがめて下さい． | ☐ Please bend forward at the waist. |
| 体を左右に曲げて下さい． | ☐ Please bend from side to side. |
| 背骨を叩きますね． | ☐ Let me tap your spinal column. |
| 痛いところがあったら言って下さい． | ☐ Let me know if you have any pain. |

## 🔵 神経の診察

> 意識状態・大脳高次機能

| | |
|---|---|
| お名前をお聞かせ下さい. | ☐ What's your name? |
| | ☐ May I have your name? |
| —何歳ですか. | — How old are you? |
| —何年生まれですか. | — When were you born? |
| | |
| いまどこにいますか. | ☐ Where are you now? |
| —なぜここにいるのですか. | — Why are you here? |
| —私はだれですか. | — Who am I? |
| —（付き添いの人を指して）この人は誰ですか. | — Who is he〔she〕? |
| | |
| 今日は何日ですか. | ☐ What day is it today? |
| —今月は何月ですか. | — What month is this? |
| —今年は何年ですか. | — What year is this? |
| | |
| 100 引く 7 はいくつになりますか. | ☐ If you take seven from one hundred, how much do you get? |
| —それから 7 を引き続けると… | — If you take seven from that number and keep going ＿＿＿? |
| | |
| 朝食に何を食べましたか. | ☐ What did you eat for breakfast? |

> 脳神経

### ▶ 嗅神経（I）

☞「鼻」（220 ページ）.

### ▶ 視神経（II），動眼神経（III），滑車神経（IV），外転神経（VI）

☞「眼」（217 ページ）.

### ▶ 三叉神経（V）

| | |
|---|---|
| 顔面〔額／頬／あご〕を触ります． | ☐ I'm going to [Let me] brush your face〔forehead/upper cheeks/jaw〕. |
| 感じ方は左右で同じですか． | ☐ Does it feel the same in both sides? |
| 歯を食いしばってください． | ☐ Please clench your teeth. |

### ▶ 顔面神経（VII）

| | |
|---|---|
| 両目をぎゅっとつぶって下さい． | ☐ Please close both your eyes tightly. |
| 眉を上げて下さい． | ☐ Raise your eyebrows. |
| 口をぎゅっとつぐんで下さい． | ☐ Please squeeze your mouth shut. |
| 「イー」と言って下さい． | ☐ Say "e." |
| 笑って下さい． | ☐ Smile. |

### ▶ 前庭蝸牛神経（VIII）

☞「耳」（219ページ）．

### ▶ 舌咽神経（IX），迷走神経（X）

| | |
|---|---|
| 口を開けて下さい． | ☐ Please open your mouth. |
| 「アー」と言って下さい． | ☐ Say "ah." |

### ▶ 副神経（XI）

肩をすくめて下さい．

☐ Please shrug your shoulders.

### ▶ 舌下神経（XII）

舌を突き出して下さい．

☐ Please stick out your tongue.

舌を左右に〔端から端へ〕動かして下さい．

☐ Move your tongue from left to right 〔from side to side〕.

舌を上にあげて下さい．

☐ Lift up your tongue.

## 運動機能

### ▶ 上肢

利き手はどちらですか．
―右利きですか，左利きですか．

☐ Which is your dominant hand?
― Are you right-handed or left-handed?

手〔手のひら／手の甲〕を見せて下さい．

☐ Let me look at your hand(s) 〔your palm(s)/the back of your hand(s)〕.

私の指を握って下さい．
―できるだけ強くぎゅっと握って下さい．
―もっと強く．

☐ Please grasp my finger(s).
― Squeeze it 〔them〕 as hard as you can.
― Harder, please.

両腕を真っ直ぐ前に伸ばして，そのままにしていて下さい．
―手のひらを上に向けて下さい．

―両腕はそのままで両目を閉じて下さい．
―はい，けっこうです．

☐ Hold both your arms out straight and keep still.
― Turn your palms up.
Hold both arms out, palms up.
― Keep both your arms still and close your eyes.
― Fine.

### ▶ 下肢

診察台の上に仰向けに〔腹ばいに〕寝て下さい．
- Please lie down on your back 〔stomach〕 on the examination table.

膝を曲げて両足を上げて下さい．
- Please bend your knees and raise both your legs.

—そのままで両目を閉じて下さい．
— Keep your legs still and close your eyes.

—はい，楽にして下さい．
— Now, please relax.

腱反射を見ます．
- Let me check your tendon reflexes.

—手足の力を抜いて下さい．
— Please relax your arms and legs.

### 感覚機能

皮膚をピン〔刷毛〕で触ります．
- I'm going to [Let me] touch you with a pin〔brush〕.

—左右で同じですか．
— Does it feel the same in both sides [in right and left]?

音叉をあてます．
- I'm going to place this tuning fork on you.

—これが振動しなくなったら教えて下さい．
— Please tell me when you cannot feel the "buzzing" feeling.

目を閉じて下さい．
- Please close your eyes.

—足のどの指を触っていますか．
— Which toe am I touching?

### 小脳機能

真っ直ぐ前を見て下さい．
- Please look straight ahead.

—自分の指で私の指に触ってから，ご自分の鼻に触って下さい．
— Touch my finger with your finger and then touch your nose.

—くり返して下さい．
— Do it again.

—もっと速くやって下さい．
— Do it faster.

| | |
|---|---|
| 両手をこのように動かして下さい． | ☐ Please move your hands like this. |
| 立って下さい．<br>―足はバランスがとりやすいように軽く開いてけっこうですよ． | ☐ Please stand up.<br>― You can stand with your feet slightly apart so that you can balance yourself. |
| 目を閉じて下さい．<br>―目を閉じたままにして下さい．<br>―じっとしていて下さい． | ☐ Please close your eyes.<br>― Keep them shut.<br>― Stand still. |
| 目を開けて下さい．<br>―足を揃えて立って下さい． | ☐ Please open your eyes.<br>― Stand up with your feet together. |
| 真っ直ぐ歩いて下さい．<br>―普通に歩いて下さい．<br>―早足で歩いて下さい．<br>―向きを変えて下さい． | ☐ Walk straight ahead.<br>― Walk as you usually do.<br>― Walk faster [at a quicker pace].<br>― Turn around. |
| このように歩いて下さい． | ☐ Please walk like this. |

### 髄膜刺激症状

| | |
|---|---|
| 診察台の上に仰向けに寝て下さい． | ☐ Please lie down on your back on the examination table. |
| 私が頭を動かしますので，首の力を抜いていて下さい．<br>―両足を真っ直ぐに伸ばして下さい．<br>―足を持ち上げると頭痛がひどくなりますか． | ☐ Let me move your head. Please relax your neck.<br>― Straighten out both your legs.<br>― Does your headache get worse when you raise your legs? |

chapter 4 身体の診察

## 診察の終了

これで終わりました．
- [ ] Now, we're finished.
- [ ] It's over now.
- [ ] That's all.

ありがとうございました．
- [ ] Thank you.

起き上がっていいですよ．
- [ ] You can [may] get up now.

服を着てもいいですよ．
- [ ] You can [may] get dressed now.

着終わってからお話しましょう．
- [ ] I'll talk with you when you are finished.

---

**名句・ことわざ**

情けは他人(ひと)の為ならず

〔英訳〕Charity [Affection] is not merely for others' sake.

この種のことわざ・名言は世界共通で数多くある．例えば，英語では "Do good; you do it for yourself."（他人に善行を施せ．それは自分ためになるのだから）や "One good turn deserves another."（他人に善行を施せば善行で報いられる）などという．

## 用語・表現ファイル

### 病院会話のヒント　その1　診察中に安心感を与える表現

| | |
|---|---|
| けっこうです. | OK [All right].<br>Fine.<br>Good.<br>Very good [Great].<br>Terrific. |
| 楽にして[体の力を抜いて]下さい. | Please relax.<br>Relax your muscles. |
| 心配しないで下さい. | Don't be afraid.<br>Don't worry. |
| 大丈夫ですか. | Are you OK?<br>Are you comfortable? |
| 痛くはありませんよ. | This won't hurt. |
| 痛みますか. | Does this hurt?<br>Do you feel the pain? |
| これは少し辛いかもしれません. | I'm sorry if this makes you a little uncomfortable. |
| ―少し痛いかもしれません. | This may hurt a little. |
| ―少し冷たいかもしれません. | This may feel a little cold. |
| ―少し押される感じがするかもしれません. | You may feel a little pressure. |
| 痛かったら[気分が悪かったら]言って下さい. | Let me know if it hurts [if you feel sick]. |
| あとちょっとで終わります. | It'll only take a moment longer.<br>It'll be over in a moment. |
| 大丈夫ですよ. | It'll be all right. |

## 車内放送のヒント その1 旅客中に受答える大きな要集

はい、そうです。                     OK. / All right. /
                                    Fine. /
                                    Good. /
                                    Very good. / Great. /
                                    Exactly.

少々お待ちください。ただ今、で確か…    Wait a moment. / Please wait. /
                                    Relax for a minutes.

恐れ入りますが…                      Don't be afraid. /
                                    Don't worry.

大丈夫ですか。                       Are you OK? /
                                    Yes, it could a ended?

お気を悪くなさらないで…              Has went bear…

よろしいですか。                     Does this arrive /
                                    Do you see the right?

ご迷惑をおかけして申し訳ござ          I'm sorry if this makes you are
いません。                            but it can no comfortable. /
ただ今お直しいたします。              This may take a time. /
少々寒くなるかと思いますが、         The place feel a little cold
ご了承ください。                      you may feel a little uncomfort-
                                    able.

お分かりいただけましたでしょうか。    I'm not know if they help by be
まだですか。                         feel help.

ちょっとしっかりしてですか。         It's only take a moment. I must
                                    be back in a moment.

                                    All readings.

chapter 5

# 診察が終わって

## Closing the Consultation

検査の説明 238
診断の説明 245
治療の説明 254
専門医への紹介 260
次回の診察予約 263

# 検査の説明

☞「検査」(269 ページ).

## ● 検査の必要がないとき

今すぐに検査を行う必要はありません.
☐ You don't need to have any test now.

症状が改善しなければ, 精密検査の予定をたてましょう.
☐ If your symptoms don't improve, we need to set up a schedule for a thorough examination.

## ● 検査が必要なとき

…が必要です.
1. 血液検査
2. 尿検査
3. 胸部 X 線
4. 心電図

☐ You need to have...
1. a blood test.
2. a urine test.
3. a chest X-ray.
4. an ECG〔electrocardiogram〕.

正確に診断するために, いくつかの検査が必要です.
☐ You need some tests for an accurate diagnosis.

胃潰瘍〔狭心症／肺がん〕の疑いがあります.
―確かめるために検査をしましょう.
―他の可能性を除外するために検査をしましょう.

☐ I suspect you have a stomach ulcer〔angina/lung cancer〕.
― We need to run some tests to be certain.
― I'd like to rule out other possibilities. So let us do〔run〕some tests.

この検査は痛みがありません.
☐ This test is painless.

この検査をするには 1 泊入院が必要です.
☐ This test requires an overnight stay in the hospital.

検査について何か質問がありますか.
☐ Do you have any questions about the test?

### 当日検査

今日は胸部 X 線をとりましょう．
☐ Today, we'd like to take a chest X-ray.

この書類を持ってレントゲン室〔心電図室／採血室〕へ行って下さい．
☐ Please take this form with you to the X-ray room 〔the ECG room/the blood collection room〕.

検査室は 1 階の廊下の突き当たりにあります．
☐ The exam room is at the end of the hallway on the first floor.

スタッフが検査室までご案内します．
☐ One of our staff is taking you there.

ご気分が悪い〔歩くのが辛い〕ようでしたら車椅子をご使用になって下さい．
☐ Please use a wheelchair if you feel sick 〔if you have difficulty walking〕.

検査が終わったら結果を持ってこちらへ戻って来て下さい．
☐ When the tests are finished, please get the results and come back here.

戻られたらスタッフに声をかけて下さい．
☐ Let one of our staff know when you are back.

結果は次回の診察のときにお話します．
☐ I'll explain the results of today's test(s) at the time of your next visit.

(インフルエンザや溶連菌など，迅速診断をするときに)
鼻〔のど〕に綿棒を入れますよ．
☐ I'm going to [Let me] insert [put in] a Q-tip into your nostril 〔throat〕.

―少しこそばゆいかもしれませんが，痛くはありませんよ．
― This may tickle a little, but it's not painful.

―すぐに結果がわかります．
― We'll get the result immediately [rapidly].

| | |
|---|---|
| 検査が終わったらもう一度こちらへ戻って来て，受付で次回の予約をして下さい．それからお帰りになってけっこうですよ． | ☐ After the tests are finished, please come back here and make an appointment for your next visit at the reception desk. Then, you can go home. |

### 予約検査

| | |
|---|---|
| 来週，腹部超音波と胃内視鏡の検査をします． | ☐ We're going to do an abdominal ultrasound and an upper (gastrointestinal) endoscopy next week. |
| お帰りの際，この用紙を受付のクラーク〔看護師〕にお渡し下さい．検査について書いておきました． | ☐ On your way out, please give this form to the clerk 〔nurse〕 at the reception desk. I've written you up for the tests. |
| 受付で予約して帰って下さい． | ☐ Please make an appointment at the reception desk before you go home. |
| クラーク〔看護師〕が同じ日に予約を入れてくれるでしょう． | ☐ The clerk 〔nurse〕 will schedule them for the same day. |
| 検査は毎週火曜日の午前に行っています． | ☐ We do [run] the tests every Tuesday morning. |
| 予約のご希望日はありますか． | ☐ What days are best for you?<br>☐ What day do you prefer? |
| 5月12日，月曜日，10時に予約を入れましたので，30分前までに来院して下さい． | ☐ I scheduled your tests for Monday, May 12th at 10:00. Please come to the hospital 30 minutes before the scheduled appointment. |
| 予約カードをお渡しします． | ☐ Here's your appointment card. |

| 検査上の注意事項が書いてありますので，お読み下さい． | ☐ Please read the instructions on the appointment card. |
|---|---|
| よろしいですか．ほかに何かありますか． | ☐ OK? Anything else? |

chapter 5 診察が終わって

---

### 名句・ことわざ

**To study the phenomena of disease without books is to sail an uncharted sea, while to study books without patients is not to go to sea at all.**

書物を読まずに疾病の現象を学ぶのは海図を持たずに航海するに等しい．患者を診ずに書物のみで学ぶのはまったく航海に出ないに等しい

カナダの医師オスラー（William Osler, 1849-1919, *Aequanimitas*）の名言．オスラーは "The good physician treats the disease ; the great physician treats the patient who has the disease."（良い医師は病気を治し，優れた医師は病む患者を治す）とも言って，ベッドサイドで患者を診ることがいかに大切であるかを説いている．

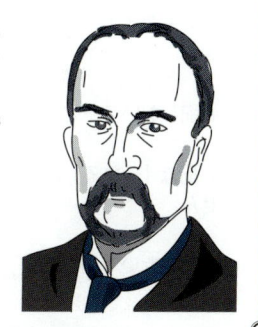

## 用語・表現ファイル

### 病院会話のヒント　その2　確認，励まし，慰め，慰労

**1. 確認**

| | |
|---|---|
| 大丈夫ですか. | Are you all right?<br>Are you OK? |
| よろしいですか. | (Is everything) all right? /OK? |
| こんなふうですか. | Like this? |
| …なのですね. | Is it correct that____? |
| 私の言うことがわかりますか. | Do you understand me [what I've just said]? |
| 私の指示がわかりましたか. | Did you understand my instructions? |
| 私の説明ではっきりしますか. | Is my explanation clear? |
| 私の言ったことを繰り返して下さい. | Can you repeat what I've just said? |
| ご質問がありますか. | (Do you have) any questions? |

**2. 励まし**

| | |
|---|---|
| 大丈夫ですよ. | You'll [It'll] be all right.<br>You're going to be just fine. |
| 心配しないで下さい. | Please don't worry. |
| 心配な[恐れる]ことはありません. | There's nothing to be afraid of. |
| あわてないで下さい. | Please don't panic. |

## 用語・表現ファイル（つづき）

| | |
|---|---|
| しばらくおそばについています． | I'll just sit with you for a while.<br>I'll be here for you for a while. |
| どうぞ楽にしていて下さい． | Please relax. |
| 気をお楽に． | Take it easy. |
| 2，3分で済みますから． | It'll be over in a few minutes. |
| あともう少しですよ． | Just a little longer. |
| もう少しで終わります． | You're almost finished. |
| 順調です［調子はいいですよ］． | You're doing fine. |
| この調子で続けて． | Keep it up. |
| その調子で頑張って． | Keep up the good work. |
| すぐに気分がよくなりますよ． | You'll feel better soon. |
| あきらめないで下さい． | Don't give up. |

### 3. 慰め

| | |
|---|---|
| それはお気の毒に． | That's too bad. |
| お気の毒に思います． | I'm sorry.<br>I'm sad for you. |
| お辛い〔辛かった〕でしょう． | This must be〔have been〕hard for you. |
| とても大変だったのですね． | You had a hard time, didn't you? |
| 何か私にできることはありますか． | What can I do for you? |

## 用語・表現ファイル（つづき）

| | |
|---|---|
| おそばにいてお話をうかがいましょう． | I'm here and I want to listen. |
| 明日またお話しましょう． | I'll talk with you tomorrow. |
| (亡くなった患者さんの家族に) お母さまは心停止されました，残念です．できるだけのことをしたのですが，力が及びませんでした． | Your mother went into cardiac arrest. I'm sorry. We did everything we could, but we weren't able to revive her. |

### 4. 慰労

| | |
|---|---|
| よく頑張りましたね． | Well done! |
| さあ，終わりましたよ．よく頑張りましたね． | It's all over. You did very well. |
| よかったですね． | Good.<br>Great. |
| よくやりましたね． | (You did a) good job. |
| ご協力ありがとうございました． | Thank you for your cooperation. |

# 診断の説明

## ● 検査結果の説明

検査結果をご説明しましょう．
- [ ] Let me explain the results of the test(s).

検査の結果，症状〔痛み〕の原因がわかりました．
- [ ] The tests show what's causing your symptom〔pain〕.

血液検査では…
1. すべてが正常です．
2. 少し貧血があります．
3. 血糖〔コレステロール／尿酸〕の数値が正常値を越えています．

- [ ] Your blood test shows that...
    1. everything is normal.
    2. you have a slight anemia.
    3. your blood sugar〔cholesterol/uric acid〕level is above normal〔high〕.

検査から判断すると…
1. 心配なところはありません．
2. 胃炎のようです．

- [ ] Judging from the tests,...
    1. you have nothing to worry about.
    2. you seem to have gastritis.

（画像を見せながら）これはあなたの脳〔胸部／腹部〕のCT〔X線〕です．
- [ ] Here're the CT〔X-ray〕images of your brain〔chest/abdomen〕.

出血している様子はありません．
- [ ] There's no sign of bleeding.

ここに異常陰影があります．
- [ ] There's an abnormal shadow here〔in this area〕.

ここを見て下さい．骨折しています．
- [ ] Here, the bone is broken.

胆嚢内に石があるようです．
- [ ] I suspect you have stones in your gallbladder.

大腸内視鏡の所見では，大腸にレーズンほどのポリープが2つあります．
- [ ] According to your colonoscopy, you have two polyps, about the size of raisins, in your lower bowel.

## ➔ 診断内容

### 異常がないとき

| | |
|---|---|
| ご心配ないでしょう. | ☐ I don't think there's anything to worry about. |
| (診察したところ)悪いところはありません. | ☐ I can't find [see] anything wrong (on my exam). |
| たいしたことはありません. | ☐ It is nothing serious. |
| …以外,特に大きな問題はありません. | ☐ I can't see anything seriously wrong here other than some＿＿＿. |
| 健康な人でもありうる症状ですよ. | ☐ Healthy people also have similar symptoms. |
| 様子をみることにしましょう. | ☐ We'll see what happens. |
| お仕事〔日常生活〕に差し支えなければ,しばらく様子をみましょう. | ☐ If you are physically fit for ordinary work〔everyday life〕, let's watch what develops for the time being. |

### 一般的な説明

グリーンさん,…の疑いがあります.

1. 風邪
2. 白内障
3. 胃潰瘍
4. 良性腫瘍
5. 骨折

☐ Mr. 〔Mrs./Ms./Miss〕Green, you seem to have...
1. a common cold.
2. a cataract.
3. a stomach ulcer.
4. a benign tumor.
5. a fracture.

血圧に問題があります.
☐ You have a problem with your blood pressure.

—やや高めです.上が150で,下が95です.
— Your blood pressure is a little high. It's 150 over 95.

| | |
|---|---|
| —めまいは急な血圧低下によるものでしょう. | — Your dizziness is probably caused by a sudden drop in a blood pressure. |
| 症状から見て片頭痛の疑いがあります. | ☐ Your symptoms seem to come from migraine.<br>☐ Migraine is a likely explanation for your symptoms. |
| 風邪が原因で気管支炎を起こしています. | ☐ The cold has developed into bronchitis. |
| 胃の痛みはストレスからくるものでしょう. | ☐ Well, I think your stomachache could be due to a great deal of stress. |
| 2週間以内にもう一度来て下さい.よくなっているかどうかをみましょう. | ☐ I'd like you to come back in two weeks, and we'll see if you are better. |
| その間,薬を飲んで下さい. | ☐ In the meantime, I'd like you to take a medication. |
| 痛みの原因はまだわかりません. | ☐ We don't know yet what is causing your pain. |
| さらに精密検査を行って調べましょう. | ☐ We need some more detailed tests for the diagnosis. |

### 深刻な説明

☞「悪い知らせの伝え方」(249ページ).

| | |
|---|---|
| 今日一緒に話を聞いてもらいたい人が来ていますか. | ☐ Is there anyone with you today whom you'd like to talk with us? |
| ご主人〔奥様／パートナー〕とご一緒がよければ,別の機会に話しましょうか. | ☐ Shall we have this discussion another time when your husband〔wife/partner〕can join us? |

| | |
|---|---|
| それでは，病気〔検査結果〕について詳しくお話しましょう．よろしいですか． | ☐ Now, I'd like to discuss the details of your disease〔test results〕with you. Would that be all right? |
| 残念ですが，悪いお知らせです． | ☐ I'm sorry but I have some bad news for you. |
| 生検や他の検査結果で胃がんの所見が見られます． | ☐ I'm sorry but your biopsy and other test results have shown signs of stomach cancer. |
| —残念ながら，悪性です． | — Unfortunately, it's malignant. |
| お母さんは心不全の状態です．<br>—お気の毒ですが，重症です． | ☐ Your mother has heart failure.<br>— I'm sorry but she is very sick〔critically ill〕. |

### 名句・ことわざ

医は生涯の業にて，とても上手名人には至らざるものと見ゆ．
己れ上手と思わば，はや下手になるの兆としるべし．

〔英訳〕Medicine is a profession which one needs to pursue throughout one's life, so it's next to impossible to master the skill. The pride of a physician who commends himself as a skillful master is a sign of becoming less skillful.

『解体新書』の翻訳で著名な江戸時代の医者・蘭学者 杉田玄白（1733-1817，『形影夜話』）の名言．英語では "Pride goes before a fall. / Pride must have a fall."（慢心はいずれ滅びる）ということわざがある．

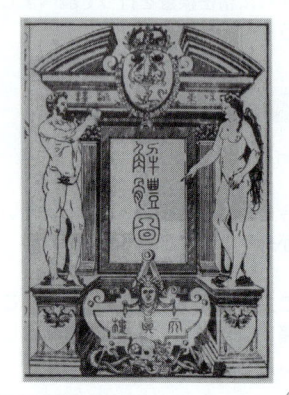

### コラム

## 悪い知らせの伝え方

　悪い知らせをどう伝えるかは，通常の診療や看護を行うときの会話と異なり，特別なコミュニケーション技術を必要とする．悪い知らせは，プライバシーや患者さんの気持ちを十分に配慮して，時と場所を選んで慎重に伝えねばならない．外国人の患者さんは一人ひとり文化背景・個性・知識レベルが異なっているし，英語が母語であるとは限らない．できれば英語のわかる第三者（家族，通訳，医療ソーシャルワーカーなど）に同席してもらうとよいだろう．言葉で伝えると同時に，患者さんとのアイコンタクトなど非言語の情報にも注意を払うことが大切である．

　ここでは肺がんの患者さんの例をあげるので参考にしていただきたい．

☞「死の伝え方」（360 ページ）．

### Step 1　本題に入る前に相手の気持ちや状態を確認する

|  |  |
|---|---|
| クロスさん，こんにちは．<br>―お待たせしました．<br>―どうぞおかけ下さい． | ☐ Hello, Mr. Cross.<br>― I'm sorry to have kept you waiting.<br>― Please sit down. |
| 医師の斎藤と看護師の森が同席してよろしいでしょうか． | ☐ Is it all right if Dr. Saito and Nurse Mori sit with me? |
| ご気分はいかがですか．<br>―夜はよく眠れますか．<br>―食欲はありますか．<br>―この部屋は少し寒く〔暑く〕ありませんか． | ☐ How are you feeling now? ★1<br>― Can you sleep well at night?<br>― Are you eating all right?<br>― Isn't it a little chilly 〔hot〕 in here? |
| あなたの病状についてかかりつけ医の林先生から何か聞いていますか． | ☐ What has Dr. Hayashi, your regular doctor, told you about your condition? ★2 |

---

★1 雑談（small talk）から入って患者さんの緊張を解きほぐし，精神状態や英語力を確かめる．
★2 患者さんがどの程度の情報をもっているかを確認する．

### コラム（つづき）

| | |
|---|---|
| —あなたはご自分の病状をどう理解していますか. | — What do you understand [know] about your condition? |

**Step 2　悪い情報を伝える**

| | |
|---|---|
| 今日はこれまでの検査結果についてお話させていただきます. | ☐ Now, let me talk about what the test results showed. |
| あなたの病状とこの先の方針についてお話したいのですが. | ☐ I'd like to talk with you about your condition and your next steps. |
| —話を一緒に聞いてもらいたい人がいますか. | — Is there anyone who you'd like to talk with? |
| —ご家族か友人で話し合いに同席してもらいたい人がいますか. | — Is there any family member or friend you would like to have with you for this discussion? |
| 実は，よくないお知らせがあるのです. | ☐ I'm afraid I have some bad news.★3 |
| 残念ですが，右肺に悪性腫瘍が見つかりました. | ☐ I'm sorry to have to tell you this, but you have a malignant tumor in the right lung. |
| 大変残念なのですが，がんが再発しています. | ☐ Unfortunately, [I'm so sorry to say but] your cancer has returned.★4 |
| 私の話がおわかりになりますか. | ☐ Do you understand what I'm telling you? |

---

★3 前置きとして，よくない知らせであることを伝える.
★4 資料（写真・データなど）を見せたり図を描いたりするなどして，病状・部位・進行度・転移の有無を説明する．その他「残念ながら」という気持ちを示す表現としては，"I'm sorry, but ....", "I'm sorry to tell you that ....", "I'm afraid that ....", "Unfortunately, ... (遺憾なのですが)", "It's hard [difficult] for me to tell you this, but ....(申し上げにくいのですが)", "To be frank with you ....(率直に申し上げると)", "As we expected, ....(予想されたように)" など.

### コラム（つづき）

| | |
|---|---|
| ご質問があればいつでも訊いて下さい. | ☐ If you have any questions, please ask [interrupt] me anytime.★5 |

#### Step 3　患者さんの気持ちに添って共感を示す★6

| | |
|---|---|
| さぞ, お辛いでしょう. | ☐ This must be terrible [awful] for you. |
| この知らせで力を落とされたことと思います. | ☐ I can see that this news is upsetting for you. |
| さぞショックなことと思います. | ☐ I understand this must be a shock for you. |
| あなたと同じ立場の人であれば誰でもこの知らせを聞くのは辛いことでしょう. | ☐ People in your situation find this very difficult to hear. |

#### Step 4　今後の治療について話す

| | |
|---|---|
| 慎重に考えて治療方針を決めましょう. | ☐ Let's think carefully and decide on your treatment plan.★7 |
| この病気の治療としては, いくつか選択肢があります. 例えば, …. | ☐ There are several treatment options for this disease, such as＿＿. |
| —まず腫瘍のサイズを小さくする〔痛みを和らげる〕方法を考えましょう. | — First, we'll try to find a way to shrink the tumor [give you some relief from pain]. |

---

★5 患者さんは医師の話をさえぎって質問しにくい. 一方的な説明にならないように, 患者さんの表情をみながら質問を受ける.

★6 共感を示す表現には注意が必要. 例えば, 日本語では「お気持ちお察しいたします」という表現をよく用いるが, 英語で "I know how you feel." と言われると, 「あなたに私の気持ちがわかるはずがない」と反発する患者さんがいるかもしれない. 英米の医師や看護師はこの表現を使わないようにとの指導を受けるという.

★7 患者さんと一緒に病気に立ち向かうという姿勢を示す.

### コラム（つづき）

| | |
|---|---|
| ―詳細については後でがんの専門医がご説明いたします． | ― We'll have a cancer specialist see you later and he will explain everything for you in detail. |
| ―長くかかるかもしれませんが，ご一緒に治療に取り組んでいきましょう． | ― This is going to be a long course, but I'd like to know that we'll be working with you through it. |

セカンドオピニオンを希望される場合には，遠慮なくおっしゃって下さい．

☐ If you'd like to get a second opinion, please don't hesitate to let me know.

### Step 5　延命治療についての意思を確認する

もし不治あるいは末期の病状になった場合，延命治療は希望されますか．例えば，…

☐ If you have an incurable and irreversible medical condition or if you have a terminal [an end-stage] condition, would you like to have life support treatment? For example,...

1. 輸液．
2. 輸血．
3. 中心静脈栄養．
4. 胃瘻などの経管栄養．
5. 昇圧剤の投与．
6. 人工呼吸器の装着．
7. 心臓マッサージ，電気ショックなどの蘇生術．

1. intravenous [IV] fluids?
2. blood transfusion?
3. total parenteral nutrition?
4. tube feeding [gastric/gastrostomy feeding]?
5. administration of vasopressors?
6. use of mechanical ventilator [breathing machine]?
7. resuscitation such as heart massage or electric shock [defibrillation]?

もし脳死状態となってしまった場合，生命維持装置を外すことを希望されますか．

☐ If you become brain dead, would you like to remove [withdraw] life support equipment?

### コラム(つづき)

| | |
|---|---|
| リビングウィルや事前指示書の書面があれば，コピーをご提出ください． | ☐ If you have a living will or advance health care directive with you, please give us a copy of it. |
| なお，延命治療についての希望はいつでも撤回・変更ができます． | ☐ You can cancel or change your wish for life support treatment at any time. |
| 苦痛を和らげる治療は最大限行うことをお約束します． | ☐ We promise that we'll try everything possible to relieve the pain and make you comfortable. |

**Step 6　最後に話を締めくくる**

| | |
|---|---|
| 今後の生活で気がかりなことはありますか． | ☐ Do you have any concerns about how this is going to affect your life? |
| ―ご要望があれば，医療ソーシャルワーカーやカウンセラーをご紹介いたします． | ― I can refer you to a medical social worker or a counselor if you'd like to have one. |
| （ここまでのお話で）何かご質問はありますか． | ☐ Do you have any questions for me (about what I've told you)? |
| ―ご質問があれば，（担当医の）関先生か私にご連絡下さい． | ― If you have any questions, please contact either Dr. Seki (your doctor in charge) or myself. |
| ―ご質問を書いておくとよいかもしれません． | ― It may be helpful to write down any questions you have. |
| それでは来週の月曜日にまたお会いしましょう． | ☐ Then, I'll see you again next Monday. |
| ―どうぞお大事に． | ― Take good care of yourself. |

# 治療の説明

## ● 治療の必要がないとき

| | |
|---|---|
| 特別な治療は必要ないでしょう. | ☐ You don't need any special treatment. |
| 2, 3日〔5, 6日〕ゆっくり休むのが一番ですよ. | ☐ Please get some good rest for a few〔several〕days. |
| 薬を飲むよりも禁煙することが重要です. | ☐ It's more important to stop smoking than to take medications. |

## ● 治療が必要なとき

今後の治療方針についてお話しましょう.　　☐ Let's talk about your future treatment plan.

### 投薬・注射

☞「薬剤投与」(297 ページ).

…ための薬を出しましょう.　　☐ I'm going to [Let me] give you something to…

1. 症状を緩和する
2. 痛みを和らげる
3. 熱を下げる
4. 落ち着く

1. make your symptoms better.
   make you feel better.
2. ease your pain.
3. bring down your fever.
4. relax [calm you down].

…を出しましょう.　　☐ I'm going to [Let me] give you…

1. 薬［内服薬］
2. 軟膏
3. 錠剤
4. 水薬
5. 坐薬
6. 湿布薬

1. a medication.
2. an ointment.
3. tablets.
4. a liquid medication.
5. a suppository.
6. a compress [poultice].

| | |
|---|---|
| 薬の使用方法，副作用については薬剤師より後ほど詳しく説明があります． | ☐ The pharmacist is going to explain how and when to take it and its side effects later. |
| これが薬の処方箋です． | ☐ Here's your prescription. |
| どこの薬局でも調剤してもらえます． | ☐ You can have it filled at any pharmacy. |
| この薬は当病院内でもらえます． | ☐ You can have it at the pharmacy in this hospital. |
| お帰りの前に薬局で受け取って下さい． | ☐ Please pick it up at the pharmacy before you leave the hospital. |
| 薬の副作用がみられたら，直ちに使うのをやめて 045–xxx–xxxx まで電話をして下さい． | ☐ If you have any side effects, stop the medication at once and call us at 045–xxx–xxxx. |
| 今日から薬が変わります． | ☐ Starting today you'll have a different kind of medication. |
| 今日から薬の量が変わります． | ☐ Starting today I'm going to [Let me] change the dose of your medication. |
| —薬の量を減らしましょう． | — I'm going to [Let me] decrease the dose. |
| —薬の量を増やしましょう． | — I'm going to [Let me] increase the dose. |
| 注射をしましょう． | ☐ I'm going to [Let me] give you an injection. |
| 消毒用アルコールにアレルギーはありますか． | ☐ Are you allergic to rubbing alcohol? |
| これは痛み止めの注射です． | ☐ This shot will help ease your pain. |
| —刺しますよ．チクリとします． | — Here we go. You may feel a prick. |

chapter 5 診察が終わって

| | |
|---|---|
| 腕〔手〕がしびれませんか. | ☐ Is your arm〔hand〕numb? |
| これは点滴です. | ☐ This is to feed you intravenously. |
| — 2 時間くらいかかります. | — It'll take about two hours. |
| —先にトイレを済ませてきて下さい. | — Please go to the toilet before we start it. |
| —気分が悪いとき〔刺入部が痛むとき〕はこのコールボタンを押して知らせて下さい. | — If you feel sick〔If the site of the injection hurts〕, please let us know by pressing this call button. |
| 輸血をする必要があります. | ☐ You need to have a transfusion. |

### 外科的処置

| | |
|---|---|
| 縫合する必要があります. | ☐ We need to stitch your wound. |
| 痛み止めの注射をしますね. | ☐ Let me give you a shot for pain. |
| —ちょっと痛いかもしれません. 痛いときは教えて下さい. | — This may be a little painful. Let me know when it hurts. |
| — 2, 3 分で終わります. | — It'll take only a few minutes. |
| 今日は抜糸をしましょう. | ☐ I'm going to [Let me] remove the stitches from the wound today. |
| この糸は抜糸が不要です. | ☐ This suture doesn't have to be removed. |
| 傷口をみましょう. | ☐ I'm going to [Let me] look at your wound. |
| —よくなっています. | — It has healed over. |
| —化膿しています. | — It has formed pus. |
| 傷口の処置をしましょう. | ☐ I'm going to [Let me] treat your wound. |
| 消毒をしましょう. | ☐ I'm going to [Let me] cleanse the wound with an antiseptic. |

| | |
|---|---|
| 包帯を取替えましょう. | ☐ I'm going to [Let me] change the dressing. |
| 傷口をかかないで下さい.<br>―包帯をとらないで下さい.<br>―包帯を濡らさないで下さい. | ☐ Please don't scratch the wound.<br>― Don't remove the bandage.<br>― Don't get the bandage wet. |
| (腕に) ギプス包帯をする必要があります. | ☐ You need a cast (on your arm). |
| 今日はギプスをはずしましょう. | ☐ I'm going to [Let me] take your cast off today. |

### リハビリテーション

☞「リハビリテーション」(401 ページ).

| | |
|---|---|
| リハビリのために…を受ける必要があります.<br>　1. 理学療法<br>　2. 作業療法<br>　3. 言語療法 | ☐ You need to have some…for your rehabilitation.<br>　1. physical therapy<br>　2. occupational therapy<br>　3. speech therapy |
| しばらく…のために通院して下さい.<br>　1. 頸椎牽引<br>　2. マッサージ<br>　3. 温熱療法<br>　4. 電気療法 | ☐ Please come here [to the hospital] for…for some time.<br>　1. cervical traction<br>　2. massage<br>　3. heat therapy<br>　4. electrotherapy |
| リハビリ室までスタッフがご案内します. | ☐ One of our staff is taking you to the rehabilitation room. |

### 入院

☞「入院」(337 ページ).

| | |
|---|---|
| あなたは…入院する必要があります.<br>　1.　今すぐ<br>　2.　近日中に〔近い将来〕 | ☐ You need to be admitted to the hospital...<br>　1.　immediately.<br>　2.　soon〔in the near future〕. |
| 腎臓に問題があるようなので，入院して精密検査〔治療〕することをお勧めします. | ☐ You have a possible kidney problem. I suggest you stay in the hospital and have a more thorough examination〔have some treatment〕. |
| 入院期間はほぼ5日間になるでしょう. | ☐ You'll have to be in the hospital for about 5 days. |
| 入院受付係で入院の予約をして下さい. | ☐ Please make an appointment for hospitalization at the admitting office. |
| 入院費や手続きについては病院事務で訊いて下さい. | ☐ Please ask about your hospital bill and the procedure for admission at the hospital business office. |

### 手術

☞「手術」(323 ページ).

| | |
|---|---|
| あなたは…胆嚢の手術をする必要があります.<br>　1.　今すぐ<br>　2.　近日中に〔近い将来〕 | ☐ You need to have surgery on your gallbladder...<br>　1.　immediately.<br>　2.　soon〔in the near future〕. |
| …という理由で手術が必要です.<br>　1.　生検の結果，悪性細胞が認められた | ☐ You need to have surgery because...<br>　1.　your biopsy has shown signs of malignant cells. |

| | |
|---|---|
| 2. 良性ポリープとがんとの鑑別が困難 | 2. we have difficulty distinguishing between benign polyps and cancer. |
| 3. ポリープががん化する可能性がある | 3. your polyps may change into cancer. |
| 4. 他の治療〔保存的治療〕では症状のコントロールができない | 4. any other nonsurgical 〔conservative〕 treatment makes symptom control difficult. |

| | |
|---|---|
| あなたの場合，手術か薬による治療か，2つの可能性が考えられます． | ☐ In your case, there're two possible courses you can take, either surgery or management with medication. |
| この手術にはリスクが伴います． | ☐ There are possible risks involved with this surgery. |
| 外科医に診察してもらう必要があります． | ☐ You need to see a surgeon. |
| 手術については外科医が後でご説明いたします． | ☐ The surgeon is going to explain and talk with you later. |

## 専門医への紹介

肺の専門医に診察してもらう必要が
あります．

☐ You need to see a lung specialist.

診察のために心臓の専門医をご紹介
しましょう．

☐ I'm going to [Let me] refer you [give you a referral] to a heart specialist for consultation.

他の病院〔診療所〕をご紹介しま
しょう．

☐ I'm going to [Let me] refer you to another hospital〔clinic〕.

紹介状を書きましょう．

☐ I'd be happy to write a referral letter.

セカンドオピニオンを希望される場
合には，遠慮なくおっしゃって下さ
い．

☐ If you'd like to have〔get/obtain〕a second opinion, please don't hesitate to let me know.

## 用語・表現ファイル

### 専門医

|  |  |
|---|---|
| 内科医 | internist |
| 外科医 | surgeon |
| 一般外科医 | general surgeon |
| 小児科医 | pediatrician |
| 小児外科医 | pediatric surgeon |
| 循環器科医 | heart specialist, cardiologist |
| 心臓血管外科医 | cardiovascular surgeon |
| 呼吸器科医 | lung specialist, pulmonologist |
| 消化器科医 | gastroenterologist |
| 血液内科医 | hematologist |
| 腎臓内科医 | nephrologist |
| リウマチ科医 | rheumatologist |
| 内分泌科医 | endocrinologist |
| 泌尿器科医 | urologist |
| 乳腺外科医 | breast surgeon |
| 神経科医 | neurologist |
| 脳神経外科医 | neurosurgeon |
| 精神科医 | psychiatrist |
| 整形外科医 | orthopedic surgeon, orthopedist |
| 形成外科医 | plastic surgeon |
| 婦人科医 | gynecologist |
| 産科医 | obstetrician |
| 皮膚科医 | dermatologist |
| 眼科医 | ophthalmologist |
| 耳鼻咽喉科医 | ENT doctor, otolaryngologist |
| 放射線診断医 | diagnostic radiologist |
| インターベンション（放射線）治療医 | interventional radiologist |
| 放射線療法医 | radiotherapist |
| リハビリテーション科医 | rehabilitation physician, physiatrist |
| 麻酔科医 | anesthesiologist |
| 腫瘍専門医 | oncologist, tumor specialist |
| 感染対策専門医 | infection control doctor, infectious disease specialist |
| アレルギー専門医 | allergist |
| 睡眠専門医 | sleep disorder specialist |

## 用語・表現ファイル(つづき)

| | |
|---|---|
| ホスピス・緩和ケア専門医 | hospice and palliative medicine specialist |
| 救急医療専門医 | emergency medicine specialist |
| スポーツ医 | sports physician [doctor], sports medicine specialist |
| 産業医 | occupational health physician |
| 老年病専門医 | geriatrician, gerontologist |
| 病理医 | pathologist |
| 歯科医 | dentist |
| 歯科矯正医 | orthodontist |
| 口腔外科医 | oral [dental] surgeon, maxillofacial surgeon |
| 一般開業医 | general practitioner |

☞「病院関係者」(89 ページ).

---

### 名句・ことわざ

**Physician, heal [cure] thyself.**

**医者よ,まず自分の病気を治せ**

聖書由来のことわざで,'thyself' は 'yourself' を意味する.日本の「医者の不養生」に相当する.

## 次回の診察予約

症状がよくなればもう来なくてけっこうですよ.
- [ ] You don't have to come again if your symptoms are getting better.

…ときは再度受診して下さい.
1. 症状［具合］がよくならない
2. 症状が前よりひどい
3. 症状が再発する
4. 薬がなくなった
5. 必要がある

- [ ] Please come back again...
  1. if your symptoms haven't improved.
     if you don't feel better.
  2. if your symptoms get worse.
     if you feel worse.
  3. if your symptoms have returned.
  4. after your medication has run out.
  5. when you feel a need to.

しばらく定期的に通院して下さい.
- [ ] Please come here [to the hospital] regularly for a while.

週〔月〕に一度通院して下さい.
- [ ] Please come here [to the hospital] once a week〔month〕.

再検査〔診察〕のため6か月以内にもう一度お出で下さい.
- [ ] Please come again in six months to have a follow-up test〔examination〕.

…ときには03–xxxx–xxxxに電話を下さい.
1. 薬が合わない［副作用がある］
2. 具合が悪くて緊急に受診したい
3. 何かご質問がある

- [ ] Please call us at 03–xxxx–xxxx...
  1. if you have any side effects.
  2. if you need to see me urgently because you feel sick.
  3. if you have any questions.

外に出られたら，窓口のクラーク〔看護師〕が手続きをしてくれます.
- [ ] If you go outside, the clerk [the nurse] at the reception desk will take care of you.

| | |
|---|---|
| 次回の予約は6月8日，午前9時です．それでよろしいですか． | ☐ Your next appointment is June 8, at 9 in the morning. Is that all right with you? |
| 今のところ6月末まで予約がつまっています．7月5日はいかがですか． | ☐ I'm afraid I'm fully booked until the end of June. How about July 5? |
| …から次回の予約券を受け取って下さい．<br>1. クラーク<br>2. 看護師<br>3. 受付係 | ☐ Please get your appointment card for your next visit from the...<br>1. clerk.<br>2. nurse.<br>3. receptionist. |
| 診察券をお返しします． | ☐ Let me give you back your hospital ID card. |
| どうぞお大事に． | ☐ Take (good) care of yourself.<br>☐ Take care! |
| それではまた来週〔来月〕． | ☐ (I'll) see you next week 〔month〕. |
| さようなら． | ☐ Goodbye. |

---

### 名句・ことわざ

**A disease known is half cured.**

病気は原因がわかれば［診断がつけば］半分治ったに等しい

日本には「病を知れば癒ゆるに近し」ということわざがある．

## 用語・表現ファイル

## 日常生活への指示

### 1. 安静,睡眠

| | |
|---|---|
| 従来通りの生活でけっこうです. | You may go about your normal daily routines. |
| 活動を少し制限して下さい. | You should restrict your activities slightly. |
| ―仕事は休んで,しばらく休養して下さい. | — You shouldn't go to work. Please rest for a while. |
| ―制限つきで仕事をしてもよいでしょう. | — You may work with some restrictions. |
| ―軽い家事をしてもけっこうです. | — You can do some light housework. |
| 睡眠と休息をとって下さい. | Please get your sleep and rest. |
| 無理はしないで[過労は避けて]下さい. | Don't work too hard. Avoid overwork. |

あなたは…必要があります.
1. 安静にしている
2. もっと多く睡眠をとる
3. 疲れ過ぎないようにする

You need to...
1. stay in bed.
2. sleep more.
3. avoid getting overly tired.

長い間立ちっぱなしでいたり,重い荷物を持ったりしないようにして下さい.

Please don't stand on your feet for a long time or lift heavy things.

### 2. 運動

きつい[激しい]運動はしないで下さい.

Please avoid hard [strenuous] exercise.

あなたは…必要があります.
1. もっと運動する
2. 定期的に運動する
3. 軽い運動をする

You need to...
1. get more exercise.
2. get regular exercise.
3. do some light exercise.

## 用語・表現ファイル(つづき)

| | |
|---|---|
| 4. 運動を制限する | 4. get less exercise. |

| | |
|---|---|
| できるだけ散歩をお勧めします. | I recommend that you take a walk whenever you can. |
| 新しい運動を始める前には私に尋ねて下さい. | Please check with me before starting any new exercise. |

### 3. 食事

| | |
|---|---|
| 規則正しい食生活をして下さい.<br>―バランスよく食べて下さい.<br>―適量を食べて下さい.<br>―食事を抜かないで下さい. | Please eat your meals regularly.<br>— Eat a well-balanced diet.<br>— Eat in moderation.<br>— Don't skip meals. |

あなたは…必要があります.　　　　You need to...

| | |
|---|---|
| 1. 水分を多くとる | 1. drink lots of water. |
| 2. 水分を控える | 2. cut down on your water. |
| 3. 塩分〔糖分〕を制限し,塩気が強い食品〔菓子類〕を避ける | 3. limit salt〔sugar〕and avoid eating salty foods〔sweets〕. |
| 4. 脂っこい〔香辛料のきいた〕食品を制限する | 4. limit fatty〔spicy〕foods. |
| 5. 繊維を含んだ食品,例えば,野菜や果物を食べる | 5. eat foods high in fiber like vegetables and raw fruits. |
| 6. カフェインが入った飲み物,例えば,コーヒー,お茶,コーラなどを避ける | 6. avoid caffeinated beverages like coffee, tea, or cola. |

| | |
|---|---|
| 質問があれば栄養士か私に尋ねて下さい. | If you have any questions, please ask a dietitian or me. |

### 4. その他

| | |
|---|---|
| 禁煙するよう努力して下さい. | Please try to stop smoking. |

## 用語・表現ファイル（つづき）

| | |
|---|---|
| アルコールは適量であればかまいません． | You can drink alcohol in moderation. |
| ―アルコールを飲まないよう努力して下さい． | ― Please try to stop drinking alcohol. |
| 運転はけっこうでしょう． | You can drive. |
| ―運転はしないで下さい． | ― Please don't drive. |
| 性行為はしてかまいません． | You can continue your sexual activities. |
| ―性行為は制限して下さい． | ― Please restrict your sexual activities. |
| 気持ちを楽にして，動揺しないようにして下さい． | Please relax and avoid getting upset. |

---

### 名句・ことわざ

#### 笑う門には福来たる

〔英訳〕**Good fortune comes to a laughing [merry] home.**

英語には "Laughter will make one fat."（笑い声は人を肥らせる）や "Laugh and be [grow] fat."（笑って肥れ）など類似のことわざがある．

chapter 6

# 検査

## Diagnostic Tests

**検査一般** 270
**各種検査** 275
血液検査 275
尿検査 276
心電図検査 276
トレッドミル負荷心電図検査 277
ホルター心電図検査 278
X線検査 280
CT/MRI検査 282
超音波検査（エコー） 283
内視鏡検査 285
呼吸機能検査 286
マンモグラフィ検査 287
乳房の自己検診 288
視力検査 289
聴力検査 290

## 検査一般

☞「検査の説明」(238 ページ).

### ● インフォームド・コンセント

| | |
|---|---|
| これは正確な診断結果を出すために必要な検査です. | ☐ You need this test for an accurate diagnosis. |
| 検査を行うためには同意が必要です. | ☐ I need your consent to do this test. |
| 検査に伴うリスクとしては薬剤によるアレルギー,出血などがあります. | ☐ There are possible risks involved with this test, such as allergic reactions to the medications, bleeding and others. |
| 非常にまれですが,死に至る重篤な合併症が生じることもあります. | ☐ Very rarely, serious complications can occur, including death. |
| 死亡率は 10,000 人に 1 人です. | ☐ The mortality rate for this test is one in ten-thousand patients. |
| この同意書をよく読んで,サインして下さい. | ☐ Please read this (informed) consent form carefully and sign it. |

☞「インフォームド・コンセントのサンプル」(429 ページ).

| | |
|---|---|
| どなたか同意書にサインして下さる人はいますか. | ☐ Do you have anyone who can sign the consent form for you? |
| ご質問がありますか. | ☐ (Do you have) any questions? |

## ➲ 検査前に

### 検査日以前

#### ▶ 飲食への注意

| | |
|---|---|
| 検査前夜の夕食後から検査までは何も口にしないで下さい. | ☐ Please don't drink or eat anything after supper the night before, up until your test. |
| 夜の 12 時を過ぎてからは何も口にしないで下さい. | ☐ Don't eat or drink anything after midnight. |
| 検査前 8 時間は何も口にしないで下さい. | ☐ Don't eat or drink anything for 8 hours before the test. |
| 当日は軽い朝食〔昼食〕にして,検査前 2 時間は食べたり飲んだりしないで下さい. | ☐ Have a light breakfast〔lunch〕, but don't eat or drink anything for 2 hours before the test. |
| 薬を少しの水で飲むのはかまいません. | ☐ You may take your medications with a small sip of water. |
| 検査前は特別食以外食べないで下さい. | ☐ Don't eat anything except for the special diet before the test. |
| 検査前夜に下剤を服用して下さい. | ☐ Please take a laxative the night before the test. |
| この検査に特別な準備は必要ありません. | ☐ No preparation is necessary for this test. |

#### ▶ 予約取り消し

| | |
|---|---|
| 予約の日に来られない場合は,直ちに電話して下さい. | ☐ If you can't keep your appointment, please call us as soon as possible. |

**検査当日**

| | |
|---|---|
| 順番がきたらお名前をお呼びします． | ☐ We'll call your name when your turn comes. |
| ―呼ばれるまでここでお待ち下さい． | ― Please wait here till your name is called. |
| ―呼ばれたら3番の部屋に入って下さい． | ― When your name is called, enter room 3. |
| ブラウンさん，お入り下さい． | ☐ Mr.〔Mrs./Ms./Miss〕Brown, please come in. |

☞検査中の体位・動作の指示については「各種検査」(275ページ)．

## ➡ 検査後に

| | |
|---|---|
| 検査後はふだん通りの食事や生活をしてけっこうです． | ☐ After the test, you can have your regular meals and go about your normal daily routine. |
| 1時間は飲食しないで下さい． | ☐ Please don't eat or drink anything for an hour. |
| 検査後食べてもけっこうですが，軽い食事にして下さい． | ☐ You may eat after the test. Try light meals. |
| 水分をたくさんとって下さい． | ☐ Please drink plenty of fluids. |
| 24時間はお酒を飲まないで下さい． | ☐ You shouldn't drink alcohol for 24 hours. |
| 今日は運転しないで下さい． | ☐ Please don't drive today. |
| シャワーはけっこうですが，お風呂には入らないで下さい． | ☐ You can take a shower, but avoid taking a bath. |
| 2，3日のどがいがらっぽいかもしれません． | ☐ Your throat may be scratchy for a few days. |
| 軽い腹痛があるかもしれません． | ☐ You may have mild cramping. |

| | |
|---|---|
| (内診後に) ごく少量の出血かおりものがあるかもしれません. | ☐ You may notice slight bleeding or discharge. |
| 熱や痛みがあるときには電話をして下さい. | ☐ Please call us if you have any fever or pain. |
| 検査結果は来週出ます. | ☐ We'll have the results next week. |
| お帰りになる前に再診の予約をして下さい. | ☐ Before you leave the hospital, please make a return appointment. |
| 受付で予約カードをもらって下さい. | ☐ Please go to the reception desk and get your appointment card. |

## 用語・表現ファイル

### 病院会話のヒント　その3　場所の表現

| | |
|---|---|
| 超音波検査室への行き方がわかりますか．…にあります．<br>　1. 2階<br>　2. 地下<br>　3. この廊下の突き当たり<br>　4. 臨床検査室の隣<br>　5. 角<br>　6. 角を曲がったところ<br>　7. 右〔左〕側<br>　8. ここ〔そこ／あそこ〕 | Do you know how to get to the ultrasound room? It's…<br>　1. on the second floor.<br>　2. in the basement.<br>　3. at the end of this hallway.<br>　4. next to the laboratory.<br>　5. on the corner.<br>　6. around the corner.<br>　7. on the right 〔left〕.<br>　8. here 〔there/over there〕. |
| 20メートル直進して下さい． | Go straight for 20 meters. |
| 右〔左〕に曲がって下さい． | Turn right 〔left〕. |
| 2つめの角を右に曲がると，ちょうど正面にあります． | Turn right at the second corner, and you'll find it right ahead of you. |
| エレベーターに乗って5階に行って下さい． | Take the elevator to the fifth floor. |
| エスカレータをご利用下さい． | Please use the escalator. |
| お連れしましょう．ご一緒にどうぞ． | I'll show you where it is. Please come (along) with me. |

## 各種検査

☞「確認,励まし,慰め,慰労」(242ページ).

### ➡ 血液検査

| | |
|---|---|
| 採血をしましょう. | ☐ I'm going to [Let me] take a blood sample. |
| お座り下さい. | ☐ Please sit down. |
| 腕を出して袖をまくって下さい. | ☐ Please put out your arm and roll up your sleeve. |
| —腕に駆血帯を巻きましょう. | — Let me put this tourniquet [elastic band] on your arm. |
| —手を握って下さい. | — Please make a fist. |
| —こんなふうに. | — Do like this. |
| —楽にして下さい. | — Please relax. |
| —体の力を抜くようにして下さい. | — Try to let your body go limp. |
| アルコール消毒でかぶれることがありますか | ☐ Do you ever get a skin rash from using alcohol wipes [swabs]? |
| ちょっとチクンとしますよ. | ☐ There'll be a little prick. |
| さあ,終わりました. | ☐ Now, you're finished. |
| バンドエイドを腕に貼りますから,2,3分押さえていて下さい. | ☐ I'll just put this Band-Aid on your arm, so hold it for a few minutes. |
| 耳〔親指〕から血をとります. | ☐ I'm going to [Let me] prick your ear lobe〔thumb〕. |

## ● 尿検査

| | |
|---|---|
| 検尿が必要です. | ☐ We need a sample of your urine. |
| このコップに尿をとって下さい. | ☐ Please use this cup to collect your urine. |
| まずトイレに少し尿を出して下さい. | ☐ First, urinate a small amount into the toilet. |
| 次に,コップに少量の尿—およそ3分の1くらいまで入れて下さい. | ☐ Then, a small amount into the cup—about one-third. |
| (尿がとれたら) このテーブルの上に置いて下さい. | ☐ Please put the cup on this table. |
| 管を入れて膀胱から尿をとります. | ☐ I'm going to drain the urine from your bladder with this tube. |

## ● 心電図検査

| | |
|---|---|
| 心電図の検査をしましょう. | ☐ I'm going to [Let me] take your electrocardiogram [ECG]. |
| シャツを脱いで下さい. | ☐ Please take off your undershirt. |
| 靴下〔ストッキング〕も脱いで下さい. | ☐ Please take off your socks 〔stockings〕, too. |
| 台の上に仰向けに寝て下さい. | ☐ Please lie on your back on the table. |
| 楽にして動かないで下さい. | ☐ Please relax and don't move. |
| 2,3分で終わります. | ☐ It'll be finished in a few minutes. |
| さあ,終わりました. | ☐ Now, you're finished. |
| もう洋服を着てけっこうです. | ☐ You can get dressed now. |

## → トレッドミル負荷心電図検査

### 検査日以前

トレッドミル心電図検査を行いましょう.
- [ ] We're going to do a treadmill ECG.

トレッドミル心電図検査は運動中の心電図を記録する検査です.
- [ ] A treadmill ECG is an ECG that is recorded during exercise.

食事は,検査の1時間前までに軽く済ませておいて下さい.
- [ ] Please eat a light meal at least an hour before the test.

動きやすい服装とウォーキングシューズでおいで下さい.
- [ ] Wear comfortable clothes and walking shoes.

### 検査当日

胸に電極を貼ります.
- [ ] I'm going to put [place/attach] electrodes on the skin of your chest.

それではこのトレッドミルの上を歩いて下さい.
- [ ] Now, walk on this treadmill.

—最初はゆっくりですが,徐々にトレッドミルの速度と傾斜が増してゆきます.
— You'll start walking slowly, but gradually the speed and slope of the treadmill are increased.

トレッドミルの上を歩いている間,血圧と心電図を注意深くモニターします.
- [ ] While you walk on the treadmill, we're closely monitoring your blood pressure and ECG.

心配しないで下さい. 検査の間はおそばについていますよ.
- [ ] Don't worry! We'll be here beside [for] you during the test.

胸が痛んだり,圧迫感や違和感を覚えたりしたら言って下さい.
- [ ] Let me know if you have any chest pain, or feel pressure or discomfort.

(その他の負荷心電図検査)

|  |  |
|---|---|
| この自転車はエルゴメータといって，運動中の心電図を記録します． | ☐ This bicycle is called an ergometer that records the ECG during exercise. |
| 自転車をこいで下さい．<br>―ペダルが徐々に重くなっていきますよ． | ☐ Please pedal the bike.<br>— The pedals will gradually become heavier. |
| マスター二階段（昇降）試験をしましょう． | ☐ We're going to do [conduct] a Master two step (exercise) test. |
| この踏み段をメトロノームの音に合わせて昇り降りして下さい． | ☐ Please walk up and down these steps matching your pace to the beats of the metronome. |

## ホルター心電図検査

### 検査日以前

|  |  |
|---|---|
| ホルター心電図をとりましょう． | ☐ We're going to do a Holter ECG. |
| ホルター心電図検査は24時間かけて心電図を記録する検査です． | ☐ A Holter ECG is a test that records your ECG for 24 hours. |
| 入院する必要はありません． | ☐ You don't need to be hospitalized. |
| 食事やお薬はいつも通りでけっこうです． | ☐ You can have your regular meals and continue with your current medication. |
| 前もってお風呂やシャワーは済ませて下さい． | ☐ Take a shower or a bath beforehand. |
| 前開きのシャツやブラウスなど，ゆったりした服装でおいで下さい． | ☐ Wear loose-fitting clothes, such as a shirt or blouse that buttons in front. |

### 検査当日

ホルター心電計についてご説明いたします.
- 胸に電極を貼ります.

- この小さなポーチを 24 時間ずっと腰に付けて〔首にかけて〕いただきます.

その間ふだん通りの行動を続けて下さってけっこうです.

シャワーやお風呂は避け,電極を濡らさないで下さい.

これがホルター記録紙です.

- 検査中の行動や症状を正確に記録して下さい.

- 胸痛,息切れ,動悸,めまいなどの症状を自覚した時には,症状が起きた正確な時刻,その時に何をしていたか,例えば睡眠中,食事中,歩行中,テニスをしていたなどを,記録して下さい.

- 何らかの症状を自覚した時には,記録計についているボタンを押して下さい.

明日の午前中〔午後〕のこの時間に機器を外しますのでご来院下さい.

---

- [ ] Let me tell you [explain] about the Holter monitor.
  - I'm going to put [place/attach] electrodes on the skin of your chest.
  - You need to wear this small pouch around your waist [neck], continuously for 24 hours.

- [ ] During this period, you can carry on with your normal activities.

- [ ] You shouldn't take a shower or bath, or get the electrodes wet.

- [ ] Here's a Holter monitor diary form.
  - Keep an accurate diary of your activities and symptoms during the test.
  - If you feel symptoms such as chest pain, shortness of breath, palpitations or dizziness, note in your diary the exact time of day they began, and what you were doing such as sleeping, eating, walking, or playing tennis.
  - Press the button on the recorder when you have some kind of symptoms.

- [ ] Please come to the hospital to have the device removed tomorrow morning [tomorrow afternoon] about this time.

| | |
|---|---|
| 記録されたデータを医師が解析します．検査結果は次回の診察時にお話しします． | ☐ The recorded data will be analyzed and interpreted by a doctor. We'll have the results on your follow-up appointment. |
| 詳しくは，このパンフレットをお読み下さい． | ☐ For further information, please read this brochure. |
| ご質問や何か困ったことがありましたら，遠慮なくご連絡下さい． | ☐ If you have any questions or problems, feel free to call [contact] us. |

## → X線検査

| | |
|---|---|
| …のレントゲンをとりましょう． | ☐ I'm going to [Let me] take an X-ray of your... |
| 1. 胸部 | 1. chest. |
| 2. 腹部 | 2. abdomen. |
| 3. 頸椎〔首〕 | 3. cervical spine〔neck〕. |
| 4. 腰椎 | 4. lumbar spine. |
| 5. 頭部 | 5. head. |
| 6. 乳房 | 6. breasts. |
| 7. 胃 | 7. stomach. |
| 8. 腸 | 8. bowels. |
| 9. 腎臓 | 9. kidneys. |
| 上半身の服を脱いで下さい． | ☐ Please take off your clothes from the waist up. |
| 装飾品もぜんぶ取って下さい． | ☐ Remove all of your jewelry as well. |
| この検査着を着て下さい． | ☐ Put on this exam gown. |
| 前を向いて真っ直ぐ立って下さい． | ☐ Please stand with your head facing the front. |
| 手を横に置いて下さい，こんなふうに． | ☐ Put your arms by your side, like this. |

|  |  |
|---|---|
| 大きく息を吸って，止めて下さい． | Take a big breath in, and hold it. |
| 楽にして下さい． | Relax, please. |
| 今度は，横を向いて下さい． | Stand sideways, this time. |
| この液〔バリウム〕を飲んで下さい． | Please swallow this special drink 〔barium mixture〕. |
| コップの中身を一気に飲んで下さい． | Empty the cup in one gulp. |
| ゲップをしないで我慢して下さい． | Don't belch. Hold on to the air. |
| この台の上に横になって下さい． | Lie down on this table. |
| 台はいろいろな方向に動きます． | The table will move you into different positions. |
| 少し圧迫される感じがするかもしれません． | You may feel some pressure. |
| 痛かったらおっしゃって下さい． | Let me know when it hurts. |
| さあ，終わりました． | Now, you're finished. |
| もう洋服を着てけっこうです． | You can get dressed now. |
| 便秘をしないように，水分をたくさんとって下さい． | Please drink plenty of fluids to prevent being constipated. |
| 下剤を飲んでもいいですよ． | It may be helpful to take a laxative. |

## ⇒ CT/MRI 検査

…の CT〔MRI〕検査をしましょう.

1. 頭部
2. 胸部
3. 心臓
4. 腹部

☐ I'm going to〔Let me〕take the CT scan〔MRI〕of your...

1. head.
2. chest.
3. heart.
4. abdomen.

検査はだいたい 2, 3 分〔30 分〕かかります.

☐ It'll take about a few〔30〕minutes to complete the test.

検査は痛くありませんから心配しないで下さい.

☐ The test is painless, so don't worry.

これまでに造影剤でアレルギー反応を起こしたことはありますか.

☐ Have you ever had any allergic reactions from a contrast medium?

これまでにペースメーカー, クリップ, 人工関節などの金属を体内に埋め込む手術をしたことがありますか.

☐ Have you had any metal implants inserted in your body, such as a pacemaker, clips, or artificial joints?

眼鏡, 時計, 装飾品, ヘアピン, 入れ歯などすべての金属製品をとって下さい.

☐ Please remove all metallic objects, such as glasses, watch, jewelry, bobby pins, dentures, and others.

上半身の服を脱いで下さい.

☐ Please take off your clothes from the waist up.

この検査着を着て下さい.

☐ Put on this exam gown.

検査部位をはっきりさせるために造影剤を注射します.

☐ I'm going to give you a contrast medium to highlight the area to be examined.

| | |
|---|---|
| この台の上に仰向けに寝て下さい． | ☐ Please lie on your back on this table. |
| この器具をつけますが，痛くありませんから． | ☐ I'll set up this equipment for you. It won't hurt you. |
| 楽にして動かないで下さい． | ☐ Please try to relax and don't move. |
| 検査が済むまでじっとしていて下さい． | ☐ Keep still until the test is finished. |
| 検査の間，音楽を聴いて楽にしていて下さい． | ☐ You can listen to music during the test, and try to relax. |
| 検査中，機械がブーン〔カチカチ〕という音を出しますが，心配いりません． | ☐ The machine makes a whirring 〔knocking〕 noise, but don't worry. |
| 台がゆっくり動いていきます． | ☐ The table will be moving slowly. |
| 大きく息を吸って下さい．<br>―息を止めて下さい．<br>―楽にして下さい． | ☐ Please take a big breath in.<br>— Hold it.<br>— Relax. |
| さあ，終わりました． | ☐ Now, you're finished. |
| もう洋服を着てけっこうです． | ☐ You can get dressed now. |

## ❯ 超音波検査（エコー）

| | |
|---|---|
| …の超音波検査をしましょう．<br><br>　1．腹部<br>　2．甲状腺<br>　3．乳房<br>　4．心臓 | ☐ I'm going to [Let me] perform the ultrasound on your...<br>　1．abdomen.<br>　2．thyroid.<br>　3．breasts.<br>　4．heart. |
| この検査はおよそ 15 分ほどかかります． | ☐ This test usually takes about 15 minutes. |

| | |
|---|---|
| 上半身の服を脱いで下さい． | ☐ Please take off your clothes from the waist up. |
| 台の上に仰向けに寝て下さい． | ☐ Please lie on your back on the table. |
| スカート〔ズボン〕をさげてお腹を出して下さい． | ☐ Please roll your skirt〔pants〕down from your abdomen. |
| お腹にゼリーを塗りますよ． | ☐ I'm going to spread gel on 〔apply gel to〕your abdomen. |
| 多少押される感じがしますが，痛くはありません． | ☐ You may feel a little gentle pressure, but it's not painful. |
| どうぞ…<br>1. お腹をふくらませて下さい．<br>2. お腹をひっこめて下さい．<br>3. 普通に息をして下さい．<br>4. 大きく息を吸って下さい．<br>5. 息を止めて下さい．<br>6. 楽にして下さい． | ☐ Please...<br>1. inflate [push out] your stomach.<br>2. suck in your stomach.<br>3. breathe like you usually do.<br>4. take a big breath in.<br>5. hold it.<br>6. relax. |
| 両手を頭の上に上げて下さい． | ☐ Please raise both your hands above your head. |
| 右向き〔左向き〕に寝て下さい． | ☐ Please lie on your right〔left〕side. |
| さあ，終わりました． | ☐ Now, you're finished. |
| ゼリーを拭き取りましょう．ペーパータオルをお使い下さい． | ☐ Let's wipe off the gel. Use these paper towels. |
| もう洋服を着てけっこうです． | ☐ You can get dressed now. |

## ◯ 内視鏡検査

|  |  |
|---|---|
| 上部消化管内視鏡〔大腸内視鏡〕検査をしましょう. | ☐ I'm going to [Let me] perform an upper endoscopy 〔colonoscopy〕. |
| 検査はだいたい30分かかります. | ☐ It'll take about 30 minutes to complete the test. |
| 上半身〔下半身〕の服を脱いで下さい. | ☐ Please take off your clothes from the waist up 〔from the waist down〕. |
| この検査着を着て下さい. | ☐ Put on this exam gown. |
| 腕に注射をします. | ☐ I'm going to give you an injection in the arm. |
| のどに麻酔をしますから,合図するまでこの液体を口の中に含んでおいて下さい. | ☐ I'm going to anesthetize your throat. Please keep this liquid in your mouth till I say "OK." |
| 管をごくんと飲んで下さい. | ☐ Swallow this tube in one gulp. |
| 体の力を抜くようにして下さい。 | ☐ Try to let your body go limp. |
| 空気を入れますから,しばらくゲップ〔おなら〕を我慢して下さい. | ☐ I'm going to insert air (to expand your GI tract), so please don't belch 〔pass gas〕. |
| 念のために胃〔腸〕の生検をします. | ☐ I'm going to perform a biopsy of your stomach 〔colon〕 to be certain. |
| さあ,終わりました. | ☐ Now, you're finished. |
| もう洋服を着てけっこうです. | ☐ You can get dressed now. |

## ➲ 呼吸機能検査

| | |
|---|---|
| 呼吸機能検査をしましょう. | ☐ I'm going to [Let me] perform a spirometric test. |
| どうぞお座り下さい. | ☐ Please sit down. |
| 鼻にクリップをつけます. | ☐ Let me apply the nose clip. |
| マウスピースを口にくわえて唇をしっかり閉じて下さい. | ☐ Please put the mouthpiece in your mouth with your lips tightly closed. |
| 肩の力を抜いて楽にしていて下さい. | ☐ Please relax the muscles of your shoulders. |
| 普通に呼吸をして下さい. | ☐ Breathe normally [like you usually do]. |
| ―それでは,ゆっくり息を吐いて,吐いて,吐いて,全部吐いて! 息をゆっくり吸いましょう.できるだけ大きく吸って,吸って,胸いっぱい吸って! さあ,思いっきり早く吐いて,吐いて,吐いて,もっと,最後まで吐ききって! | ― Now slowly blow out...out...out...all the way! Take a slow deep breath...as deep as you can...breathe in...in...deeper. Now blow as hard and as fast as you can,...blow out...out...more...get it all out! |
| はい,けっこうです.楽にして下さい. | ☐ Good [OK], you're doing fine. Please relax. |
| マウスピースを口から外してもいいですよ.鼻のクリップは付けたままにしておいて下さい. | ☐ You can take the mouthpiece out of your mouth, but leave the nose clip attached. |
| では,もう一度やってみましょう. | ☐ Now let's do it one more time. |
| さあ,終わりました.よく頑張りましたね. | ☐ It's all over. You did very well! |
| このティッシュペーパーでお口を拭いて下さい. | ☐ Here's the tissue to wipe your mouth. |

## ➡ マンモグラフィ検査

| | |
|---|---|
| マンモグラフィ検査は初めてですか. | ☐ Is this your first mammogram? |
| マンモグラフィ検査をしましょう. | ☐ I'm going to [Let me] perform the mammogram. |
| ―上半身の服を脱いで下さい. | ― Please take off your clothes from the waist up. |
| ―この機械の前に立って下さい. | ― Stand in front of this machine. |
| ―プレートの上に右の乳房を載せて下さい. | ― Place your right breast on the plate. |
| ―右腕を上げてこの取っ手を握って,左腕を下げて,顔を左に向けて下さい. | ― Lift your right arm up and grasp this lever, then put your left arm down, and turn your face to the left. |
| ―乳房を2つのプラ板に挟んで圧迫します. | ― I'm going to compress the breast between the two plates. |
| 押される感じがしますよ. | ☐ Now you'll feel squeezed. |
| 痛かったらおっしゃって下さい. | ☐ Let me know if it hurts. |
| 辛かったらごめんなさい.でもすぐ終わりますから. | ☐ I'm sorry if this makes you a little uncomfortable, but it'll be over in a minute. |
| では,息を止めて,少しの間動かないで下さい. | ☐ Hold your breath, and remain still just a second. |
| けっこうです.楽にして下さい. | ☐ Good. Relax. |
| 今度は,左の乳房を撮りましょう. | ☐ This time, I'm going to [Let me] take the picture of your left breast. |
| さあ,終わりました. | ☐ Now, you're finished. |
| もう洋服を着てけっこうです. | ☐ You can get dressed now. |

## 🔵 乳房の自己検診

| | |
|---|---|
| 乳房の自己検診の仕方をお教えしましょう. | ☐ I'm going to [Let me] tell you how to do a breast self exam [BSE]. |
| 上半身の服を脱いで下さい. | ☐ Take off your clothes from the waist up. |
| まず右乳房を調べます.<br>―仰向けに寝て,枕を右肩の下に入れます.(→ a)<br>―左手の指先の腹で乳房全体をまんべんなく軽く触れながら,しこりがないかをチェックします.(→ b) | ☐ First, check your right breast.<br>— Lie on your back and put a pillow under your right shoulder.<br>— With the pads of your left fingers, go over the entire area, touching gently to feel for the presence of any lumps. |
| それから脇の下をチェックします. | ☐ Then, check your armpit. |
| 乳首を軽く絞るようにしてつまみ,分泌物が出ないかをチェックします. | ☐ Squeeze the nipple gently to observe for the presence of liquid drainage. |
| 左乳房を同様の手順で調べます. | ☐ Repeat the process on the left breast. |
| 両手を腰に当てて鏡の前に立ち,乳房の形や大きさが左右対称になっているかどうかチェックします.(→ c) | ☐ Stand in front of a mirror with your hands on your hips and see if your breasts are symmetrical in appearance. |
| ふだんとは違う変化,例えば,皮膚のへこみや隆起した個所はないかをチェックします. | ☐ See if there are any unusual changes, such as dimples or bumps around the skin. |
| 乳首がへこんでいないかチェックします. | ☐ Check your nipples to see if they are turned in or inverted. |

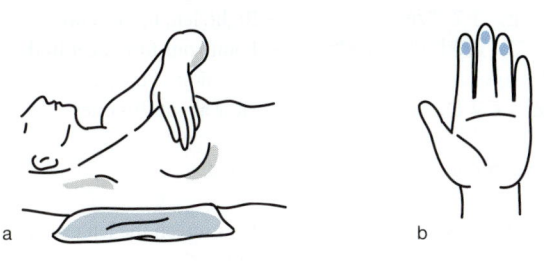

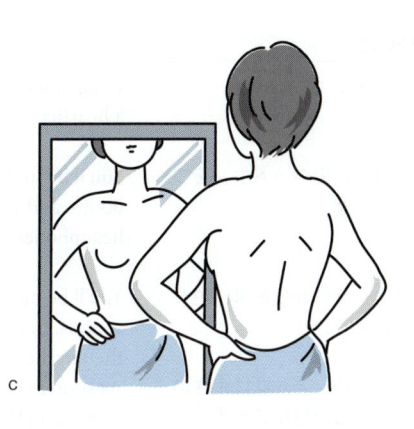

## ● 視力検査

| 視力検査をしましょう. | ☐ I'm going to [Let me] perform a visual acuity test. |

前を向いて視力表を見て下さい.　　☐ Please look at the eye chart with your head facing the front.

まず右目を調べましょう.　　☐ Let's screen the right eye first.
—この遮眼子で左目を隠して下さい.　　— Cover the left eye with this occluder.
—リングに透き間が開いています.　　— The rings have gaps.

| | |
|---|---|
| —このリングはどっちの方向に開いていますか. | — Which direction is the gap in this ring? |
| —右，左，上，下ですか. | — Right, left, up or down? |
| —人差し指で，透き間の方向を指して下さい. | — Point your forefinger in the direction of the gap. |
| —これはどうですか. | — How about this one? |
| はい，けっこうです. | ☐ Good. |
| 今度は，左目を調べましょう. | ☐ Let's screen the left eye, this time. |

## ➔ 聴力検査

| | |
|---|---|
| 聴力検査をしましょう. | ☐ I'm going to [Let me] perform a hearing [audiometry] test. |
| 防音室に入ってこのヘッドホンをつけていただきます. | ☐ You'll be in the soundproof booth, and wear these headphones. |
| 最初は右耳に，それから左耳に色々な音が聞こえます. | ☐ You'll be hearing a variety of sounds, first in the right ear and then in the left. |
| —音が聞こえたら，どんなに小さい音でも聞こえるたびにこのボタンを押して下さい. | — As soon as you hear a sound, even though it is very quiet, please press this button. |
| —音が消えるまでボタンを押し続けて下さい. | — Keep it pressed until the sound goes away. |
| 用意はよろしいですか. | ☐ Are you ready? |
| では腰かけてヘッドホンをつけて下さい. | ☐ Please sit down, and put on the headphones. |

## コラム

# 視力の測り方の違い

　日本で視力検査に使われるのは Landolt C eye chart（形が C に似たランドルト環視力表）だが，これは必ずしも万国共通ではない．米国ではアルファベットを読ませて計測する Snellen eye chart（スネレン視力表）を使用する．表記の仕方も小数で示す日本の視力検査と違い，分数で示す．分子は被検者と視力表までの距離を示し，米国では一般に 20 フィート離れた所から視力測定するので 20 となる．分母は，被検者が 20 フィートの位置から識別できる文字の大きさを，標準視力の人であればどのくらい離れて識別することが可能かを表す．標準視力 20/20（twenty-twenty vision）は日本でいう視力 1.0 に相当し，例えば，20/40 は標準視力の人であれば 40 フィート離れた所から識別できる文字を 20 フィートの所でないと見えないということを示し，日本でいう視力 0.5 に相当する．メートル法を使う国では 6/6 vision のように 6 m を基準にする．英語で "You have 20/20 [6/6] vision. / Your visual acuity is 20/20 [6/6]." は直訳すると「あなたの視力は 1.0 です．」となるが，慣用的に「あなたの視力は正常です」という意味に用いられる．

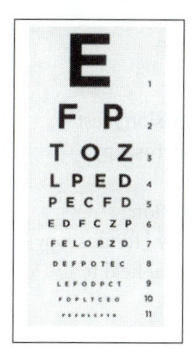

| 米国（例） | 日本 |
|---|---|
| 20/10 | 2.0 |
| 20/20 | 1.0 |
| 20/40 | 0.5 |
| 20/200 | 0.1 |

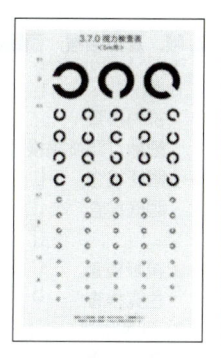

# 用語・表現ファイル

## 検査項目

### 1. 一般検査

| | |
|---|---|
| 血液検査 | blood test |
| 尿検査 | urine test [urinalysis] |
| 便検査 | stool test |
| X線検査 | X-ray |
| CT [コンピュータ断層撮影] | CT [computed tomography] scan |
| MRI [磁気共鳴断層撮影] | MRI [magnetic resonance imaging] |
| 超音波検査 | ultrasound |
| 内視鏡検査 | endoscopy |
| 細菌検査 | bacteriological examination |
| (痰／尿／血液) 培養検査 | (sputum/urine/blood) culture |
| 病理検査 | pathological examination |
| 細胞診 [組織診] | cytology [histology] |
| アレルギー検査 | allergy test |

### 2. 眼, 耳鼻咽喉, 頭頸部

1) 眼

| | |
|---|---|
| 視力検査 | visual acuity [vision] test |
| 細隙灯顕微鏡検査 | slit lamp biomicroscopy |
| 眼圧検査 | tonometry |
| 眼底検査 | fundal examination, ophthalmoscopy [funduscopy] |
| 視野検査 | perimetry [visual field test] |
| 色覚検査 | color vision test |

2) 耳鼻咽喉

| | |
|---|---|
| 聴力検査 | audiometry [hearing test] |
| ティンパノメトリー | tympanometry |
| 鼻咽喉内視鏡検査 | nasopharyngoscopy, rhinolaryngoscopy |
| 副鼻腔X線 [CT／MRI] | sinus X-ray [CT/MRI] |
| 平衡機能検査 | balance and vestibular function test |
| 嗅覚検査 | olfactometry [smell test] |
| 味覚検査 | gustometry [taste test] |

## 用語・表現ファイル（つづき）

    嚥下造影検査                           barium swallowing study
3) 頭頸部
    甲状腺超音波検査                   thyroid ultrasound
    甲状腺シンチグラフィ             thyroid scan

### 3. 呼吸器系

  喀痰検査                              sputum test
  呼吸機能検査                         PFT〔pulmonary function test〕
  ツベルクリンテスト               tuberculin skin test
  動脈血ガス分析                     arterial blood gas analysis
  胸部Ｘ線〔CT／MRI〕           chest X-ray〔CT/MRI〕
  気管支鏡検査                         bronchoscopy
  胸腔鏡検査                           thoracoscopy
  胸腔穿刺〔胸水検査〕           thoracentesis〔pleural fluid analysis〕
  肺血流シンチグラフィ           pulmonary perfusion scan
  終夜睡眠ポリグラフィ           polysomnography〔sleep test〕

### 4. 心臓，血管系

  心電図                                  ECG〔electrocardiography〕
  ホルター心電図                     Holter ECG recording〔24hr ECG〕
  運動負荷検査                         exercise stress test
  心臓超音波検査                     echocardiography
  経食道心臓超音波検査           TEE〔transesophageal echocardiography〕
  頸動脈超音波検査                 carotid ultrasound
  心臓カテーテル検査             cardiac catheterization study
  冠動脈造影検査                     coronary angiography
  大動脈造影検査                     aortography
  （下肢）静脈造影検査           venography（of lower limbs）
  心筋血流シンチグラフィ         myocardial perfusion scan

### 5. 消化器系

  腹部超音波検査                     abdominal ultrasound

## 用語・表現ファイル(つづき)

|  |  |
|---|---|
| 上部消化管内視鏡検査 | upper endoscopy, EGD [esophagogastroduodenal endoscopy] |
| 大腸内視鏡検査 | colonoscopy |
| 超音波内視鏡検査 | ultrasonic endoscopy |
| 腹部X線〔CT／MRI〕 | abdominal X-ray〔CT/MRI〕 |
| 上部消化管造影検査 | upper GI [gastrointestinal] series, upper gastrointestinal radiography |
| 注腸造影検査 | barium enema |
| 内視鏡的逆行性胆管膵管造影検査 | ERCP [endoscopic retrograde cholangiopancreatography] |
| 磁気共鳴胆管膵管造影検査 | MRCP [magnetic resonance cholangiopancreatography] |
| 腹腔穿刺〔腹水検査〕 | abdominal paracentesis〔ascitic fluid analysis〕 |

### 6. 腎,泌尿器,男性生殖器系

|  |  |
|---|---|
| 尿流測定 | uroflowmetry |
| 膀胱内圧測定 | cystometry |
| 尿道括約筋筋電図 | urethral sphincter EMG [electromyography] |
| 腹部〔経直腸〕超音波検査 | abdominal〔transrectal〕ultrasound |
| 尿道膀胱鏡検査 | cystourethroscopy |
| 静脈性腎盂造影検査 | IVP [intravenous pyelography] |
| 逆行性腎盂造影検査 | retrograde pyelography |
| (逆行性)膀胱造影検査 | (retrograde) cystography |
| (逆行性)尿道造影検査 | (retrograde) urethrography |
| 排尿時膀胱尿道造影検査 | voiding cystourethrography |
| 腎シンチグラフィ | renal scan |
| 精液検査 | semen analysis |

### 7. 乳房,女性生殖器系

|  |  |
|---|---|
| 乳房超音波検査 | breast ultrasound |
| 乳房X線検査 | mammography |
| 基礎体温測定 | basal body temperature charting |

## 用語・表現ファイル（つづき）

| 妊娠試験 | pregnancy test |
| --- | --- |
| 経腟超音波検査 | transvaginal ultrasound |
| 子宮頸部擦過細胞診 | Pap smear |
| 子宮内膜組織診 | endometrial biopsy |
| 腟拡大鏡検査 | colposcopy |
| 子宮鏡検査 | hysteroscopy |
| 腹腔鏡検査 | laparoscopy |
| 子宮卵管造影検査 | hysterosalpingography |
| 羊水穿刺 | amniocentesis |
| 染色体検査 | chromosome analysis |
| 性交後試験（ヒューナーテスト） | post coital test |

### 8. 内分泌系

| ブドウ糖負荷試験 | GTT [glucose tolerance test] |
| --- | --- |

### 9. 血液系

| 骨髄穿刺 | bone marrow aspiration |
| --- | --- |
| 骨髄生検 | bone marrow biopsy |
| リンパ節生検 | lymph node biopsy |

### 10. 骨，関節，運動器

| 脊髄腔造影検査 | myelography |
| --- | --- |
| 骨密度測定 | bone density test |
| 骨シンチグラフィ | bone scan |

### 11. 神経，筋

| 頭部 X 線 | skull [head] X-ray |
| --- | --- |
| 脳 CT [MRI] | brain CT [MRI] |
| 脳血管造影検査 | cerebral angiography |
| 磁気共鳴血管造影検査 | MRA [magnetic resonance angiography] |
| デジタル減算血管造影検査 | DSA [digital subtraction angiography] |

## 用語・表現ファイル（つづき）

| | |
|---|---|
| 脳血流 SPECT | brain SPECT [single photon emission computed tomography] |
| 腰椎穿刺〔髄液検査〕 | lumbar puncture〔cerebrospinal fluid analysis〕 |
| 脳波検査 | EEG [electroencephalography] |
| 筋電図検査 | EMG [electromyography] |

**12. その他**

| | |
|---|---|
| ガリウムシンチグラフィ | Gallium scan |
| 陽電子放出断層撮影 | PET [positron emission tomography] |

chapter 7

# 薬剤投与

## Medications

薬の処方箋 298
薬剤の服用歴 300
用法・用量 303
服薬・使用上の注意 313
保管上の注意 317
副作用 318

## 薬の処方箋

治療のための薬をさしあげます．

- ☐ I'm going to [Let me] give you medication for your illness.★

薬は…でお出しします．
1. 錠剤
2. 丸薬
3. 粉薬［散剤］
4. 水薬
5. 軟膏
6. 坐薬
7. 目薬［点眼薬］
8. 舌の下に入れる薬［舌下錠］
9. 湿布薬

— この薬は…日〔週〕分です．

— 2種類の飲み薬がでています．

- ☐ I'm going to [Let me] give you...
    1. some tablets.
    2. some pills.
    3. powder.
    4. a liquid medication.
    5. an ointment.
    6. a suppository.
    7. eyedrops.
    8. a medication under your tongue.
    9. a compress [poultice].

— This medication is for＿＿＿days〔weeks〕.

— You'll take two kinds of medication.

この薬はジェネリック医薬品［後発医薬品］にすることができます．

— ジェネリックをお使いになりますか．

— ジェネリック医薬品はブランド医薬品［先発医薬品］と安全性や効果の点で変わりありません．

— 日本ではこの薬のジェネリック医薬品はありません．

- ☐ Generic forms of this medication are available.

— Would you like to use generic medications?

— Generic medications are as safe and effective as the brand name products.

— Generic forms of this medication are not available in Japan.

これが薬の処方箋です．

— 処方箋はどこの調剤薬局へ持って行ってもいいですよ．

— 薬は病院内の薬局でもらって下さい．

- ☐ This is a prescription for your medication.

— You can have the prescription filled at any outside pharmacy.

— Please get your medication from the hospital pharmacy.

---

★ 一般的には medicine, drug ともいう．しかし医療関係者は medication のほうを多く用いる．

| | |
|---|---|
| ―処方箋を薬局の窓口にお出し下さい. | ― Give the prescription at the counter of the pharmacy. |
| ―会計を済ませてから,薬局で薬をもらって下さい. | ― Pay at the cashier's window, and then pick up your medication at the pharmacy. |

もし…ときは連絡して下さい.　　　　☐ Please call me〔us〕…
1. (2, 3日たっても) 症状が改善しない
2. 症状が前よりひどくなる
3. 予期しない副作用がみられる
4. 何かご質問がある

1. if your symptoms don't improve (within a few days).
2. if your symptoms become worse.
3. if you notice any unexpected side effects.
4. if you have any questions.

今日は薬がありません.　　　　☐ You don't need any medication today.

(患者さんが日本では認可されていない薬を要求した場合) その薬は日本では手に入りません.　　　　☐ That medication is not available in Japan.

---

### 名句・ことわざ

#### Bitter pills may have blessed effects.
#### 苦い薬はよく効く

"Good medicine is bitter in the mouth [tastes bitter to the mouth]." (よい薬は口に苦い) ともいう. 日本の「良薬口に苦し」に相当する.

## 薬剤の服用歴

### ⇒ 使用中の薬

| | |
|---|---|
| 現在，薬を飲んで〔使って〕いますか． | ☐ Are you now taking 〔using〕 any drugs or medications? |
| 最近2, 3週間の間に飲んだ〔使った〕薬が何かありますか． | ☐ Have you taken 〔used〕 any drugs or medications in the past few weeks? |
| その薬は…ですか．<br>　1．処方薬<br>　2．市販薬 | ☐ Are they...<br>　1．prescription medications?<br>　2．over-the-counter medications? |
| どこで〔どの病院で〕処方してもらいましたか． | ☐ Where 〔In which hospital〕 did you get the prescription? |
| その薬をお持ちでしたら，見せて下さい． | ☐ If you have them with you now, please show them to me. |
| お薬手帳を持っていますか． | ☐ Do you have your personal medication record? |
| ―持っていたら見せて下さい． | ― If you have it with you now, please show it to me. |
| この薬をなぜ飲んで〔使って〕いるのですか． | ☐ Why are you taking 〔using〕 this medication? |
| 飲み〔使い〕始めてどのくらいになりますか． | ☐ How long have you taken 〔used〕 it? |
| 何回くらい飲んで〔使って〕いますか．<br>　1．1日1回．<br>　2．1日2回．<br>　3．1日3回．<br>　4．もっと多い回数で． | ☐ How often do you take 〔use〕 it?<br>　1．Once a day?<br>　2．Twice a day?<br>　3．Three times a day?<br>　4．More often? |

|  |  |
|---|---|
| 1回にどのくらいの量を飲み〔使い〕ますか. | How much do you take〔use〕at one time? |
| 時々飲む〔使う〕薬がありますか. | Is there any medication you take〔use〕only once in a while? |

## ● 補完代替医療品（サプリメント）

現在サプリメントを使って〔飲んで〕いますか.
Do you currently use〔drink〕any dietary [nutritional] supplements?

—それは何ですか.
— What is it?
1. ビタミン剤.
2. ミネラル.
3. カルシウム.
4. 食物繊維.
5. 薬草.
6. その他.

1. Vitamins?
2. Minerals?
3. Calcium?
4. Dietary fiber?
5. Herbs?
6. Other?

## ● 処方する薬について

|  |  |
|---|---|
| この薬を飲んだ〔使った〕ことがありますか. | Have you ever taken〔used〕this medication before? |
| それはいつのことですか. | When? |
| 何のためでしたか. | For what? |
| 1日にどのくらいの量を飲み〔使い〕ましたか. | How much did you take〔use〕a day? |
| どのくらいの期間でしたか. | For how long? |
| その薬は効果がありましたか. | Did it help? |
| 副作用がありましたか. | Did you have any side effects from it? |

## → アレルギーについて

薬に対するアレルギーがあります か．
―どの薬に対するアレルギーですか．
―どんな症状を起こしますか．

☐ Are you allergic to any medications?
— Which medications?
— What happens to you?

以前に発疹，蕁麻疹，呼吸困難，めまいなどのアレルギーを起こしたことがありますか．

☐ Have you ever had any allergic reaction, such as a rash, hives, breathing difficulties, or dizziness?

これまでに薬の副作用はありましたか．
―その薬の名前を教えてください．

―どんな副作用でしたか．

☐ Have you ever had any side effects after taking medications?
— What's the name of the medication?
— What kind of side effects?

---

**名句・ことわざ**

An apple a day keeps the doctor away.
1日1個のりんごで医者いらず

## 用法・用量

☞「頻度の表現」(321 ページ).

### ➔ 一般的な説明

| | |
|---|---|
| 薬の説明書をお渡しいたしますので，よく読んで下さい． | ☐ Here are the instructions on your medication. Please read them carefully. |
| この薬はきちんと［規則正しく］飲んで〔使って〕下さい． | ☐ Please take〔use〕this medication regularly. |
| この薬は指示されたとおりに飲んで〔使って〕下さい． | ☐ Please take〔use〕this medication exactly as directed. |
| この薬は検査の説明書に従ってお飲み下さい． | ☐ Please take this medication according to the printed instructions on your test. |

### ➔ 内服薬

この…飲んで下さい．
 1. 錠剤は 1 回…錠
 2. 丸薬は 1 回…粒
 3. カプセルは 1 回…カプセル
 4. 粉薬は 1 回…包み
 5. シロップは 1 回…目盛り

☐ Please take...
 1. ____tablet(s) each time.
 2. ____pill(s) each time.
 3. ____capsule(s) each time.
 4. ____packet(s) each time.
 5. ____portion(s) of syrup each time.

この薬は…飲んで下さい．
 1. 1 日…回
 2. …時間おきに

☐ Please take this medication...
 1. ____times a day.
 2. every____hours.

この薬は…飲んで下さい．
 1. 起床時に
 2. 食前…分に
 3. 食直前に
 4. 食事と一緒に
 5. 食直後に

☐ Please take this medication...
 1. when you get up.
 2. ____minutes before meals.
 3. right before meals [food].
 4. with meals.
 5. right after meals [eating].

| | |
|---|---|
| 6. 食後…分に | 6. ____minutes after meals. |
| 7. 朝食後〔昼食後／夕食後〕 | 7. after breakfast 〔lunch/supper〕. |
| 8. 食間に | 8. between meals. |
| 9. 寝る前に | 9. before you go to bed. |
| 10. 運動の前に | 10. before you exercise. |
| 11. 朝…時頃 | 11. about____o'clock in the morning. |
| 12. 空腹時〔食事の1時間前か2時間後〕に | 12. on an empty stomach 〔1 hour before or 2 hours after meals〕. |

| | |
|---|---|
| この薬は…に飲んで〔使って〕下さい. | ☐ Please take 〔use〕 this medication… |
| 1. 痛みがあるとき | 1. when you feel pain. when you are in pain. |
| 2. …℃より高い熱が出たとき | 2. when you have a fever over ____degrees Celsius. |
| 3. 胸が重苦しいとき | 3. when you feel pressure in your chest. |
| 4. 咳がひどいとき | 4. when you have a bad cough. |
| 5. 吐き気があるとき | 5. when you feel sick to your stomach. when you're nauseated. |
| 6. 下痢をしたとき | 6. when you have diarrhea. |
| 7. 便秘しているとき | 7. when you're constipated. |
| 8. 発作を起こしたとき | 8. when you have an attack. |
| 9. かゆいとき | 9. when you feel itchy. |
| 10. 眠れないとき | 10. when you can't sleep. |
| 11. ひきつけを起こしたとき | 11. when you have seizures. |
| 12. 本当に必要なとき(この薬には習慣性があるからです) | 12. when you really need it (because it may be habit-forming). |

| | |
|---|---|
| この薬は1回飲んだ〔使った〕ら,次回までかならず…時間あけて下さい. | ☐ Please be sure to wait for____hours before taking 〔using〕 another dose. |

| | |
|---|---|
| このお薬は…飲んで下さい. | ☐ Please take this medication… |
| 1. コップ一杯の水で | 1. with a (full) glass of water. |
| 2. 多めの水で | 2. with a lot of water. |

3. 噛むか口の中で溶かしながら

この薬は割ったり，つぶしたり，噛んだりしないで下さい．
―この薬は噛んでもいいですよ．
―飲みにくいときは，つぶして…に混ぜてもいいですよ．

1. お湯
2. やわらかい食べ物

この粉薬が飲みにくいときはアップルジュースやアイスクリームに混ぜてお飲み下さい．
―乳酸飲料〔スポーツ飲料〕に混ぜると苦くなります．

―食べ物や飲み物に混ぜないでお飲み下さい．
―飲みにくいときはオブラートに包んでお飲み下さい．

―スポイトを使うと飲みやすいです．

この薬と一緒に…を飲まないで下さい．
1. アルコール
2. 紅茶，緑茶，コーヒー
3. 牛乳

この薬と一緒に…を食べないで下さい．
1. グレープフルーツ
2. 納豆
3. ブロッコリーやホーレン草など緑黄野菜

3. by chewing or dissolving in the mouth.

☐ Please don't break, crush, or chew this medication.
— You can chew this medication.
— If you can't swallow this medication, you can crush and mix it...
1. in warm water.
2. in soft food.

☐ If you can't swallow this powder, you can mix it with apple juice or ice cream.
— If you mix it with a lactic acid beverage〔sports drink〕, it'll become bitter.
— Please take this powder without mixing it with food or drinks.
— If you can't swallow this powder, you can wrap it up in wafer paper and take it.
— It'll be easy to take the medication if you use a dropper.

☐ Please don't drink...with this medication.
1. alcohol
2. black tea, green tea, or coffee
3. milk

☐ Please don't eat...with this medication.
1. grapefruit
2. natto
3. green vegetables like broccoli or spinach

chapter 7 薬剤投与

## ● 舌下錠

| | |
|---|---|
| この錠剤は舌の下に入れたまま溶かして下さい. | ☐ Please dissolve this tablet under your tongue. |
| この錠剤は噛んだり,飲み込んだりしないで,溶けるまでそのまま舌の下に入れておいて下さい. | ☐ Don't chew or swallow this tablet but keep it under your tongue until it melts. |
| 薬を使用すると少しふらふらするので,座った状態で服用して下さい. | ☐ You may feel a little dizzy, so please sit down while taking this medication. |
| 舌に入れると少しひりひりするでしょう. | ☐ You should feel some burning when it's under your tongue. |
| 1,2分で効果が現れます. | ☐ The medication will start working in a minute or two. |
| 5分しても胸の痛みがあるときはもう1錠追加してみて下さい. | ☐ If you still have chest pain after 5 minutes, you can take one more tablet. |
| それでも激しい痛みが続くようであれば,こちらに連絡するか病院の救急外来を受診して下さい. | ☐ If severe pain still persists, contact us or go to the emergency room in the hospital. |

## 🔵 うがい薬

1 目盛りを約 60 ml の水で薄めて下さい.
☐ Please dilute one unit of this solution in about 60 milliliter water.

1 包を約 100 ml の水〔ぬるま湯〕で溶かして下さい.
☐ Please dissolve one packet in about 100 milliliter water 〔lukewarm water〕.

うがいして 1, 2 分口の中に含んでいて下さい.
☐ Gargle and hold it in your mouth for 1 to 2 minutes.

飲み込まないようにして下さい.
☐ Be careful not to swallow it.

## 🔵 吸入薬

吸入器を軽く 3, 4 回振って下さい.
☐ Please shake the inhaler gently 3 to 4 times.

息をゆっくり,十分に吐いて下さい.
☐ Breathe out slowly, all the way.

吸入口 [マウスピース] を…下さい.
☐ Put the mouthpiece (of the inhaler)…

1. 開けた口から 3, 4 cm 離して
2. 口にくわえ唇をしっかり閉じて

1. 3 to 4 centimeters away from your open mouth.
2. in your mouth with your lips closed tightly around it.

ゆっくり息を吸い込むのと同時に吸入器を押して下さい.
☐ Breathe in slowly and push down on the inhaler at the same time.

吸入後は約 10 秒間息を止めて下さい.
―これで薬が気道にとどまるでしょう.
☐ Hold your breath for about 10 seconds.
― This will allow the medication to settle into your airways.

マウスピースをはずして,ゆっくり息を吐いて下さい.
☐ Take the mouthpiece away from your mouth and breathe out slowly.

chapter 7 薬剤投与

| | |
|---|---|
| 吸入後はうがいをして下さい． | ☐ Gargle after using your inhaler. |
| 吸入器は1日〜回，…吸入ずつ，定期的に使用して下さい． | ☐ Use the inhaler regularly, and take____puffs 〜 times a day. |
| 発作時のみ吸入器を使用して下さい． | ☐ Use the inhaler only when you have attacks. |
| 使用間隔は…時間あけて下さい． | ☐ Wait____hours before using it again. |
| 1日…回まで使用できます． | ☐ You can use it____times a day. |

## ● 点眼・点耳・点鼻薬

| | |
|---|---|
| 1日〜回，…に1, 2滴さして下さい． | ☐ Please put one or two... 〜 times a day. |
| 1. 目薬［点眼薬］を片目〔両目〕 | 1. （eye）drops in one eye〔both eyes〕 |
| 2. 点鼻薬を片方〔両方〕の鼻孔 | 2. （nose）drops in one nostril〔both nostrils〕 |
| 3. 点耳薬を片耳〔両耳〕 | 3. （ear）drops in one ear〔both ears〕 |
| 1度に1滴ずつさして下さい． | ☐ Put one drop at a time. |
| 2種類以上の目薬を使用するときは5分以上たってから点眼して下さい． | ☐ When you use more than two kinds of eye drops, wait about 5 minutes between each kind. |
| 目から流れ出た点眼液はふき取って下さい． | ☐ Wipe off extra drops trickling down your cheeks. |
| 容器の先端が目に触れないようにして下さい． | ☐ Be careful not to allow the tip of the eyedropper to touch your eyes. |

## ◯ 坐薬

| | |
|---|---|
| この坐薬は肛門に挿入して下さい. | ☐ Please insert this suppository into your anus.★ |
| —できれば排便後に入れて下さい. | — Insert it after you have had a bowel movement, if possible. |
| —直腸の中へ深く押し込んで下さい. | — Push it deeply into the rectum. |
| —できれば少なくとも1時間,排便をがまんして下さい. | — Try not to empty your bowels for at least an hour, if possible. |
| 1度挿入したら,次の挿入まで…時間待って下さい. | ☐ Once inserted, please wait＿＿ hours before inserting another suppository. |
| 浣腸薬は体温よりやや高め〔40℃程度〕に温めて下さい. | ☐ Please warm the enema solution slightly above body temperature 〔about 40 degrees Celsius〕. |
| —肛門部分にオリーブ油〔ワセリン／コールドクリーム〕をたっぷり塗って下さい. | — Lubricate your anal area with a generous amount of olive oil 〔vaseline/cold cream〕. |
| —肛門にノズルをゆっくり押しながら挿入して下さい. | — Insert the nozzle into the anus with gentle pressure. |

---

★ anus という語に不快感をもつ患者さんもいる.その場合には,直腸を表す rectum,または rectal opening を用いるとよい.

## ➔ 軟膏・クリーム・ローション

| | |
|---|---|
| 使用する前に,患部を石鹸と水で洗い,すっかり乾かして下さい. | ☐ Before applying this medication, please wash the affected area with soap and water, and dry thoroughly. |
| この軟膏〔クリーム〕を患部に1日…回塗って下さい. | ☐ Please apply this ointment〔cream〕to the area＿＿times a day. |
| ―患部に薄く塗って下さい. | ― Apply a thin layer of this ointment〔cream〕to the area. |
| ―軽く〔よく〕擦り込んで下さい. | ― Rub in the ointment〔cream〕gently〔well〕. |
| このローションを患部に1日…回2,3滴つけて下さい. | ☐ Please apply a few drops of this lotion to the area＿＿times a day. |
| ―ビンはよく振ってから使って下さい. | ― Shake the bottle well before using it. |
| ―ローションが見えなくなるまで軽く擦り込んで下さい. | ― Rub in the lotion gently until it disappears. |
| この薬は目や目の周りには使わないで下さい. | ☐ Please don't use this medication in or around the eyes. |

## ➔ 湿布薬

温〔冷〕湿布を…に貼って下さい．
1. 足
2. 肩
3. 背中
4. 腰

☐ Please apply a hot〔cold〕 compress to...
1. your leg(s).
2. your shoulder(s).
3. your back.
4. your lower back.

湿布は1日に1，2回貼って下さい．

☐ Apply the compress once or twice a day.

---

### 名句・ことわざ

**Charity begins at home.**
愛はわが家から始まる

「すべては身近なところから（しかしそこで終わってはいけない）」という意味．英国の医師であり文人としても名高いブラウン（Sir Thomas Browne, 1605-1682）は著書『医師の信仰 *Religio Medici*』にこのことわざを引用して，自分を含め身近な人を愛さずして「他人に対して愛を注ぐことなど期待できるはずがない」と述べた．charity は「慈愛・思いやり・寛容さ」などの意味を含む．

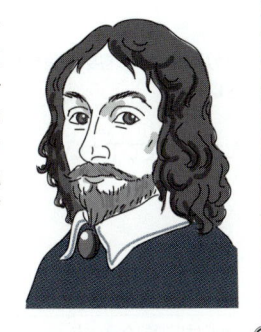

## ➡ 注射薬

| | |
|---|---|
| 注射をしましょう. | ☐ I'm going to [Let me] give you an injection [a shot].★ |
| …をしましょう.<br>　1. 皮下注射<br>　2. 筋肉内注射<br>　3. 静脈内注射<br>　4. 点滴 | ☐ I'm going to [Let me] give you…<br>　1. a subcutaneous injection.<br>　2. an intramuscular injection.<br>　3. an intravenous injection.<br>　4. an intravenous drip. |
| 場所は…にします.<br>　1. 右〔左〕腕<br>　2. お腹<br>　3. 太もも | ☐ I'm giving the injection in…<br>　1. your right〔left〕arm.<br>　2. your abdomen.<br>　3. your thigh. |
| アルコール消毒でかぶれることがありますか. | ☐ Do you ever get a skin rash from using alcohol wipes [swabs]? |
| それでは注射をしますね. ごめんなさい. ちょっとチクンとしますよ. | ☐ Here we go. Sorry. I know it stings. |
| 腕を楽にして下さい. 緊張しないで下さい. | ☐ Just relax your arm. Don't tense up. |
| 手を握ったり開いたりして下さい. | ☐ Make a fist, and then open it. |
| 点滴は約2時間かかります. | ☐ This (intravenous) drip will take about 2 hours. |
| ご自分で点滴の速度を調節しないで下さい. | ☐ Please don't adjust the drip rate yourself. |
| 痛んだら教えて下さい. | ☐ Let me know when it hurts. |

---

★ "shot" は口語的な言い方.

# 服薬・使用上の注意

## ➔ 一般的な注意

この薬を飲んで〔使って〕いる間は…下さい.
1. 運転しないで
2. 危険があるような作業はしないで
3. お酒は控えて
4. 授乳しないで

☐ While taking〔using〕this medication, please...
1. don't drive your car.
2. don't perform potentially dangerous tasks.
3. don't drink alcohol.
4. don't breast-feed.

この薬は 4, 5 日〔週／月〕間飲み〔使い〕続けて下さい.

☐ Please continue taking〔using〕this medication for several days〔weeks/months〕.

この薬は…週間〔日〕以内に飲みきって〔使いきって〕下さい.

☐ You have to take all of〔use up〕this medication within＿＿＿ weeks〔days〕.

症状がよくなっても最後まで飲み〔使い〕続けて下さい.

☐ Please continue taking〔using〕this medication for the full course of treatment even if your symptoms have disappeared.

ご自分の判断でやめないで下さい.

☐ Don't quit taking〔using〕this medication on your own.

他の人に薬をあげないで下さい.

☐ Don't give your medication to others.

他の人に処方された薬は絶対に飲まないで〔使わないで〕下さい.

☐ Never take〔use〕someone else's prescription medications.

## ⊃ 飲み忘れ・飲みすぎ

| | |
|---|---|
| 飲むのを忘れないで下さい. | ☐ Please don't miss any doses. |
| 飲み忘れたときには，すぐに飲んで下さい. | ☐ If you miss a dose of this medication, take it as soon as possible. |
| 次の服用が近いときには飲み忘れた分はとばして下さい. | ☐ Skip the missed dose if it is almost time for your next dose. |
| 次回から元のスケジュールに戻して下さい. | ☐ Go back to your regular dosing schedule next time. |
| 1回飲んだら，次のときまで最低…時間あけて下さい. | ☐ Be sure to wait for at least ____ hours before taking another dose. |
| 1度に2回分を飲まないで下さい. | ☐ Please don't take 2 doses at the same time. |

## ⊃ 妊娠・授乳

| | |
|---|---|
| 妊娠していますか．何週ですか． | ☐ Are you pregnant? How many weeks? |
| 妊娠を考えていますか． | ☐ Are you planning to become pregnant? |
| 授乳していますか． | ☐ Are you breast-feeding? |
| この薬は妊娠中〔授乳中〕でも服用〔使用〕できます． | ☐ You can take 〔use〕 this medication while you are pregnant 〔breast-feeding〕. |
| この薬は妊娠中〔授乳中〕には服用〔使用〕できません． | ☐ You must not take 〔use〕 this medication while you are pregnant 〔breast-feeding〕. |
| ―授乳〔妊娠〕を控えて下さい． | ― Please refrain from breast-feeding 〔becoming pregnant〕. |

## ● 医師・看護師への相談

私達〔医師／看護師〕に…相談して下さい.
1. 処方薬,市販薬をとわず,新たな薬を飲む〔使う〕前には
2. 妊娠したときには
3. 妊娠を考えているときには

☐ Please check with us〔the doctor/the nurse〕…
1. before you begin taking〔using〕any new medication, either prescription or over-the-counter.
2. if you become pregnant.
3. if you are planning to become pregnant.

もし…ときは連絡して下さい.
1. 症状が改善しない
2. 症状が前よりひどくなった
3. 予期しない副作用がみられる
4. 何かご質問がある

☐ Please call me〔us〕…
1. if your symptoms don't improve.
2. if your symptoms become worse.
3. if you notice any unexpected side effects.
4. if you have any questions.

薬がなくなったらおいで下さい.

☐ After your medication has run out, please see me〔us〕again.

---

名句・ことわざ

**Sleep is better than medicine.**
睡眠は薬にまさる

## ● 緊急用カード・携行品

| | |
|---|---|
| 緊急用カードを所持して下さい. | ☐ Please carry your medical alert card with you. |
| (糖尿病の患者さんへ) 必ず…を所持して下さい.<br>1. 糖尿病 ID カード<br>2. あめ,砂糖,ブドウ糖錠剤 | ☐ Please always carry...with you.<br>1. your diabetic ID card<br>2. candies, sugar, or glucose tablets |
| (アレルギーの患者さんへ) アナフィラキシーへの初期対応のため,必ず自己注射用エピネフリンを所持して下さい. | ☐ Please always carry self-injectable epinephrine for first-aid management of anaphylactic reaction. |

## 保管上の注意

この薬は…保管して下さい．
1. 室温で
2. 冷蔵庫の中に
3. 強い熱や直射日光の当たらない所に
4. 涼しく，乾燥した所に
5. 小児の手の届かない所に

この薬は…日〔週／月〕以上たったら捨てて下さい．

☐ Please keep this medication...
1. at room temperature.
2. in the refrigerator.
3. away from excessive heat and direct light.
4. in a cool, dry space.
5. out of the reach of children.

☐ Please throw away this medication after____days 〔week(s)/month(s)〕.

## 副作用

この薬はいくらか副作用があります．
□ This medication has some side effects.

この薬の副作用は軽い〔まれ〕です．
□ The side effects of this medication are rather mild 〔rare〕.

副作用は飲み続けるかぎり続くかもしれません．
□ The side effects may continue as long as you take the medication.

体が薬に慣れるにつれて副作用はなくなるでしょう．
□ The side effects will go away as your body adjusts to the medication.

副作用は人によって異なります．
□ Side effects vary from person to person.

この薬を飲んで副作用が続いたり，辛かったりする場合には，私達〔医師〕にご相談下さい．
□ If the side effects of the medication continue or are bothersome, please check with us 〔the doctor〕.

## → 緊急を要する場合

…ときには，ただちに薬の使用を中止して，すぐに私達〔医師〕に連絡して下さい．

1. 呼吸困難が起こる
2. 息切れがする
3. ぜいぜいする
4. 胸が締めつけられる
5. 胸がドキドキする［異常な動悸を感じる］
6. まぶた，唇，舌，のどがひどく腫れる
7. 発疹や蕁麻疹が出る
8. 広範囲にわたるかゆみがある
9. 強いめまいがする
10. 吐き気と嘔吐がある
11. 気を失う［意識をなくす］
12. ひきつけや痙攣を起こす
13. 不安発作を起こす
14. その他の重い症状がある

☐ Please stop the medication at once and call us〔the doctor〕if you have…

1. difficulty breathing.
2. shortness of breath.
3. wheezing.
4. squeezing pain in your chest.
5. pounding of your heart [abnormal palpitations].
6. severe swelling of your eyelids, lips, tongue, or throat.
7. a rash or hives.
8. extensive itchiness.
9. severe dizziness.
10. nausea and vomiting.
11. loss of consciousness.
12. seizures or convulsions.
13. an anxiety attack.
14. other serious symptoms.

---

### 名句・ことわざ

**Knowledge comes, but wisdom lingers.**
知識の習得はたやすい，知恵の修得には時がかかる

英国の詩人テニスン（Alfred Tennyson, 1809-1892, "Locksley Hall"）の名句．

## ● 副作用の一般的な症状

この薬を飲む〔使う〕と，時には…のような症状が出るかもしれません．

1. 食欲不振
2. 胃の不調
3. 腹部の膨満感
4. 吐き気
5. 下痢
6. 便秘
7. ガス
8. 頭痛
9. めまい，ふらふら感
10. 眠気，うとうと感
11. 口の渇き
12. 湿疹
13. かゆみ
14. 多毛
15. 脱毛
16. 体重増加
17. 体重減少
18. 不規則な月経
19. 頻尿
20. 尿の色の変化
21. 疲労感
22. 筋肉痛
23. 動悸
24. 手の震え
25. 咳
26. 出血傾向

☐ With this medication you may sometimes have such symptoms as...

1. loss of appetite.
2. upset stomach.
3. a feeling of fullness in the abdomen.
4. nausea.
5. diarrhea.
6. constipation.
7. gas.
8. headache.
9. dizziness or lightheadedness.
10. sleepiness or drowsiness.
11. dry mouth.
12. skin rash.
13. itching.
14. hair growth.
15. hair loss.
16. weight gain.
17. weight loss.
18. irregular menstrual periods.
19. frequent urination.
20. change of the color of urine.
21. fatigue.
22. muscle pain.
23. palpitations.
24. shaky hands.
25. coughing.
26. a tendency to bleed.

## 用語・表現ファイル

### 頻度の表現

#### 1. よく使う表現

| | |
|---|---|
| 毎時間 | every hour |
| 毎日 | every day |
| 6時間ごと | every six hours |
| 4時間に1回 | once every four hours |
| 1日おき | every other day |
| 3日に1回 | every three days |
| 1日〔週〕1回〔2／3回〕 | once〔twice / three times〕a day〔week〕 |
| | |
| 朝に | in the morning |
| 食前に | before meals |
| 食後に | after meals |
| 食間に | between meals |
| 就寝時に | at bedtime |
| 必要に応じて | when you need it |

#### 2. 頻度を表わす副詞

"How often...?" と尋ねた場合，患者の表現には個人差があり，主観的要素が含まれるが，おおよその目安として頻度の高い順にあげると，

always → usually → often [frequently] → sometimes →
いつも　　たいてい　　頻繁に　　　　　　　　時々

occasionally → rarely [seldom] → never
たまに　　　　　まれに　　　　　一度もない

# chapter 8

# 手術

## Surgical Consultation

インフォームド・コンセント　324
手術の説明　325
麻酔の説明　327
手術当日　330
手術後　331
自宅ケア　333

## インフォームド・コンセント

| | |
|---|---|
| 現在の症状を改善させるには〔皮膚がんを除去するには〕手術が必要です． | ☐ You need to have surgery to relieve your present symptoms 〔to remove your skin cancer〕. |
| この手術を行うためにあなたの同意が必要です． | ☐ I need your consent to do this surgery. |
| 他の治療法としては抗がん剤や放射線治療がありますが，根治が望めない可能性もあります． | ☐ There are other treatments besides surgery, such as chemotherapy〔anticancer drugs〕or radiotherapy, but a complete cure may not be obtained. |
| 手術に伴う合併症としては薬剤によるアレルギー，出血，感染などがあります． | ☐ There are possible complications involved with this surgery, such as allergic reactions to the medications, bleeding, or infection. |
| 輸血を行う場合もあります． | ☐ You may need a blood transfusion. |
| この同意書をよく読んで，サインして下さい． | ☐ Please read this (informed) consent form carefully and sign it. |
| —どなたかサインしてくれる人はいますか． | — Do you have anyone who can sign it for you? |
| ご質問がありますか． | ☐ (Do you have) any questions? |

☞「インフォームド・コンセントのサンプル」(429 ページ)．

## 手術の説明

手術は…を予定しています．

1. 白内障手術
2. 鼓室形成術
3. 肺葉切除術
4. 冠動脈バイパス術

5. 虫垂切除術
6. 腹腔鏡下胆嚢摘出術
7. 乳房温存術
8. 広汎子宮全摘術
9. 経尿道的膀胱腫瘍切除術

10. 脳動脈瘤クリッピング
11. アキレス腱縫合術

水曜日午前に手術の予定です．

—手術の前に血液検査，心電図，胸部X線検査，それに呼吸機能検査が必要です．
—現在飲んでいる処方薬をすべて病院へ（来院するときに）持ってきて下さい．

手術の3日前から特別な食事になります．

—（胃の中を空にするため）夜の12時を過ぎてからは，何も口にしないで下さい．
—これは手術中に吐いたり，胃の中のものを吸い込んだりしないために重要です．

—薬を少しの水で飲むのはかまいません．

☐ Your surgery is...
☐ You're having...
 1. cataract surgery.
 2. tympanoplasty.
 3. lobectomy.
 4. heart bypass surgery [coronary artery bypass grafting].
 5. appendectomy.
 6. laparoscopic cholecystectomy.
 7. breast conserving surgery.
 8. radical hysterectomy.
 9. transurethral resection of the bladder tumor.
 10. cerebral aneurysm clipping.
 11. Achilles tendon repair.

☐ Your surgery is scheduled for Wednesday morning.

— Before surgery you need a blood test, an ECG, chest X-rays, and a pulmonary function test.
— Please bring all your prescription medications with you (when you come to the hospital).

☐ You have to go on a special diet 3 days before the surgery.
— Don't eat, drink, or chew anything after midnight (to keep your stomach empty).
— This is important to prevent vomiting and breathing (in) stomach contents during the surgery.
— You can take your medication with a small sip of water.

— 腸の中を空にするための下剤をさしあげます．
— 手術前の 24 時間はアルコール類を飲まないで下さい．
— 手術前は禁煙して下さい．

— I'm going to give you laxative drugs to empty your bowel.
— Don't drink any alcohol within 24 hours of the surgery.
— Please stop smoking before the surgery.

10 日間ほどの入院が必要です．

☐ You have to stay in the hospital for about 10 days.

退院可能であると判断した場合には〔麻酔が覚めたら〕手術当日の夕方家に帰ることができます．

☐ You can go home the evening of your surgery if we think that you are ready for discharge〔if you have recovered from the anesthesia〕.

ご家族かお友達で…がいますか．

1. 病院への送り迎えのできる人

2. 手術後 1 週間世話をしてくれる人

☐ Do you have someone in your family or a friend...

1. who can come with you to the hospital and take you home?

2. who can look after you for the first week after surgery?

麻酔については，後で麻酔医から詳しい説明があります．

☐ Your anesthesiologist is going to give you the details of the anesthesia later.

## 麻酔の説明

| | |
|---|---|
| こんにちは，ヒルさん．麻酔医の佐野です． | ☐ Hello [Hi], Mr. [Mrs./Ms./Miss] Hill. I'm Dr. Sano, an anesthesiologist. |
| 麻酔についてご説明しましょう． | ☐ Let me tell you about your anesthesia. |
| 麻酔方法は…を予定しています．<br>　1. 全身麻酔〔吸入麻酔／静脈麻酔〕<br>　2. 局所麻酔〔脊椎麻酔／硬膜外麻酔〕 | ☐ You'll be given...<br>　1. general anesthesia 〔inhalation anesthesia/intravenous anesthesia〕.<br>　2. local anesthesia 〔spinal anesthesia/epidural anesthesia〕. |
| 全身麻酔ですので，手術中は眠っていて何も感じないでしょう． | ☐ You'll have general anesthesia, so you'll sleep and won't feel anything during the surgery. |
| —いつのまにか手術が終わって，目を覚ますことになりますよ． | — The surgery will be over before you know it and you'll be waking up again. |
| 局所麻酔なので手術中目が覚めているでしょう． | ☐ You'll have local anesthesia, so you'll be awake during the surgery. |
| これから少し質問させていただきます． | ☐ I'd like to ask a few questions [get some information from you]. |
| これまでに何か（大きな）病気をしたことがありますか． | ☐ Have you ever had any major illnesses? |
| 今どんな薬を飲んでいますか． | ☐ What medications are you now taking? |

| | |
|---|---|
| これまでに何か手術をしたことがありますか. | ☐ Have you ever had surgery? |
| —どんな手術ですか. | — What kind of surgery was it? |
| —それはいつでしたか. | — When was it? |
| —どこの病院ですか. | — In what hospital? |
| —麻酔は全身麻酔でしたか,局所麻酔でしたか. | — Was the anesthesia general or local? |
| —そのとき,何か問題が起こりましたか. | — Did you have any problems at that time? |
| 麻酔薬やその他の薬にアレルギーがありますか. | ☐ Do you have any allergies to anesthetics or other medications? |
| —どんな薬でアレルギー反応が起きましたか. | — What medications caused the allergic reactions? |
| —いつですか. | — When was it? |
| —どのような反応が起きましたか. | — What kind of reactions did you have? |
| —ご家族のどなたかに麻酔で問題が起こった人はいますか. | — Do you know if anyone in your immediate family has had problems with anesthesia? |
| ぐらぐらする歯がありますか. | ☐ Do you have any loose teeth? |
| 入れ歯やコンタクトレンズをしていますか. | ☐ Do you wear any dentures or contact lenses? |
| 入れ歯やコンタクトレンズ,指輪は手術前にはずして下さい. | ☐ Please take out your dentures or contact lenses, or take off your rings before the surgery. |
| 明日の手術の(具体的な)スケジュールをお話しましょう. | ☐ I'm going to [Let me] tell you about the schedule of tomorrow's surgery. |
| 明日の朝,リラックスできるように薬をさしあげます. | ☐ I'm going to give you some sedation that will make you feel relaxed tomorrow morning. |

| | |
|---|---|
| 8時に手術室へ移動していただきます． | You'll be escorted [transferred] to the operating room at 8 o'clock. |
| まず，心電計と血圧計などのモニターを装着します． | First, I'll attach ECG, blood pressure, and other monitors to your body. |
| それから腕に点滴します． | Then, I'm going to give you intravenous fluids. |
| その後，麻酔を開始します． | After that, I'm going to start giving you an anesthetic medication. |
| 心配しないで下さい．手術中はずっとおそばで診ていますから． | Please don't worry. I'll be with you the whole time for your care during the surgery. |
| 手術後は少し不快感をもたれるでしょうが，それは時間が経つにつれなくなります． | You'll have some discomfort after the surgery, but it will go away over time. |
| 手術後，2, 3日の間，のどが痛かったり，声が嗄れたりするかもしれません． | For a few days after the surgery, you may have throat pain or a hoarse voice. |
| 何かご質問がありますか． | (Do you have) any questions? |

# 手術当日

☞「確認,励まし,慰め,慰労」(242 ページ).

## ➡ 手術直前

| | |
|---|---|
| 準備のためにお腹の部分の毛を剃りましょう. | ☐ To prepare for your surgery, I'm going to [Let me] shave your abdomen. |
| 注射をします.眠くなりますよ. | ☐ I'm going to give you an injection. It will make you sleepy. |
| ―ご気分が悪くなったら手を上げて知らせて下さい. | ― If you feel sick, please let us know by raising your hand. |
| ―少しふらふらする感じがあるかもしれませんが,心配はいりません. | ― You might feel a little dizzy, but don't worry. |
| 顔にこのマスクをかけます. | ☐ I'm going to put this mask over your face. |
| ―楽な気持ちで,いつものように息をして下さい. | ― Just relax, and please breathe like you usually do. |

## ➡ 手術直後

| | |
|---|---|
| グレイさん,手術は終わりましたよ. | ☐ Now, you're finished, Mr. [Mrs./Ms./Miss] Gray. |
| 目〔口〕を開けて下さい. | ☐ Please open your eyes〔mouth〕. |
| 私の手を握って下さい. | ☐ Grasp my hand. |
| 深呼吸して下さい. | ☐ Take a deep [big] breath. |
| 手術はうまくいきましたよ. | ☐ Your surgery was successful. |
| 辛かったでしょうが,よく頑張りましたね. | ☐ You had a hard time, but you've made it. |
| 30 分ほどしてからお部屋に戻れます. | ☐ You can go back to your room in 30 minutes or so. |

## 手術後

ご気分はいかがですか．

□ How are you feeling now?

痛みますか．
―痛み始めたらすぐ教えて下さい．

―痛み止めの薬をさしあげましょう．

□ Are you in pain?
— Just let me know right away if it starts to hurt.
— I'm going to [Let me] give you pain medication.

深呼吸をしてみて下さい．
―始めに，手をお腹の上において下さい．
―鼻からできるだけ大きく息を吸い込んで下さい．お腹がもち上がるのがわかりますよ．
―ゆっくりと口から息を吐いてから体の力を抜いて楽にして下さい．
―目が覚めている間，これを１時間に５回以上繰り返して下さい．

□ Please try to take a deep breath.
— First, place your hand(s) on your abdomen.
— Breathe in through your nose as deeply as possible. You'll notice that your abdomen will rise.
— Breathe out through your mouth slowly, and relax.
— Repeat more than 5 times an hour while awake.

咳をしてみて下さい．

□ Please try to cough.

今は何も飲めません．

―口をゆすいであげましょう．

―ガスが出たら知らせて下さい．

―少しお腹が痛むかもしれません．

□ You can't drink anything at the moment.
— I'm going to [Let me] give you mouth wash.
— Please let us know when you have passed gas.
— You may have slight abdominal pain.

食事は流動食から始め，徐々に固形食になります．
―普通食が食べられます．

□ You can slowly progress from a liquid diet to solid food.
— You can eat regular meals now.

| | |
|---|---|
| 体の向きを変えるのをお手伝いしましょう. | I'm going to [Let me] help you change your position. |
| ―ご自分でも体の向きを変えて下さい. | — Try to turn from side to side yourself. |
| ―できるだけ早く歩くようにして下さい. | — Try to walk as soon as you can. |
| ―2時間ごとに起き上がって歩いて下さい. | — Try to get up and walk every two hours. |
| ―体を早く動かしていただくと,それだけ回復は早まります. | — The sooner we have you on the move, the quicker you'll start to heal. |
| 傷が治りしだい退院できます. | Once the wound has healed satisfactorily, you can leave the hospital. |
| ホッチキスの針をとりましょう. | I'm going to [Let me] take out the staples now. |
| 抜糸をしましょう. | I'm going to [Let me] take out the stitches. |
| 痛むかもしれませんが,ほんの一瞬ですよ. | This might hurt, but only for a second. |
| 抜糸は必要ありません. | We don't have to take out the stitches. |

---

### 名句・ことわざ

### All is well that ends well.
### 終わりよければすべてよし

英国の劇作家・詩人ヘイウッド (John Heywood, 1497? - 1580? *Be Merry Friends*) に由来することわざ. シェイクスピア (William Shakespeare) の喜劇のタイトルにもなっている. 大切なのは結末で, 目的が達成されれば, 途中の失敗・挫折・心配などは忘れ去られてしまうという意味.

## 自宅ケア

しばらくの間，切開した所が痛んだり，痒くなったり，感覚がなくなったりするかもしれません．
― 1，2 日，少し出血するかもしれません．
― 傷を閉じたテープ〔糸／留め金〕は乾いた状態にして 24 時間そのままにして下さい．
― シャワーを浴びるときは，傷口をぬるま湯と石鹸でそっと洗って下さい．
― 傷口をこすらないで下さい．

― 抗生物質の軟膏をぬってから，傷口に新しい包帯を巻いて下さい．

― 消毒は必要ありません．

アルコールは当分飲まないで下さい．

タバコは控えて下さい．

運転は 24 時間しないで下さい．

明日からシャワーを使うことができます．

お風呂もけっこうです．

☐ Your incision may be sore, itchy, or numb for a while.
― You may notice slight bleeding for a day or two.
― Please keep the strips of tape 〔sutures/staples〕 dry and intact for the first 24 hours.
― When you shower, gently wash your incision with warm water and soap.
― Avoid any rubbing on the wound.
― Please apply the antibiotic ointment and place a clean bandage over the wound.
― You don't have to sterilize the wound.

☐ You shouldn't drink alcohol for a while.

☐ You shouldn't smoke.

☐ You shouldn't drive your car for 24 hours.

☐ You can take a shower tomorrow.

☐ You can take a bath, too.

| 帰宅された当初は，とても弱って気が滅入るかもしれませんが，それはごく普通のことです． | ☐ When you first return home, you may feel very weak and depressed. This is quite normal. |
|---|---|
| ―心配はいりませんが，もしそのような状態が続くようであればお知らせ下さい． | ― Don't worry, but if that continues, let us know. |
| 日中は頻繁に休息をとって下さい． | ☐ Please try to rest frequently during the day. |
| 2，3日〔週間〕したら元に戻れますよ． | ☐ You're likely to feel back to normal within a few days〔weeks〕. |
| 1週間くらいしたら仕事に戻れます． | ☐ You can go back to work about a week or so later. |
| 術後の性生活は今までどおりでけっこうです． | ☐ The surgery shouldn't interfere with your sexual relations. |
| 次のような場合は03–xxxx–xxxxまで電話をして下さい． | ☐ Please call us at 03–xxxx–xxxx... |
| 1. 腫れ，強い痛み，膿などの感染の徴候が出たら． | 1. if you have any signs of infection, such as swelling, severe pain, or drainage. |
| 2. 38℃より高い熱が1日以上続いたら． | 2. if you have a fever over 38 degrees for more than a day. |
| 3. 術後2，3日，便通がなかったら． | 3. if you have no bowel movements within a few days of surgery. |
| 4. 激しい頭痛，息切れがあったら． | 4. if you have a severe headache or shortness of breath. |
| 5. その他，気になる症状があるとき． | 5. if you have any other symptoms which you're worried about. |
| 経過観察のため，退院後1週間くらいしたら外科外来へおいで下さい．そのときまでには検査結果が出ていますから． | ☐ Please come to the Surgical Outpatient Department for a follow-up visit about one week or so after you leave the hospital. The results from the laboratory will be ready [back] by then. |

# 用語・表現ファイル

## 病院会話のヒント その4 相づち

### 1. 同意・賛成を表して

| | |
|---|---|
| はい. | Yes. |
| ("May I...?" と訊かれて) ええ, どうぞ. | Certainly. |
| | Sure. |
| | Yes, of course. |
| 承知しました. | All right. |
| | OK/Okay. |
| けっこうです. | Fine. |
| | Good. |
| わかりました. | I see. |
| | I understand. |
| | I got you [it]. |
| もちろん喜んで (いたします). | With pleasure. |
| | Certainly. |
| | Sure. |
| そのとおり [そう] です. | (That's) right. |
| | Exactly. |
| あなたの言うとおりです. | You're right. |
| 私もそう思います. | I think so, too. |
| そうだといいですね. | I hope so. |
| (残念ながら) そうらしいです. | I'm afraid so. |
| それをうかがって嬉しく思います. | I'm glad to hear that. |

### 2. 反対・否定を表して

| | |
|---|---|
| いいえ. | No. |
| いや, 残念ですが. | No, I'm afraid not. |
| ("May I...?" と訊かれて) いいえ, いけません. | No, you may not. |
| そうは思いません. | I don't think so. |
| 残念ながら私にはできません. | I'm sorry, but I can't. |
| 賛成できません. | I don't agree (with you). |

## 用語・表現ファイル（つづき）

### 3. あいまいな言い方

| | |
|---|---|
| 多分［おそらく］そうです． | Maybe. |
| | Perhaps. |
| | Probably. |
| 場合によりますね． | That [It] depends. |
| 確かではありません． | I'm not quite sure. |
| ご意向にそえるとよいのですが，そのことについては担当医に相談しましょう． | I wish I could. I'll check with your doctor about that. |

### 4. 軽い受け答え★

| | |
|---|---|
| ええ［うんうん］ | Uh-huh. |
| | I see. |
| そうですか．本当ですか． | Is that so? |
| | Really? |
| | Oh? |
| | Well. |
| そうですねぇ［ええっと］． | Let me see. |
| | Let's see. |
| （お礼に対して）どういたしまして． | You're welcome. |
| （謝罪に対して）いいんですよ． | That's all right. |
| | That's OK. |

★ 日本人は話の途中で半ば無意識に相づちを打つ傾向があるため，外国人はそれをYesと誤解することがある．患者さんの目を見ながら話を聞き，ある程度の区切りのところで，あるいは話が終わったときにUh-huh/Really?などと言葉をはさむとよい．

chapter 9

# 入院

## Hospital Admission

入院前 338
入院当日 342
患者さんへの指示（安静度・移動） 352
患者さんへの対応 353
退院 359

## 入院前

入院受付係で入院の予約をして下さい．
☐ Please make an appointment for hospitalization at the admitting office.

入院費や手続きについては病院事務で尋ねて下さい．
☐ Please ask about your hospital bill and the procedure for admission in the hospital business office.

この入院説明書をお読み下さい．
☐ Please read this brochure on admission.

―持ってくるもの，面会時間などの説明がのっています．
― You'll find information about what to bring, visiting hours, and so on [etc.].★

入院手続きの用紙です．記入して下さい．
☐ Here's an admission form. Please fill it out.

―どなたか保証人が必要です．
― You need someone who can guarantee you.

―ご家族以外で保証人になる方が必要です．
― You need someone who can guarantee you other than your family.

―その方に署名をお願いできますか．
― Could you ask him [her] to sign this form?

日本語の通訳をしてくれる人がいたら，お名前と電話番号を書いて下さい．
☐ If you have someone who could interpret for you, please write his [her] name and telephone number.

緊急連絡先を書いて下さい．
☐ Please write your emergency contact number.

---

★ etc. は主に書きことばに用いる．

| 診察券,保険証,洗面用具,寝間着,バスローブ,スリッパ,湯のみ,箸〔フォークとスプーン〕を持ってきて下さい. | ☐ Please bring your hospital ID, insurance card, toiletries, pajamas, a bathrobe, slippers, a teacup, and chopsticks 〔a fork and a spoon〕. |
|---|---|
| ―お持ちでない場合は売店で買うことができます. | ― If you don't bring these items, you can buy them at the gift shop in the hospital. |
| ―寝間着は病院で貸し出すことが可能です.1日700円になります. | ― We have pajamas for rent. You have to pay 700 yen per day. |
| このほか必要なものをお持ち下さい. | ☐ Besides these items, you can bring what is necessary for you during your hospital stay. |
| 持ち物にはすべて名前をつけて下さい. | ☐ Mark all items with your name. |
| 現在飲んでいる薬をお持ち下さい. | ☐ Please bring any medications you are taking. |
| 少額のお金のほか貴重品は持ってこないで下さい. | ☐ Please don't bring valuables, other than a small amount of money, to the hospital. |
| 当病院では付き添いは必要ありません〔必要です〕. | ☐ Having someone stay with you isn't necessary 〔is necessary〕 in this hospital. |
| 当院では母子同室です. | ☐ This hospital has a rooming-in policy. |
| その他,入院についてご質問がありましたら,入院受付係にお尋ね下さい. | ☐ If you have any other questions about your admission, please ask 〔call〕 the admitting office. |

chapter 9 入院

## 用語・表現ファイル

### 病院会話のヒント　その5　入院患者さんへのあいさつ

☞「診察室でのあいさつ」(16 ページ).

#### 1. 会ったとき

| | |
|---|---|
| ガーナーさん，おはようございます． | Good morning, Mr.〔Mrs./Ms./Miss〕Garner. |
| マイクさん，こんにちは． | Hello〔Hi〕, Mike.★ |
| 調子はどうですか． | How are you doing? |
| 今日〔今朝〕はご気分いかがですか． | How are you feeling today〔this morning〕? |
| ご気分はよくなっていますか． | Are you feeling better? |
| ゆうべはよく眠れましたか． | Did you sleep well last night? |

#### 2. 別れるとき

| | |
|---|---|
| もう行かなくてはなりません．失礼します．すぐに〔1 時間以内に〕戻ってまいります． | Well, I must be going now. Excuse me. I'll be back in a minute〔within one hour〕. |
| ケインさん，さようなら． | Good-by(e), Mr. Cain. |
| それでは，またあとで． | (I'll) see you later. |
| ブラウンさん，お休みなさい． | Good night, Mrs. Brown. |
| 明日〔月曜日に〕またお会いしましょう． | See you tomorrow〔on Monday〕. |
| お大事に． | Take care (of yourself). |

#### 3. 紹介のあいさつ

| | |
|---|---|
| はじめまして，ハリスさん． | Nice to meet you, Mrs. Harris. How do you do, Mrs. Harris? |
| 私は… | I'm... |
| 1. 医師の岸です． | 1. Dr. Kishi. |
| 2. 担当医の加藤です． | 2. Dr. Kato, your doctor in charge. |
| 3. 看護師の前田です． | 3. Ms. Maeda, a nurse. |
| 4. 看護師の佐々木です．前田さんから引き継いで担当します． | 4. Mr. Sasaki. I'll be your nurse after Ms. Maeda. |

## 用語・表現ファイル（つづき）

―夜間担当します． ― I'm going to work the night shift [work on the night shift].

こちらは…
1. 同室の鈴木さんです．
2. 麻酔医の庄司先生です．

This is...
1. Mr. Suzuki, your roommate.
2. Dr. Shoji, an anesthesiologist.

★ "Hello", "Hi" は朝，昼，夜にかかわらず1日中使える．

---

### 名句・ことわざ

**It may seem a strange principle to enunciate as the very first requirement in a Hospital that it should do the sick no harm.**

**病院本来の目的からすれば奇妙なことではあるが，病院は少なくとも患者に害を与えてはならない**

看護教育の生みの親であるナイチンゲール (Florence Nightingale, 1820-1910, *Notes on Hospitals, Preface*) の名言．病院本来の目的は患者を救い，治療し，そして社会復帰させることにあるはずだが，過密状態や衛生状態の劣悪さのため，その病院が感染症の温床になって却って患者を死亡させてしまう，とナイチンゲールは嘆いた．

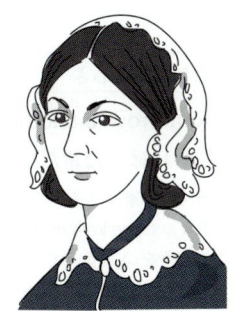

## 入院当日

### → あいさつ

| | |
|---|---|
| こんにちは，クロスさん． | ☐ Hello, Mr.〔Mrs./Ms./Miss〕Cross. |
| 担当医の中村です． | ☐ My name is Dr. Nakamura. I'm your doctor. |
| 担当看護師の和田です． | ☐ My name is Ms.〔Mr.〕Wada. I'm your nurse. |
| それでは寝間着に着替えて下さい． | ☐ Please change into your pajamas. |
| これはあなたのIDバンドです．手首につけましょう． | ☐ Here's your identification band. I'm going to〔Let me〕attach it to your wrist. |
| ―入院中はずさないで下さい． | ― Please don't remove it during your stay. |

---

### 名句・ことわざ

**Tomorrow is another day.**

明日にはまた新たな日がやってくる（明日は明日の風が吹く）

米国の作家ミッチェル（Margaret Mitchell, 1900-1949）の小説『風と共に去りぬ *Gone With the Wind*』の中の最後の台詞．女主人公スカーレットはこの言葉をつぶやいて，くじけそうになっている心を奮い立たせた．初出は16世紀前半のことわざ．

## 用語・表現ファイル

### 病院案内

| | |
|---|---|
| 1階 | 1st floor |
| 2階 | 2nd floor |
| 3階 | 3rd floor |
| 4階 | 4th floor |
| 地下 | basement |
| 本館 | main building |
| 新館 | new building |
| 中央病棟 | central wing |
| 東〔西／南／北〕病棟 | east〔west/south/north〕wing |
| 外来棟 | outpatient wing★ |
| 入院棟 | inpatient wing★ |

#### 1. 外来

| | |
|---|---|
| 事務室 | business office |
| 　総合案内 | 　general information（desk） |
| 　新患受付 | 　first visit reception（desk） |
| 　再来受付 | 　regular reception（desk） |
| 　会計受付 | 　billing and payment（window）, cashier's office |
| 　入院受付 | 　admitting window〔office〕 |
| 内科外来 | internal medicine outpatient |
| 外科外来 | surgery outpatient |

☞「診療部門」(52ページ).

| | |
|---|---|
| 診察室 | (doctor's) office/consulting room |
| 救命救急室 | emergency room［ER］ |
| 薬局 | pharmacy |
| カフェテリア［食堂］ | cafeteria |
| 喫茶室 | coffee shop |
| 売店 | gift［hospital］shop |
| 自動販売機 | vending machine |
| ATM | ATM |
| 郵便受け | mailbox |
| 理容室 | barbershop |
| コインランドリー | Laundromat |

## 用語・表現ファイル（つづき）

| | |
|---|---|
| 玄関ホール | entrance hall |
| 　夜間・休日出入口 | 　night and holiday entrance |
| 　救急入口 | 　emergency entrance |
| ロビー | lobby |
| 洗面所 | restroom, rest room |
| 公衆電話 | public telephone, pay phone |
| ロッカー | locker (room) |
| 警備室 | guard station |
| 駐車場 | parking lot |

### 2. 検査部

| | |
|---|---|
| 採血室 | blood collection [phlebotomy] room |
| 臨床検査室 | (clinical) laboratory |
| 内視鏡室 | endoscopy room |
| 超音波検査室 | ultrasound room |
| 心電図室 | ECG room |
| 呼吸機能検査室 | pulmonary function testing room |
| 放射線部 | radiology department |
| 　レントゲン室 | 　X-ray room |
| 　CT 室 | 　CT room |
| 　MRI 室 | 　MRI room |
| 　核医学検査室 | 　nuclear medicine imaging room |

### 3. 手術

| | |
|---|---|
| 手術室 | operating room [OR] |
| 回復室 | recovery room |
| 待合室 | waiting room |

### 4. 病棟

| | |
|---|---|
| 集中治療部 | intensive care unit [ICU] |
| 冠動脈疾患集中治療部 | coronary care unit [CCU] |
| 新生児集中治療部 | neonatal [newborn] intensive care unit [NICU] |

## 用語・表現ファイル（つづき）

|  |  |
|---|---|
| 内科病棟 | medical ward [floor/unit] |
| 外科病棟 | surgical ward [floor/unit] |
| 小児科病棟 | pediatric ward [floor/unit] |
| 整形外科病棟 | orthopedic ward [floor/unit] |
| 婦人科病棟 | gynecological ward [floor/unit] |
| 産科病棟 | maternity ward [floor/unit] |
| 　陣痛室 | labor room |
| 　分娩室 | delivery room |
| 　新生児室 | nursery |
| 隔離病棟 | isolation unit [ward] |
| 緩和ケア病棟 | palliative [hospice] care unit |
| ナースステーション | nurses' station |
| 個室 | private [single] room |
| 2人部屋 | double room |
| 4〔8〕人部屋 | four〔eight〕-bed room |
| ラウンジ | lounge |
| 面談室 | interview room |
| 面会室 | visitors' room |

### 5. その他

|  |  |
|---|---|
| 透析センター〔室〕 | dialysis center〔room〕 |
| リハビリテーションセンター | rehabilitation center |
| 　理学療法室 | physical therapy room |
| 　作業療法室 | occupational therapy room |
| 　言語（聴覚）療法室 | speech (-language-hearing) therapy room |
| 訪問看護部 | department of home visiting nurses |
| 医療福祉相談室 | medical social work room [office] |
| 栄養相談室 | nutrition counseling room |
| 臨床治験室 | clinical trials room |
| 図書室 | medical library |
| チャペル | chapel |
| 霊安室 | hospital morgue |
| 健診センター | Health Screening Center |

\* center, unit, department, division など, 病院によって名称は異なる.

## Patient Room(病室)

- oxygen outlet(酸素プラグ差し込み口)
- telephone(電話)
- bedside table(床頭台)
- IV pole(点滴台)
- overbed light(オーバーベッドライト)
- call bell(コールベル)
- hospital gown(病室着)
- chair(いす)
- overbed table(オーバーベッドテーブル)
- bed(ベッド)
- closet(クローゼット)
- toilet(トイレット)
- sink(洗面台)
- emergency bell(非常用ベル)
- 入口

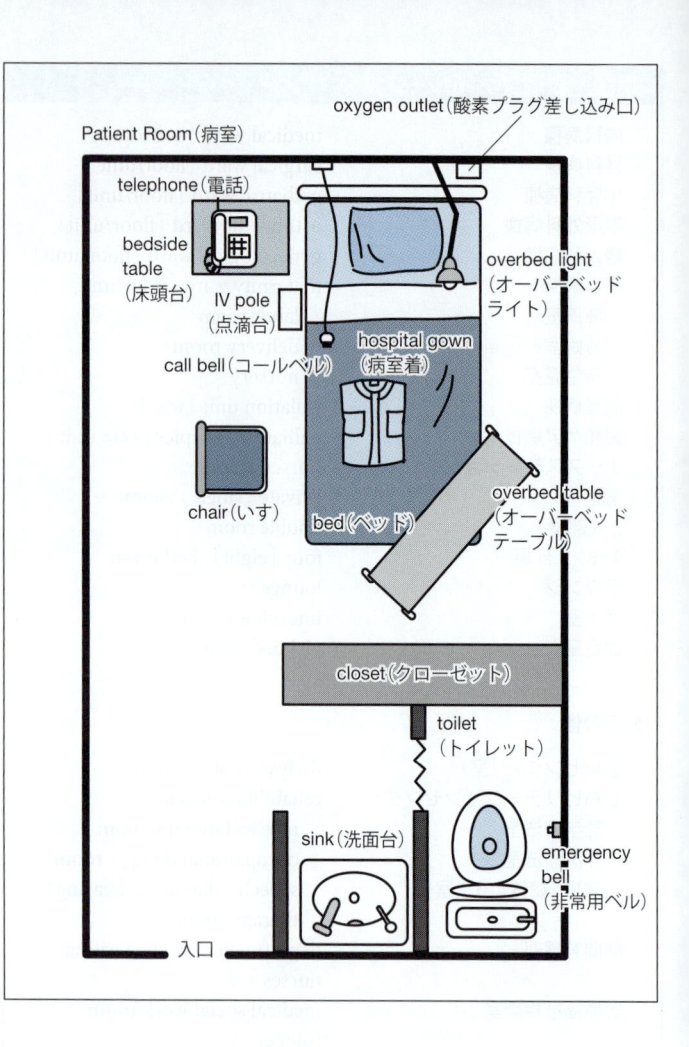

## ● 病室・病棟案内

| | |
|---|---|
| あなたの病室は 325 号室です. | ☐ You'll be in room 325.★ |
| それでは病室〔病棟〕をご案内しましょう. | ☐ I'll show you your room 〔the floor〕. |
| 同室の方をご紹介しましょう. | ☐ Let me introduce you to your roommate. |
| ―こちらは山口さんです. | ― This is Mr.〔Mrs./Ms./Miss〕Yamaguchi. |
| これがあなたのベッドです. | ☐ This is your bed. |
| ―この調整つまみを使うと，ベッドを下げることができます. | ― You can use this control to lower your bed. |
| ―このボタンを押すと，ベッドの枕元を上げることができます. | ― You can raise the head of the bed by pressing this button. |
| コールボタンはここ枕元にあります. | ☐ Here's the call button by the pillow. |
| ―用事があるときには，ボタンを押して看護師を呼んで下さい. | ― Please press the button to call the nurse when you need help. |
| この床頭台とあそこのロッカーを使って下さい. | ☐ Please use this bedside table and that locker. |
| 貴重品は病室に置かないで下さい. | ☐ Please don't keep valuables in the room. |
| ―どうしても貴重品を持ってくるときには… | ― If you must bring valuables with you,... |
| 1. ご家族の方にお預け下さい. | 1. leave them with a member of your family. |
| 2. 入院受付にお預け下さい. | 2. keep them in the admitting office. |

---

★ 数字の部分の読み方は "three hundred and twenty-five", "three twenty-five", "three-two-five". ☞「数字の読み方」(214 ページ).

| | |
|---|---|
| 3. 病院備え付けの金庫に入れて下さい．出し入れは午前8時半から午後5時半までになっています． | 3. keep them in the hospital safe, which is accessible for deposits and withdrawals from 8:30 am to 5:30 pm. |
| 入室・退室の際は，備え付けの消毒薬で手指を消毒して下さい． | ☐ Please clean〔wipe〕your hand and finger surfaces with the hand sanitizer provided when entering and leaving the room. |
| トイレはナースステーションの隣にあります． | ☐ The toilet is next to the nurses' station. |
| 浴室は廊下の突き当たりにあります．<br>―入浴〔シャワー〕時間は，月・水・金曜日の午後1時から9時までの間です． | ☐ The bathroom is at the end of the hallway.<br>— You can take a bath〔shower〕between the hours of 1:00 pm and 9:00 pm on Mondays, Wednesdays and Fridays. |
| 売店，カフェテリア，ポスト，ATMは地下にあります． | ☐ The gift shop, the cafeteria, the mailbox, and ATM are in the basement. |
| 自動販売機はカフェテリアの隣にあって24時間使えます． | ☐ The vending machines, open 24 hours a day, are located next to the cafeteria. |
| 入院中の洗濯はコインランドリー〔コイン式洗濯機と乾燥機〕をご利用になれます．<br>―コインランドリーは地下にあります．<br>―当院では有料の洗濯サービスがあります．<br>―病棟のクラークにその旨をお伝え下さい． | ☐ If you have washing to do during your hospital stay, you can use the Laundromat [coin-operated washers and dryers].<br>— The Laundromat is [The coin-operated washers and dryers are] located in the basement.<br>— Laundry services are available at an additional charge.<br>— Tell a ward clerk of your interest in the service. |

## ⤵ 病院生活

食事時間は朝食は 7 時半から 8 時，昼食は 12 時から 1 時，夕食は 5 時から 6 時です．

― ご希望があればパンをお出しすることができます．
― ご家族やお友達が持ってきた食べ物は，看護師に相談してから食べて下さい．
― 当院でお出しする食事以外は何も召しあがらないで下さい．

消灯時間は午後 9 時です．
― 消灯後は静かにして下さい．

面会時間は，平日は午後 3 時から 8 時，日曜・祭日は午前 10 時から午後 8 時までです．

― 面会室は各階の廊下の突き当たりにあります．
― お子さんを連れてこられる場合は，看護師か医師の許可を受けて下さい．
― 家族以外の方の面会は医師の許可がないとできません．

携帯用テレビを借りることができます．病棟のクラークに頼んで下さい．
― テレビはカード式です．
― ほかの患者さんのことを考えて，テレビやラジオの音量はさげて下さい．

☐ Breakfast is served between 7:30 am and 8:00 am, lunch between 12:00 am and 1:00 pm, and dinner between 5:00 pm and 6:00 pm.

— We can serve you bread, if you like.
— Please check with your nurse before eating foods brought in by your family or friends.
— Please don't eat anything other than food provided by the hospital.

☐ Lights are turned off at 9:00 pm.
— Please be quiet after lights are turned off.

☐ Visiting hours are from 3:00 pm to 8:00 pm on weekdays, and from 10:00 am to 8:00 pm on Sundays and holidays.

— The visitors' room is at the end of the hallway on each floor.
— Please check with the charge nurse or your doctor before bringing children.
— Visitors other than your family are not allowed without your doctor's permission.

☐ You can rent a portable television. Please ask a clerk on the floor.
— You can watch TV with a card.
— Please keep television or radio volume low in consideration of other patients.

| | |
|---|---|
| —ラジオやテレビを聞くときは，イヤホンを使用して下さい． | — When listening to radio or watching television, use the earphones provided. |
| 冷蔵庫はカード式です． | ☐ You can use the refrigerator with a card. |
| 携帯電話は院内では禁止されています． | ☐ The use of cell phones isn't allowed anywhere in the hospital. |
| —携帯電話は病室では使わないで下さい． | — Please don't use cell phones in the room. |
| —1階に通話可能な指定の場所があります． | — There's a designated area where cell phones can be used on the first floor. |
| —病院内専用の携帯電話を借りることができます． | — You can rent a cell phone for use in this hospital only. |
| 公衆電話はロビーにあります． | ☐ Public telephones are located in the lobby. |
| 当病院は禁煙になっております． | ☐ This hospital is a smoke-free institution. |
| —院内では，患者・見舞い客にかかわらず禁煙になっています． | — Smoking is not allowed by patients or visitors anywhere in the hospital. |
| —1階に指定の喫煙所があります． | — There's a designated smoking area on the first floor. |
| 外出〔外泊〕される時には，必ず担当医の許可を得て下さい． | ☐ When you are going out of the hospital〔staying out overnight〕, be sure to check with your doctor and get his〔her〕 permission. |
| 担当医が午後の2時ごろ診察に来ます． | ☐ Your doctor will be coming to see you about two in the afternoon. |
| —まもなく回診があります． | — The doctors will be making their rounds soon. |

| ご質問がありますか. | □ (Do you have) any questions? |
| --- | --- |
| 何か用事がありましたら,私に知らせて下さい. | □ Please let me know if you need any help. |

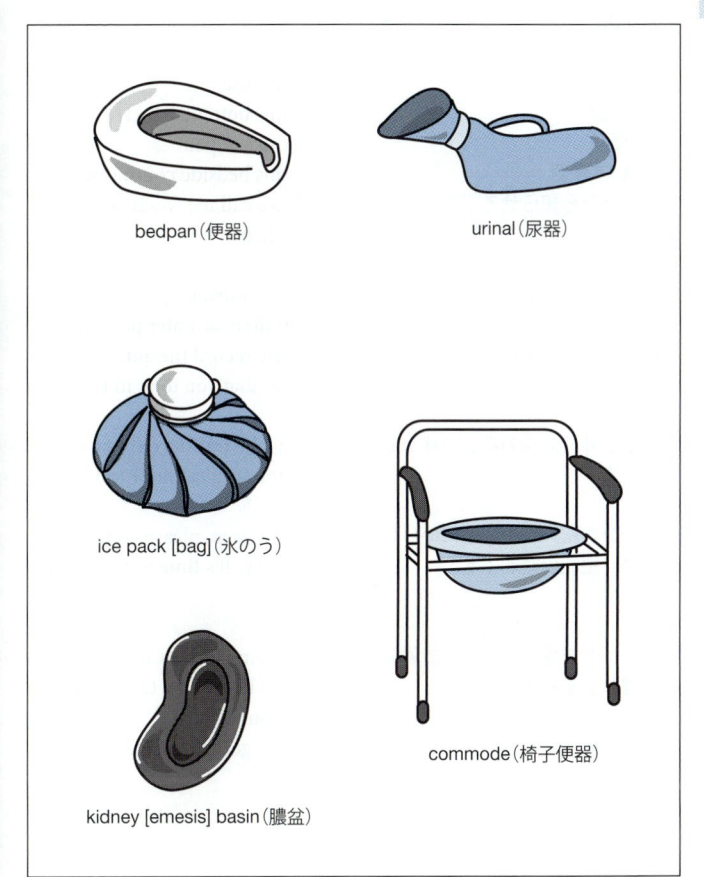

bedpan(便器)

urinal(尿器)

ice pack [bag](氷のう)

commode(椅子便器)

kidney [emesis] basin(膿盆)

## 患者さんへの指示(安静度・移動)

病院内〔病棟内〕を自由に移動してもいいですよ。
― トイレに行くとき以外はベッド上で安静にしていて下さい.
― ベッドから降りないで下さい.
― トイレにはまだ行けません.
― ベッドの上で起き上がってもいいですよ.

この…を使って下さい.
1. 尿器
2. 便器
3. いす便器
― 終わったら知らせて下さい.

水分は1日に…ml まで摂取できます.
― 飲んだ水分量をこの用紙に記入して下さい.

今日から外科病棟の病室に移っていただきます.

グリーンさん,新生児室にいらして下さい. 授乳の時間です.

レントゲンを撮りますから放射線科へお連れしましょう.
― この車椅子に乗って下さい.

☐ Please feel free to walk [move] around the hospital [floor].
― Please stay in bed except when you go to the toilet.
― Please don't get out of bed.
― You're not allowed to walk to the toilet.
― You can sit up in bed.

☐ Please use...
1. this bottle [urinal].
2. this bedpan.
3. this bedside commode.
― Please call me when you have finished.

☐ You can drink up to _____ milliliters of water per day.
― Please record the amount of water that you took in this form.

☐ You'll be transferred to a room on the surgical floor today.

☐ Mrs. Green, please go to the nursery. It's time to feed your baby.

☐ I'm going to [Let me] take you to the Radiology Department for your X-ray.
― Please get in this wheelchair.

# 患者さんへの対応

## ● 投薬・処置

キムさん, …

1. お薬ですよ.
   —これは痛み止めの薬です.

2. 酸素マスク〔カニューラ〕です.
   —鼻と口にかけましょう.

   —楽に普通に息をしていて下さい.

☐ Mr.〔Mrs./Ms./Miss〕Kim, here's...
1. your medication.
   — This medication will help ease your pain.
2. an oxygen mask〔a cannula〕.
   — I'm going to [Let me] slip it over your nose and mouth.
   — Just relax and breathe like you usually do.

グレイさん, …の時間です.

1. 検温
2. 注射
3. 安静
4. 授乳
5. リハビリテーション
6. 入浴

☐ Mr.〔Mrs./Ms./Miss〕Gray, it's time...
1. to take your temperature.
2. to give you an injection.
3. for you to stay in bed [for your bedrest].
4. for you to feed your baby.
5. for your rehabilitation training.
6. for you to take a bath.

これから…しましょう.
1. 熱〔血圧／脈拍〕を測る
2. 注射をする
3. 点滴をする
4. 傷口をみる
5. 傷口の処置をする
6. 包帯を取り替える
7. 管を入れて膀胱からお小水をとる
   —(女性患者に) 膝を立てて, 足を開いて下さい.

☐ I'm going to [Let me]...
1. take your temperature〔blood pressure/pulse〕.
2. give you an injection.
3. feed you intravenously.
4. look at your wound.
5. treat your wound.
6. change your dressing.
7. drain the urine from your bladder with this tube.
   — Please put your knees up and legs apart.

―（男性患者に）寝たまま足をひろげて下さい．
  8. 浣腸をする
　　―横になって膝を胸にひきよせて下さい．

  9. 体の向きを変える
　　―体の向きを変えるときは，私がお手伝いしましょう．
　　―こちら〔あちら〕を向いて下さい．
　　―ごろんと転がって下さい．
　　―床ずれができないように体の向きを頻繁に変えて下さい．

  10. 清拭をする［身体をふく］
  11. シーツ〔リネン〕を交換する

さあ終わりました．

　　— Please lie with your legs flat and legs apart.
  8. give you an enema.
　　— Please lie down with your knees pulled toward your chest.

  9. change your position.
　　— I'll help you turn when you change your position.
　　— Please turn over this 〔that〕 way.
　　— Please roll over.
　　— Please change your position frequently to prevent bedsores.

  10. give you a bed bath.
  11. change your sheets 〔linens〕.

☐ It's over now.
☐ That's all.

## ➔ 患者さんのケア

（あなたは）…したいですか．
  1. お水を飲む
  2. 痛み止めをもらう
  3. お小水をする
  4. 便をする
  5. トイレに行く
  6. 体の向きを変える

（私が）…しましょうか．
  1. シーツをなおす
  2. もう1枚毛布をかける
  3. 背中〔足／腕〕をマッサージする
  4. ここに冷湿布〔温湿布〕をする
  5. 窓を開ける〔閉める〕
  6. 明かり〔テレビ〕を消す〔つける〕

☐ Would you like to...
  1. drink some water?
  2. have some pain medication?
  3. urinate?
  4. have a bowel movement?
  5. go to the toilet?
  6. change your position?

☐ Shall I...
  1. straighten your sheets?
  2. give you one more blanket?
  3. rub your back 〔leg(s)/arm(s)〕?
  4. apply a cold 〔hot〕 pack here?
  5. open 〔close〕 the window?
  6. turn off 〔on〕 the light 〔TV〕?

| | |
|---|---|
| 7. ブラインドを上げる〔下ろす〕 | 7. pull up〔down〕the shade? |

(私が)…してもよいですか.
1. トレイを下げる
2. この新聞を片付ける

☐ May I...
1. take your tray?
2. put this paper away?

ご気分はいかがですか. ☐ How do you feel now?

昨夜はよく眠れましたか. ☐ Did you sleep well last night?

夕食〔昼食〕はいかがでしたか. ☐ How did you enjoy your dinner〔lunch〕?

お風呂に入ってさっぱりしましたか. ☐ Do you feel refreshed after the bath?

ご用のあるときは,遠慮しないで… ☐ If you need any help, don't hesitate to...

1. 私を呼んで下さい.
2. コールボタンを押して下さい.

1. call me.
2. press the call button.

何かご用はありませんか. ☐ Can I help you?

お手伝いしましょう. ☐ Let me help you.

## ● 患者さんから呼ばれて

ケインさん,お呼びですか. ☐ Mr.〔Mrs./Ms./Miss〕Cain, how can I help you?

—すぐにまいります. — I'm coming.
　　　　　　　　　　　　　　　I'll be right there.

(病室に入るとき) 失礼します. ☐ May I come in?

お待たせしました. ☐ I'm sorry to have kept you waiting.

遅れてごめんなさい. ☐ Sorry I'm late.

| | |
|---|---|
| どうされましたか. | ☐ What can I do for you? |
| | ☐ What's the matter? |
| —痛みますか. | — Do you have any pain? |
| | — Is it painful? |
| —苦しいですか. | — Are you uncomfortable? |
| —ご気分が悪いのですか. | — Do you feel sick? |
| —胸が苦しいのですか. | — Do you feel pressure in your chest? |
| —ご心配なことがありますか. | — Do you have any worries? |
| —お困りのことがありますか. | — Do you have any trouble? |
| ドクターを呼びましょう. | ☐ I'll call your doctor for you. |
| —ドクターがすぐまいります. | — Your doctor will be here soon. |

## 用語・表現ファイル

### 病院会話のヒント　その6
### 一般的な話題（患者さんの気持ちを和らげるために）

| | |
|---|---|
| あなたの生まれ故郷について話して下さい． | Please tell me about your hometown. |
| ―市の規模はどのくらいですか． | — How big is your city? |
| ―気候はどうですか． | — What's the climate like there? |

ご家族についてお聞かせ下さい．　Please tell me about your family.
―皆さんお国にいらっしゃるのですか．　— Does everyone live in your country?
―ご家族は何人ですか．　— How many people are there in your family?

―ご家族のみなさんはお元気ですか．　— How's your family?
―お子さんがいますか．　— Do you have any children?
―お子さんは何人いますか．　— How many children do you have?

―何歳ですか．　— How old are they?
―ごきょうだいがいますか．　— Do you have any brothers or sisters?

―ごきょうだいは何人いますか．　— How many brothers or sisters do you have?

日本に来てからどのくらい経ちますか．　How long have you been in Japan?
―日本へ来られた理由は何ですか．　— What brought you to Japan?
―日本にどのくらいご滞在の予定ですか．　— How long are you going to stay in Japan?
―どこかへ旅行しましたか．　— Have you traveled anywhere?

日本の食べ物では何が一番好きですか．　What kind of Japanese food do you like best?
―苦手な食べ物がありますか．　— Is there any Japanese food you don't care for?

## 用語・表現ファイル（つづき）

| | |
|---|---|
| 趣味についてお聞かせ下さい． | Please tell me about your hobby. |
| —どんなご趣味をおもちですか． | — What hobbies do you have? / What are your hobbies? |
| —暇なときには何をして過ごしますか． | — How do you spend your leisure time? / What do you do in your spare time? |
| —休みの日にはどう過ごしますか． | — How do you spend your holidays? / What do you do on holidays? |
| あなたのお好きなテレビ番組は何ですか． | What's your favorite TV program? |
| あなたのお好きな歌手〔すもうとり〕はだれですか． | Who is your favorite singer 〔sumo wrestler〕? |
| …についてどう思いますか． | What do you think about____? / How do you like ____? |

---

### 名句・ことわざ

**If Winter comes, can Spring be far behind?**
**冬来たりなば春遠からじ**

英国のロマン派詩人シェリー（Percy Bysshe Shelley, 1792-1822, "Ode to the West Wind"）の名句．

## 退院

| | |
|---|---|
| スミスさん，おめでとうございます． | ☐ Mr. [Mrs./Ms./Miss] Smith, congratulations! |
| 今日ご退院ですね． | ☐ You're leaving the hospital today. |
| これは家で飲んでいただく薬です． | ☐ Here's your medication to take home. |
| 薬は指示どおりに飲んで下さい． | ☐ Please take your medication as instructed. |

…と感じたら休息をとって下さい．
1. 体が弱っている
2. 体がだるい

☐ Please rest...
1. if you feel weak.
2. if you feel tired.

…時には電話をして下さい．
1. 処方した薬〔鎮痛薬〕がきかずに痛みが続く
2. 熱が 38℃以上ある
3. 繰り返し吐いた
4. 傷口から臭いのする分泌物が出た
5. 縫った傷口が開いた
6. 異常な症状が出たり，心配な症状が長引いたりする

☐ Please call us if...
1. there is persistent pain not relieved by the medication prescribed [painkillers].
2. you have a fever of 38 degrees Celsius or higher.
3. you have repeated vomiting.
4. you have foul-smelling discharge from the wound.
5. the stitches come open.
6. you have any other abnormal or prolonged symptoms which cause concern.

―連絡先〔電話番号〕は 03–xxxx–xxxx です．

― Our telephone number is 03–xxxx–xxxx.

☞「数字の読み方」(214 ページ)．

| | |
|---|---|
| 会計窓口で支払いを済ませて下さい． | ☐ Please pay at the cashier counter [window]. |
| ―自動精算機も使えます．"English" のボタンを押して下さい． | ― You can also use the automatic bill payment machine. Press the English selection button. |

―当病院ではクレジットカードによる支払いに応じます．
— We accept [Our hospital accepts] payment by credit card.

診察券をお返ししましょう．
☐ Let me give you back your hospital ID.

これは次に外来にいらっしゃる時の予約券です．
☐ This is your appointment card for your next visit.

6月8日，火曜日，午前10時に外来へ来て下さい．
☐ Please come to the outpatient department at ten in the morning, Tuesday, June 8.

どうぞお大事に．
☐ Please take good care of yourself.

---

### コラム

## 死の伝え方

最愛の人の死，または命が終わろうとしている，あるいは終わった―その事実に直面する家族の悲しみは大きい．ましてや，異国の地で最期を迎えねばならないとすれば，その辛さ・心細さは計り知れないものがある．死をどう伝えるかは医療者にとって辛い仕事であり，医療コミュニケーションの中でもとりわけ難しい技術を要する．慰めるつもりでいった言葉が，かえって深い悲しみにある家族の心を傷つけてしまうかもしれない．

以下に例をあげるが，これはあくまでも1つの参考例として，個別の状況に合わせて対応していただきたい．

#### ●危篤の知らせ

（病室で）
残念ですが，ヒルさんの容体が急変しました．
☐ Unfortunately, Mr. Hill's condition took a sudden turn for the worse.

彼は危篤状態です．
☐ I'm afraid he has fallen into critical condition.
☐ He is critically ill.

### コラム（つづき）

| | |
|---|---|
| 彼の容体はかなり深刻です． | ☐ His condition is serious. He is in serious condition.★ |
| ―必要があれば，他のご家族にも連絡して下さい． | ― Please let other family members know it if necessary. |
| 明日までもたない [命を保てない] かもしれません． | ☐ He may not last [live] until tomorrow. |
| ―ご家族，友人，牧師など，最後のお別れをするために会わせたい人がいますか． | ― Is there any family member, friend or clergy you would like to have with you to say final goodbyes to him? |

（電話で）

| | |
|---|---|
| もしもし，ヒルさんの主治医〔金沢病院の看護師〕の加藤です． | ☐ Hello, I'm Dr. Kato, Mr. Hill's doctor〔Ms. Kato, a nurse at Kanazawa Hospital〕. |
| 残念ですが，先ほどヒルさんの容体が急変しました． | ☐ I'm sorry, Mr. Hill's condition took a sudden turn for the worse a short while ago. |
| ―会いにいらしていただけますか． | ― Could you come to the hospital to visit him? |
| ―病院に到着されましたら5階のナースステーションにお出で下さい． | ― When you get to the hospital, please come to the nurses' station on the fifth floor. |

### ●死を告げる

病室に入る前に，まず家族が付き添っているかどうかを確認する．家族と離れて来日している外国人の場合，友人や会社の同僚が緊急連絡先になっているかもしれない．患者さんにとってのキーパーソンが付き添っている状況で死を告げることが望ましい．

（臨終の場に居合わせた家族に）

| | |
|---|---|
| 担当医の伊藤です． | ☐ I'm Dr. Ito, his attending physician. |

### コラム（つづき）

（担当医でない場合）

呼吸器専門医の林です．
- [ ] I'm Dr. Hayashi, a lung specialist.

それでは，診察をさせていただきます．
- [ ] Let me examine Mr. Hill.

残念ですが，お別れです．
- [ ] I'm sorry to say it's time to say your goodbyes.

お亡くなりになりました［ご臨終です］．5 時 20 分です．
- [ ] He passed away [died]. It's five twenty [It's twenty minutes past five].

―大変残念です．
― I'm very sorry for your loss.

―外でお待ちしていますので，もしよろしければしばらく傍にいてあげて下さい．
― Please stay with him for a while, if you wish. We'll be waiting outside.

―ご用のあるときには声をかけて下さい．
― When you need assistance, let us know.

―必要な手配をいたしましょう．看護師か医療ソーシャルワーカーがお手伝いいたします．
― We'll make the necessary arrangements. A nurse or a medical social worker will be glad to help you.

―何かご質問はありませんか．
― Do you have any questions?

★ さらに付け加えて "We have tried everything possible to save his life." "There's nothing more that we can do other than to make him comfortable." "We know that he is nearing the end of his life." などと述べて遺憾の意を表すこともできる．

chapter 10

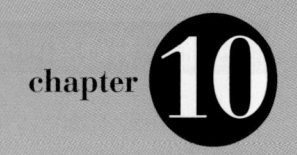

# 妊娠・分娩

## Pregnancy and Delivery

妊娠歴・分娩歴・その他の病歴　364
妊娠　367
分娩　375

## 妊娠歴・分娩歴・その他の病歴

それぞれの妊娠，分娩についてお話し下さい．
- [ ] Please tell me about each of your past pregnancies and deliveries.

### ➡ 妊娠歴

これまでに何回妊娠しましたか．
- [ ] How many times have you been pregnant?

妊娠中に何か問題がありましたか．
―どんな問題でしたか．
―いつ起こりましたか．
―どんな治療を受けましたか．
- [ ] Have you had any problem during your pregnancy?
— What was the problem?
— When did it occur?
— How was it treated?

### ➡ 分娩歴

お子さんを何人生みましたか．
―お子さん達の性別と年齢を教えて下さい．
- [ ] How many babies have you had?
— Please let me know the sex and age of your children.

これまでに流産や妊娠中絶をしたことがありますか．
―いつのことですか．
―何回しましたか．

―妊娠何週目でしたか．
- [ ] Have you had any miscarriages or abortions?
— When (did you have them)?
— How many times (did you have them)?
— How many weeks pregnant were you when you had the miscarriage〔abortion〕?

分娩前，分娩中に何か問題がありましたか．
―どんな問題でしたか．
―いつ起こりましたか．
―どんな治療を受けましたか．
- [ ] Have you had any problem before or during your delivery?
— What was the problem?
— When did it occur?
— How was it treated?

| | |
|---|---|
| お産は正常分娩でしたか. | ☐ Was your delivery normal? |
| ―経腟分娩でしたか,帝王切開でしたか. | — Did you have a vaginal delivery or a Cesarean delivery? |
| ―帝王切開となった理由は何ですか. | — Why was the Cesarean delivery needed? |
| ―鉗子分娩でしたか,吸引分娩でしたか. | — Was it a forceps delivery or a vacuum extraction? |

お産にどのくらい時間がかかりましたか.
1. 最初のお子さんのとき.
2. そのあとのお子さんのとき.

☐ How long was your labor with...
1. the first baby?
2. other babies?

出産後に何か問題がありましたか.

☐ Have you had any problem after delivery?

―どんな問題でしたか.
―いつ起こりましたか.

— What was the problem?
— When did it occur?

これまでに…を生んだことがありますか.
1. 未熟児
   ―何週でしたか.

   ―何グラムで生まれましたか.

2. 巨大児
   ―何週でしたか.

   ―何グラムで生まれましたか.

3. さかご[骨盤位]のお子さん

4. へその緒が首に巻きついて生まれたお子さん
5. 先天性障害をもつお子さん

   ―どのような障害ですか.
6. 双生児
7. 死産のお子さん

☐ Have you ever had...

1. a baby that was premature?
   — How many weeks pregnant were you?
   — How many grams did the baby weigh?
2. an abnormally large baby?
   — How many weeks pregnant were you?
   — How many grams did the baby weigh?
3. a baby that was born feet first?
4. a baby that was born with a cord around the neck?
5. a baby that had congenital problems?
   — What was the problem?
6. twins?
7. a baby that was born dead?

| | |
|---|---|
| 8. 出産直後に亡くなられたお子さん<br>―亡くなられた理由をお聞かせ下さい. | 8. a baby that died shortly after birth?<br>— Please tell me what caused the death of the baby. |

## ● その他の病歴

| | |
|---|---|
| これまでに心臓病，高血圧，糖尿病，肝炎，その他の慢性疾患などの病気にかかったことがありますか. | ☐ Have you ever had a disease, such as heart diseases, hypertension, diabetes, hepatitis, or other chronic diseases? |
| ―麻疹，風疹，水痘はどうですか. | — How about measles, rubella [German measles], or chicken-pox? |
| ―かかっていなければ，予防接種を受けていますか. | — If not, have you had vaccinations for them? |
| あなたかご主人〔パートナー〕に何か遺伝性の病気がありますか. | ☐ Do you or your husband 〔partner〕have any hereditary diseases? |
| タバコを吸いますか. | ☐ Do you smoke? |
| お酒を飲みますか. | ☐ Do you drink alcohol? |
| お仕事をしていますか.<br>―どんな仕事ですか.<br>―通勤は徒歩ですか，それとも自家用車，バス，電車ですか. | ☐ Do you work?<br>— What type of work do you do?<br>— Do you walk to your office, or do you go in your own car, by bus, or by train? |
| ―通勤時間はどのくらいかかりますか.<br>―出産休暇をもらえますか.<br>　どの位の期間ですか. | — How long does it take to get to your office?<br>— Can you get maternity leave? How long? |
| 住居はアパートですか，一戸建てですか.<br>―何階ですか.<br>―エレベーターがありますか. | ☐ Do you live in an apartment or a house?<br>— What floor is your apartment on?<br>— Is there an elevator? |

# 妊娠

☞「月経」(118 ページ).
☞「妊娠・授乳」(197 ページ).

## → 問診

|  |  |
|---|---|
| 最終月経の初日はいつでしたか. | ☐ When was the first day of your last menstrual period? |
| 月経周期は通常何日ですか. | ☐ How often do you get your periods?<br>☐ How many days usually pass between your periods? |
| 妊娠検査薬はお使いになられましたか. | ☐ Did you use a home pregnancy test〔a pregnancy test kit〕? |
| あなたは…がありますか〔ありましたか〕. | ☐ Do you have〔Have you had〕… |

1. 吐き気
2. 嘔吐
3. 食欲不振
4. ある物が食べたくなる,または嫌いになるなどの嗜好の変化
5. 疲労感
6. 便秘
7. 排尿困難または頻尿
8. 腰痛
9. むくみ

1. nausea?
2. vomiting?
3. loss of appetite?
4. cravings or aversions for special foods?
5. tiredness?
6. constipation?
7. difficulty urinating or frequent urination?
8. low back pain?
9. swelling?

赤ちゃんの胎動を感じましたか.　　☐ Have you felt your baby's movement?

**コラム**

## 妊娠週数・月数の数え方

外国人の妊婦さんの中には「私の国では満期出産は9か月なのに，なんで日本は10か月もかかるの」といった疑問をもつ人がいるかもしれない．妊娠予定日はWHOの指針に従って最終月経日の初日から数えて280日で計算し，これは各国共通である．しかし週数と月数の数え方が国によって異なる場合がある．日本では最終月経の初日を0週として数え始めて妊娠初期を15週，4か月までとするが，アメリカでは最終月経の初日を1週として数え始めて第1期（1st trimester）は13週，3か月までとしている．第1期の3か月，第2期（2nd trimester）の6か月，そして第3期（3rd trimester）の8か月と9か月はそれぞれ5週間になっていて，のべ40週，9か月，280日という計算になる．

妊娠の時期を話題にするとき，最近は月数よりむしろ週数を使う人が増えてはいるが，それでも一般人はまだ月数を使うことも多いので注意したい．

| 日本 | | | 米国（例） | | |
|---|---|---|---|---|---|
| 月 | 週 | 期 | month | week | trimester |
| 1 | 0～3 | 初期 | 1 | 1～4 | 1st trimester |
| 2 | 4～7 | | 2 | 5～8 | |
| 3 | 8～11 | | 3 | 9～13 | |
| 4 | 12～15 | | 4 | 14～17 | 2nd trimester |
| 5 | 16～19 | 中期 | 5 | 18～21 | |
| 6 | 20～23 | | 6 | 22～26 | |
| 7 | 24～27 | | 7 | 27～30 | 3rd trimester |
| 8 | 28～31 | 後期 | 8 | 31～35 | |
| 9 | 32～35 | | 9 | 36～40 | |
| 10 | 36～39 | | | | |

## ◯ 検査

☞「検査」(269 ページ).

| | |
|---|---|
| 血圧を測りましょう. | ☐ I'm going to [Let me] take your blood pressure. |
| 体重を測りましょう. | ☐ I'm going to [Let me] measure your weight. |
| ― 58 kg ありますね. | ― You weigh 58 kilos. |
| ―急に体重が変化しましたか.増えましたか,減りましたか. | ― Have you noticed any sudden weight change? Have you gained or lost weight? |
| コップに尿をとって検査室に出して下さい. | ☐ Please use the cup to collect your urine and take it to the exam room. |
| ―正常です. | ― Your urine is normal. |
| ―尿にタンパク〔糖〕がでています. | ― There is protein [sugar] in your urine. |
| 今日は採血をしましょう. | ☐ I'm going to [Let me] take your blood sample today. |
| NST(ノンストレステスト)を始めましょう. | ☐ Let's start the non-stress test. |

## ● 診察

| | |
|---|---|
| 診察いたしましょう. | ☐ I'm going to [Let me] examine you. |
| このベッドに横になって下さい. | ☐ Please lie down on this bed. |
| 腹囲を測りましょう. | ☐ I'm going to [Let me] measure your abdominal circumference. |
| —…cm あります. | — It's____centimeters. |
| 超音波検査をしましょう. | ☐ I'm going to [Let me] perform an ultrasound test. |
| —赤ちゃんの体重は推定…グラムです. | — The baby is supposed to weigh about____grams. |
| —順調に大きくなっています. | — The baby is growing well. |
| —赤ちゃんは元気です. | — The baby is well and healthy. |
| —心臓も元気に拍動していますよ. | — The heart is beating strongly. |
| —さかごになっていますが, 心配することはないでしょう. | — The baby is in the breech position, but don't worry. |
| —あとで助産師がさかごを直す体位を指導してくれます. | — The midwife will show you later how to turn the baby around. |
| —お子さんの性別をお知りになりたいですか. | — Would you like to find out your baby's sex? |
| それでは, この診察台にあがって下さい. | ☐ Please lie down on the examination table. |
| —下着はすべて脱いで下さい. | — Please remove all your underwear. |
| —内診をしますので, 足を少し開いて下さい. | — Open your legs a little for the examination. |
| —お腹の力を抜いてゆっくりと深呼吸して下さい. | — Relax the muscles of your abdomen, and breathe deeply and slowly. |
| 超音波のプローブを腟の中に入れますね. | ☐ Now, I'm inserting this ultrasound probe in your vagina. |
| —ここに赤ちゃんが見えますよ. | — Look, you can see your baby. |
| —心臓が動いているのもわかります. | — You can see the baby's heart beating. |

| 残念ながら赤ちゃんは亡くなっています. | ☐ I'm sorry to tell you that the baby is dead. |

## 名句・ことわざ

All the world's a stage,
And all the men and women merely players;
They have their exits and their entrances;
And one man in his time plays many parts, ...

**全世界が一つの舞台，そこでは男女を問わぬ，人間はすべて役者に過ぎない，それぞれ出があり，引っ込みあり，しかも一人一人が生涯に色々な役を演じ分けるのだ…（福田恆存訳）**

英国の劇作家シェイクスピア（William Shakespeare, 1564-1616）『お気に召すまま *As You Like It*』に登場する皮肉屋ジェイキスの名台詞．カナダの医師オスラーによると，医師や看護師は，主役の患者が生まれてから死ぬまで生涯にわたって演じる芝居に立ち会う「かけがえのない脇役」であるという（William Osler, *Aequanimitas*）．

## ● 診察が終わって

あなたは妊娠 5 週めです．
―予定日は 8 月 23 日です．

- You are five weeks pregnant.
— Your due date is August 23.

まだ妊娠をはっきりと確認することはできません．
― 2 週間くらいするとはっきりするでしょう．

- We can't confirm your pregnancy yet.
— You'll know whether you are pregnant or not in about two weeks.

赤ちゃんの超音波写真です．
―差し上げます．

- Here's the ultrasound film of your baby.
— This is for you [You can have it].

つわりを軽くする薬を差し上げましょう．
―つわりの症状は 6 週間ほどでおさまるでしょう．
―その症状は出産するまで我慢するしかありません．

- I'll give you medication for morning sickness.
— The morning sickness will go away in about six weeks.
— You'll have to put up with the symptoms till the baby is born.

処方された薬以外は飲まないで下さい．

- Please don't take any medication unless prescribed by us.

減塩食にしたほうがよいでしょう．

- I recommend you follow a low-salt diet.

体重が増え過ぎないように注意して下さい．

- Be careful not to gain too much weight.

性行為は控えて下さい．

- Please refrain from sexual activities.

出産についてお尋ねします．
―この病院での出産を希望されますか．

- I'd like to ask you about your labor and delivery.
— Do you want to have the baby in this hospital?

―どんな方法を希望しますか. — Which type of childbirth method do you prefer?
1. 自然分娩.
2. 計画分娩.
3. 無痛分娩.
4. その他.

1. Natural delivery?
2. Planned delivery?
3. Painless delivery?
4. Any other method?

―立会い出産をご希望ですか. — Would you like to have your husband〔partner〕in the delivery room?

当院では,ラマーズ法を取り入れています.
☐ We use the Lamaze technique of controlled breathing in this hospital.

当院では母子同室です.
☐ This hospital has a rooming-in policy.

可能なら母親〔両親〕学級に参加して下さい.
☐ I recommend that you attend mothers'〔parents'〕classes, if it is possible.

帰国されるのでしたら,妊娠 30 週くらいまでのうちがよろしいでしょう.
☐ If you want to go back to your country, I recommend that you go before you are about 30 weeks pregnant.

保健所へ行って母子(健康)手帳を交付してもらって下さい.
☐ Please go to the health center and get *Boshi-techo*〔the Mother and Child Health Handbook〕.

次の検診日は 3 月 7 日,火曜日です.
☐ Your next check-up is March 7, Tuesday.

| | |
|---|---|
| 次回は（自治体の）公費負担券〔受診票〕を持ってきて下さい． | ☐ Next time you come, please bring a public payment coupon 〔a public payment consultation card〕 entitling you to free checkups (issued by the local government). |
| ―…回分，公費でまかなわれます． | ― You can have＿＿free checkups at public expense. |
| …ときは 03–xxxx–xxxx までお電話下さい． | ☐ Call us at 03–xxxx–xxxx if... |
| 　1．胎動がなくなった | 　1．the baby has stopped moving. |
| 　2．お腹の張りがつよい | 　2．your abdomen feels excessively bloated. |
| 　3．出血した | 　3．you have vaginal bleeding. |
| 　4．心配なことがある | 　4．you have any concerns. |
| ご質問がありますか． | ☐ (Do you have) any questions? |

# 分娩

## 🔵 診察室で

痛みの間隔はどれくらいですか.
- How close together are the pains [contractions]?

— 10分おきですか.
— Every 10 minutes?

—痛みはどのくらい続きますか.
— How long do they last?

—だんだん長く続き,強く,そして間隔が短くなっていますか.
— Are they longer, stronger, and closer together?

—産徴[おしるし]がありましたか.
— Have you noticed a bloody show?

—破水しましたか.
— Has your water broken?

診察しましょう.
- I'm going to [Let me] examine you.

—まだ子宮口は開いていません.
— Your cervix hasn't dilated yet.

—子宮口は6センチ開いています.
— Your cervix has dilated to 6 centimeters.

—赤ちゃんは降りてきています.
— The baby is moving down.

—あと…時間くらいで生まれるでしょう.
— The baby will be born in about ____ hours.

—生まれるまでにはしばらく時間がかかりそうです.
— It will take some time before the baby is born.

水,ジュースなど水分を十分にとって下さい.
- Please drink plenty of fluids, water, juice, and others.

トイレに行きますか.
- Do you need to go to the toilet?

陣痛室にお連れしましょう.
- I'm going to [Let me] take you to the labor room.

## 🔵 陣痛室で

それでは,浣腸します.
- Now, I'm going to give you an enema.

| | |
|---|---|
| 楽にしていて下さい．痛んだら教えて下さい． | ☐ Just relax. Please tell me when you have a pain. |
| ―呼吸はゆっくり自分のリズムで，鼻から吸い込んで口から吐いてみて下さい． | ― Try to breathe slowly and rhythmically in through the nose and out through the mouth. |
| ―しばらく辛抱して下さい． | ― You'll have to wait patiently. |
| ―痛みが強くなってきたらコールボタンを押して下さい． | ― Please press the call button when the pain becomes intense. |
| 分娩室にお連れしましょう． | ☐ I'm going to [Let me] take you to the delivery room. |

## ● 分娩室で

| | |
|---|---|
| 子宮口が全開しましたよ． | ☐ Your cervix is fully dilated. |
| 指示があったときだけ，いきんで下さい． | ☐ Please push only when you are told. |
| ―さあ，いきんで． | ― Now, bear down and push. |
| ―止めて．はい，けっこうです． | ― Stop [Hold]. Good [OK]. |
| ―いきまないで． | ― Don't push. |
| ―力をためておいて． | ― Save [Conserve] your strength. |
| ―痛みと痛みの間はゆっくり休んで下さい． | ― Relax and rest between pains [contractions]. |
| ―体の力を抜いて下さい． | ― Please relax your muscles. |
| ―では，もう一度． | ― Let's do it again. |
| 頭が出てきましたよ．がんばって．さあもう一度． | ☐ The baby's head has appeared. Hang in there! Push again. |
| ―今度は口を開けてハッハッハッと浅く息を吸ったり吐いたりして下さい． | ― Now, take shallow breaths in and out through your mouth, saying "Huh, huh, huh." |
| 胎盤を出すために，もう一度いきんで下さい． | ☐ Please give one more push to expel the placenta. |

|  |  |
|---|---|
| それでは…をしましょう． | ☐ Now, I'm going to [Let me] give you… |
| 1. 会陰切開 | 1. an episiotomy. |
| 2. 会陰縫合 | 2. stitches. |
| 陣痛促進剤を使用したほうがよいでしょう． | ☐ We should induce your labor with an ecbolic [a drug to stimulate contractions]. |
| …をしなければなりません． | ☐ You'll have to have… |
| 1. 鉗子分娩 | 1. a forceps delivery. |
| 2. 吸引分娩 | 2. a vacuum extraction. |
| 3. 帝王切開 | 3. a Cesarean section. |
| おめでとうございます．男〔女〕の赤ちゃんです． | ☐ Congratulations! It's a boy 〔girl〕. |
| ―身長は 52 cm，体重は 3,800 g です． | ― He〔She〕is 52 centimeters tall and weighs 3,800 grams. |
| ―ほら，丈夫な赤ちゃんですよ． | ― Look! He〔She〕is a healthy baby. |
| ―胸に抱いてみたいですか． | ― Would you like to hug him〔her〕to your breasts? |
| ―お乳をあげたいですか． | ― Would you like to breast-feed him〔her〕? |
| 可愛い赤ちゃんですね． | ☐ What a cute [pretty] baby (she is/he is)! |
| | ☐ How cute [pretty] (she/he is)!★ |
| 回復室にお連れしましょう． | ☐ I'm going to [Let me] take you to the recovery room. |

## ● 出産後

|  |  |
|---|---|
| 子宮が収縮するために後陣痛が起こります． | ☐ You'll have after pains as your uterus continues to contract after birth. |
| ―後陣痛は 2〜3 日続きます． | ― They'll continue for a few days. |

---

★ "cute" のかわりに "beautiful"，"handsome" などを用いてもよい．

| | |
|---|---|
| 子宮は順調に回復しています. | Your uterus is recovering well [as expected]. |
| 初乳は大事です. | ☐ The first breast milk is very important. |
| 母乳はだんだんに出てくるようになります. | ☐ Your breasts will produce more and more milk. |
| 当院では助産師による母乳指導を行っています. | ☐ The midwife in this hospital will show you how to breast-feed the baby. |
| 悪露は6週間ほどで消失するでしょう. | ☐ The vaginal discharge will disappear in about six weeks. |
| 心配なことがある時には03-xxxx-xxxxまでお電話下さい. | ☐ Please call us at 03-xxxx-xxxx when you have concerns. |
| 赤ちゃんとお母さんの1か月健診は9月7日,火曜日です. | ☐ The 1-month health checkup for you and your baby is Tuesday, September 7. |

chapter 11

# 小児

## Children

子供のプロフィール 380
現病歴 382
栄養 389
成長発達 390
既往歴 392
家族歴・ペット 397
薬剤投与 397
予防接種・健診 398

# 子供のプロフィール

## ➲ 年齢

| | |
|---|---|
| お子さんはおいくつですか. | ☐ How old is your baby 〔child〕? |
| 母子（健康）手帳をもっていますか. | ☐ Do you have *Boshi-techo* [the Mother and Child Health Handbook]? |
| —それを見せて下さい. | — Please show it to me. |
| 保育園か幼稚園に通っていますか. | ☐ Does he 〔she〕 go to a day care center [nursery school] or kindergarten?★ |

## ➲ 家族

| | |
|---|---|
| きょうだいはいますか. | ☐ Does he 〔she〕 have any brothers or sisters? |
| —何歳ですか. | — How old is he 〔she〕? |
| | — How old are they? |
| ご家族は全部で何人ですか. | ☐ How many people are there in your family? |
| —皆さんお元気ですか. | — Are they all in good health? |

☞ 父親, 母親についての情報は「患者さんのプロフィール」(1 ページ).

## ➲ 現在の健康状態

| | |
|---|---|
| これまで健康状態はどうでしたか. | ☐ How has his 〔her〕 health been up until now? |
| 1. 大変よい. | 1. Excellent? |
| 2. よい. | 2. Good? |
| 3. まあまあ. | 3. Fair? |
| 4. 悪い. | 4. Poor? |

---

★ 一般的には, nursery school は 3〜4 歳児を預かる所で, kindergarten は就学前の 5〜6 歳児が通う所をさす.

| | |
|---|---|
| 体重は予定通り増えていますか. | ☐ Is he〔she〕gaining weight at the expected rate? |
| 健康上気がかりなことがありますか. | ☐ Do you have any health concerns about him〔her〕now? |
| かかりつけの医師はいますか. | ☐ Does he〔she〕have a regular doctor? |
| ―お名前を教えて下さい. | ― Please give me his〔her〕name. |

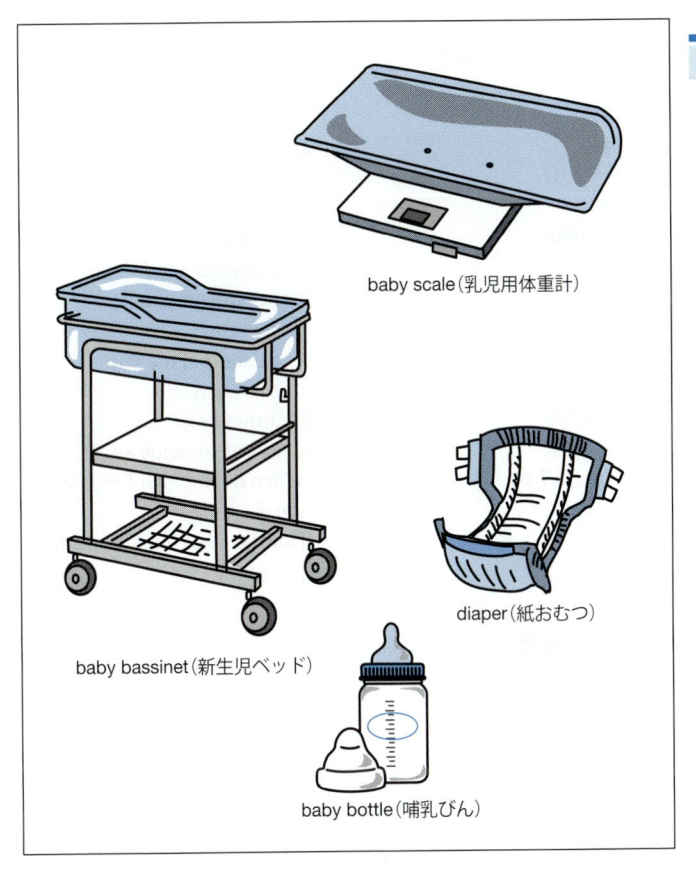

baby scale（乳児用体重計）

baby bassinet（新生児ベッド）

diaper（紙おむつ）

baby bottle（哺乳びん）

# 現病歴

☞ ここでは小児の症状に特有の表現のみをとりあげるので，詳しくは主要症状の各項目あるいは系統別レビューの各項目を参照のこと．
☞「主訴を訊く」(18 ページ)．
☞「現病歴」(24 ページ)．

## ➡ 主訴

どうなさいましたか．

☐ What's your baby's [child's] problem?

…のような症状がありますか．

☐ Does he [she] have problems, such as...

1. 高熱
2. 発疹
3. ひきつけ
4. 頭痛
5. 首の痛み
6. 腹痛
7. 排尿痛
8. 嘔吐
9. チアノーゼ
10. 嗜眠状態
11. 意識消失

1. a high fever?
2. a rash?
3. seizures [convulsions]?
4. a headache?
5. neck pain?
6. a stomachache?
7. pain on urination?
8. vomiting?
9. paleness of the skin [cyanosis]?
10. drowsiness?
11. loss of consciousness?

― いつからですか．

― When did his [her] problem start?

― どのくらい長く続いていますか．

― How long has he [she] had the problem?

## ➡ 機嫌・意識

機嫌はどうですか．
1. いつもと同じ．
2. ふだんよりぐずる．

☐ How has his [her] mood been?
1. The same?
2. More fretful than usual?

| | |
|---|---|
| 泣き方がいつもとは違ってかなり激しいですか. | ☐ Does he〔she〕cry excessively in a way that is unusual for him〔her〕? |
| 異常なほど傾眠がちですか. | ☐ Is he〔she〕abnormally drowsy? |
| 意識がはっきりしませんか. | ☐ Is he〔she〕confused? |
| 眠りすぎることがありますか. | ☐ Does he〔she〕sleep too much? |

## ● 食欲・体重

☞「食欲」(99 ページ).
☞「体重変化」(100 ページ).

| | |
|---|---|
| ミルクの飲みはどうですか.<br>　1. いつもと同じ.<br>　2. 飲みたがらない. | ☐ How does he〔she〕take the feeding〔milk〕?<br>　1. The same?<br>　2. Reluctantly? |
| ミルクを飲んだ後吐いてぐずりますか. | ☐ Does he〔she〕vomit after feedings and start to cry? |
| お子さんの食欲はどうですか.<br>　1. よい.<br>　2. かなり悪い.<br>　3. ぜんぜんない. | ☐ How has your child's appetite been?<br>　1. Good?<br>　2. Poor?<br>　3. No appetite? |
| 固形の食べ物を嫌がりますか. | ☐ Is he〔she〕reluctant to eat solid foods? |
| 食べ物をぜんぜん口にしませんか. | ☐ Is he〔she〕refusing all the foods? |
| 水分も飲みませんか. | ☐ Is he〔she〕also refusing to drink? |

体重のことがご心配ですか.

1. 標準より少ない.

2. 標準より多い.

☐ Are you concerned about his 〔her〕 weight?
1. Below the normal range for his 〔her〕 age?
2. Above the normal range for his 〔her〕 age?

## ● 系統別の病歴

### 皮膚

☞「皮膚」(159 ページ).

お子さんに皮膚の異常がありますか.
―それは何ですか.どこですか.
―引っ掻いていますか.

☐ Does he 〔she〕 have any skin problems?
— What is it? Where?
— Has he 〔she〕 been scratching?

おへそがじくじくしていますか.

☐ Is his 〔her〕 navel wet and sticky?

お子さんはオムツかぶれを頻繁に起こしますか.
―いつですか.
―どんな方策を講じていますか.

☐ Does he 〔she〕 have a diaper rash very often?
— When does he 〔she〕 have it?
— What measures are you taking?

### 耳・鼻

☞「耳鼻咽喉・頸部」(60 ページ).

耳やのどの感染症によくかかりますか.

☐ Does he 〔she〕 have frequent ear or throat infections?

どちらかの耳を引っ張りますか.

☐ Does he 〔she〕 tug at either ear?

大きな音や聞きなれない音に反応しますか.

☐ Does he 〔she〕 respond to loud or unfamiliar noises?

| | |
|---|---|
| 後ろからの呼びかけに振り向きますか. | ☐ Does he [she] turn his [her] face in the direction of the voice from behind? |
| 鼻血をよく出しますか. | ☐ Does he [she] have frequent nosebleeds? |
| 鼻汁が出ますか. | ☐ Does he [she] have any discharge from his [her] nose? |
| よく鼻がつまりますか. | ☐ Does he [she] frequently have a stuffy nose? |

### 眼

☞「眼」(54 ページ).

| | |
|---|---|
| 目をよくこすりますか. | ☐ Does he [she] often rub his [her] eyes? |
| 目つきや目の動きがおかしいと感じますか. | ☐ Do you feel that something is wrong with the expression or movement of his [her] eyes? |
| 物を見るときよく目を細めますか. | ☐ Does he [she] squint frequently to see things? |
| 物を見るときに首を傾けますか. | ☐ Does he [she] tilt his [her] head to see things? |
| テレビ画面のすぐ近くに座りますか. | ☐ Does he [she] sit very close to the TV screen? |

### 呼吸器

☞「呼吸器」(76 ページ).

| | |
|---|---|
| 出生時に呼吸に異常がありましたか. | ☐ Did he [she] have any respiratory problems at birth? |

| 息切れのためにミルクが飲めませんか. | ☐ Does shortness of breath interfere when he〔she〕takes the bottle〔nurses〕? |
|---|---|
| 咳のために目を覚ましますか. | ☐ Does he〔she〕wake up because of coughing? |

### 心・血管

☞「心・血管」(84 ページ).

| 泣くと顔が青くなりますか. | ☐ Does he〔she〕turn blue when he〔she〕cries? |
|---|---|
| ミルクを飲むのが困難ですか. | ☐ Does he〔she〕have difficulty taking the bottle〔nursing〕? |
| ―飲むのにどのくらい時間がかかりますか. | ― How long does it take for him〔her〕to take a bottle? |
| 疲れやすく,遊んでいる最中よく座ったりうずくまったりしますか. | ☐ Does he〔she〕get tired easily and often sit or squat during play? |

### 消化器

☞「消化器」(92 ページ).

| ミルクはふつうどおり飲みましたか. | ☐ Did he〔she〕take the last feeding as normal? |
|---|---|
| 授乳後ミルクを吐いて泣き始めたのですか. | ☐ Did he〔she〕vomit after feeding and start to cry? |
| 排便で困ることがありますか. | ☐ Does he〔she〕have any difficulty passing stools? |
| 便は硬めですか,やわらかめですか. | ☐ Have his〔her〕stools been rather hard or soft? |

| | |
|---|---|
| 便は何色ですか. | ☐ What's the color of his〔her〕stools? |
| お子さんは今特別なストレスを感じていますか. | ☐ Is he〔she〕under any unusual stress? |

### 泌尿器・生殖器

☞「腎・泌尿器」(103 ページ).
☞「男性生殖器」(110 ページ).

| | |
|---|---|
| 排尿で困ることがありますか. | ☐ Does he〔she〕have any difficulty urinating? |
| オムツを毎日何枚濡らしますか.<br>―最近,その枚数に変化がありましたか.<br>　1. 同じ.<br>　2. 減った.<br>　3. 増えた. | ☐ How many diapers does he〔she〕wet a day?<br>— Has the number changed recently?<br>　1. The same?<br>　2. Decreased?<br>　3. Increased? |
| 尿をするとき泣きますか. | ☐ Does he〔she〕cry when he〔she〕urinates? |
| 夜尿がありますか. | ☐ Does he〔she〕wet the bed? |
| 包茎の手術をしていますか. | ☐ Is he circumcised? |
| 泣いたり排便したりするときに陰嚢が肥大するのに気づきましたか. | ☐ Have you noticed any scrotal swelling when he cries or has a bowel movement? |

### 筋・骨格

☞「筋・骨格」(139 ページ).

| | |
|---|---|
| 手足を均等に動かすことができますか. | ☐ Can he〔she〕move his〔her〕hands, arms, feet, or legs equally well? |

| | |
|---|---|
| 首が傾いていると感じますか. | ☐ Do you feel that he〔she〕puts his〔her〕head to one side? |

### 感染症

| | |
|---|---|
| 家庭，保育園，幼稚園，学校で最近感染症にかかった人がいますか. | ☐ Has anyone around him〔her〕had recent infections at home, at day care center〔nursery school〕, at kindergarten, or at school? |

### 事故

何かを誤って口に入れましたか.

1. タバコ.
2. 薬.
3. 化粧品.
4. 洗剤.
5. 豆.
6. ボタン.
7. 硬貨.
8. その他.

☐ Did he〔she〕accidentally put something in his〔her〕mouth?
1. Cigarette?
2. Medication?
3. Cosmetics?
4. Detergent?
5. Beans?
6. Buttons?
7. Coins?
8. Something else?

## 栄養

授乳は主に何でやっていますか.

1. 母乳.
2. ミルク.
3. 混合.

―ミルクの飲みはふつう〔悪い〕ですか.
―24 時間の間に何回授乳しますか.
―毎日ミルクを何 ml 飲みますか.

水〔ジュース〕を飲みますか.

最近, 離乳食を始めましたか.

まだ哺乳瓶を使っていますか.
―コップを使って飲みますか.
―スプーンを使って食べますか.

お子さんの食欲はどうですか.
―よい〔悪い〕ですか？

食べ物に好き嫌いがありますか.

―大好きな食べ物がありますか. 甘いものやファストフードは？

―食べたがらないものがありますか.

☐ How is your baby fed?
☐ Do you feed him〔her〕…
　1. breast milk?
　2. formula milk?
　3. mixed?
― Is his〔her〕ability to suck normal〔weak〕?
― How many times do you nurse him〔her〕in 24 hours?
― How many milliliters of formula (milk) does he〔she〕take each day?

☐ Does he〔she〕take water〔juice〕?

☐ Have you recently started him〔her〕on solid foods?

☐ Does he〔she〕still bottle-feed?
― Does he〔she〕drink from a cup?
― Does he〔she〕eat with a spoon?

☐ How is your child's appetite?
― Is it good〔poor〕?

☐ Does he〔she〕have likes and dislikes about foods?

― Are there any foods he〔she〕really likes to eat? How about sweets or fast food?

― Are there any foods he〔she〕refuses to eat?

# 成長発達

## ➡ 運動・動作・生活習慣

お子さんは…ことができますか．
1. 首をあげる
2. 寝返りをうつ
3. おもちゃをつかむ
4. おすわりをする
5. はいはいする
6. つかまり立ちをする
7. つたい歩きをする
8. バイバイやコンニチハの身振りをする
9. ひとり立ちする
10. ひとりで歩く
11. ひとりで服を着る
12. 走る
13. 三輪車をこぐ
14. 排尿をコントロールする
15. 排便をコントロールする

その動作が初めてできたのは何か月〔何歳〕ごろのときですか．

☐ Is your baby [child] able to…
1. hold up his [her] head [hold his [her] head steady]?
2. roll over on his [her] own?
3. grasp toys?
4. sit up without support?
5. crawl?
6. stand with support?
7. walk holding onto something?
8. make a gesture of "bye-bye" or "hi"?
9. stand alone without support?
10. walk alone without support?
11. dress himself [herself] without support?
12. run?
13. pedal a tricycle?
14. have bladder control?
15. have bowel control?

☐ At about what month [age] was he [she] able to do that movement?

## ➡ 言語

お子さんは…しますか．
1. 声のするほうへ顔を向ける
2. 喃語を話す
3. ママ，パパなどの単純な語を口にする
4. 自分の名前が言える
5. 年齢に応じた言葉を話す

☐ Does your baby [child]…
1. turn his [her] face toward a voice?
2. babble?
3. say simple words such as Mama or Dada?
4. say his [her] own name?
5. speak appropriately for his [her] age?

| | |
|---|---|
| それが初めてできたのは何か月〔何歳〕ごろのときですか. | At about what month〔age〕was he〔she〕able to do it? |

## ● 社会性

| | |
|---|---|
| お子さんは…しますか.<br>　1. あなたや他の人を見て笑う<br>　2. 人見知りをする<br><br>　3. あなたの後を追う<br>　4. ひとり遊びをする<br>　5. 友達と遊ぶ | Does your baby [child]...<br>　1. smile at you or others?<br>　2. have stranger anxiety?<br>　　= Is he〔she〕afraid of strangers?<br>　3. seek and follow you?<br>　4. play by himself〔herself〕?<br>　5. play with friends? |
| どんな遊びが好きですか. | What are his〔her〕favorite playing activities? |
| それが初めてできたのは何か月〔何歳〕ごろのときですか. | At about what month〔age〕was he〔she〕able to do it? |
| 他に話すことがありますか. | (Is there) anything that you'd like to tell me now? |

## ● 個人特性

| | |
|---|---|
| ぬいぐるみを抱いて寝ますか. | Does he〔she〕sleep with stuffed animals? |
| 爪をかみますか. | Does he〔she〕bite his〔her〕nails? |
| おしゃぶりを使うか,指しゃぶりをしますか. | Does he〔she〕use a pacifier or suck his〔her〕thumb? |
| かんしゃくを起こしますか. | Does he〔she〕have tantrums? |
| 夜泣きをしますか. | Does he〔she〕cry in the night? |
| 夜尿がありますか. | Does he〔she〕wet his〔her〕bed? |

## 既往歴

### ➡ 出生前・出生時情報

妊娠中, あなた〔母親〕に何か異常がありましたか.

1. 妊娠高血圧症候群.
2. 高血圧.
3. 蛋白尿.
4. 浮腫.
5. 子癇.
6. 糖尿病.
7. 風疹.

妊娠中, ビタミン以外で何か薬を飲みましたか.

―何ですか.
―いつ, どのくらいの間ですか.

妊娠中, 入院を必要としましたか.

―理由は何ですか.

1. つわり.
2. 切迫流産.
3. 切迫早産.
4. 妊娠高血圧症候群.

出産時, あなた〔母親〕に何か異常がありましたか.

―合併症がありましたか.
―それについて説明して下さい.

☐ Did you〔the mother〕have any health problems during pregnancy?
1. Pregnancy-induced hypertension?
2. High blood pressure?
3. Proteinuria?
4. Edema?
5. Eclampsia?
6. Diabetes?
7. Rubella〔German measles〕?

☐ Did you〔the mother〕take any medications besides vitamins during pregnancy?

— What were they?
— When did you〔she〕take them? For how long?

☐ Were you〔Was she〕hospitalized during pregnancy?

— What was the problem? Why were you〔was she〕hospitalized?
1. Morning sickness?
2. Threatened miscarriage?
3. Threatened premature delivery?
4. Pregnancy-induced hypertension?

☐ Did you〔the mother〕have any problems during labor or delivery?

— Any complications?
— Please tell me about them.

| | |
|---|---|
| どんな分娩でしたか. | ☐ What type of delivery was it? Was it... |
| 1. 経腟分娩. | 1. a vaginal delivery? |
| 2. 鉗子分娩. | 2. a forceps delivery? |
| 3. 吸引分娩. | 3. a vacuum extraction delivery? |
| 4. 帝王切開. | 4. a Cesarean section delivery? |
| 満期産でしたか, 早産でしたか. | ☐ Was the baby born full term or premature? |
| ―何週で生まれたのですか. | ― How many weeks were you 〔was she〕 pregnant when the baby was born? |
| 出生時の体重はいくらでしたか. | ☐ How much did the baby weigh at birth? |
| 出生直後あるいは新生児初期に何か異常がありましたか. | ☐ Did the baby have any problems immediately after birth or in the early newborn stage? |
| ―すぐ泣かなかったのですか. | ― Did he 〔she〕 not cry immediately after birth? |
| ―保育器に入りましたか. | ― Was he 〔she〕 put in an incubator? |
| ―黄疸が強かったですか. | ― Did he 〔she〕 have a severe form of jaundice? |

## ● 既往症

☞「既往症」(187 ページ).

| | |
|---|---|
| お子さんはこれまでに大きな病気や怪我をしましたか. | ☐ Has your baby〔child〕ever had any serious illnesses or injuries? |
| ―何でしたか. | ― What were they? |

☞「小児に多い病気」(395 ページ).

| | |
|---|---|
| ―どんな治療を受けましたか. | ― How were they treated? |
| ―どのくらい長く続きましたか. | ― How long did the problems last? |
| ―何か後遺症は残っていますか. | ― Does he〔she〕still suffer from the aftereffects of the problems? |
| 意識を失ったことがありますか. | ☐ Has he〔she〕ever lost consciousness? |
| ひきつけを起こしたことがありますか. | ☐ Has he〔she〕ever had a seizure? |
| ―それは発熱に伴ったものでしたか. | ― Did a fever accompany it? |
| 入院したことがありますか. | ☐ Has he〔she〕ever been hospitalized? |
| なにか手術を受けたことがありますか. | ☐ Has he〔she〕ever had surgery of any kind? |
| ―何の手術でしたか. | ― What was it? |
| ―その時何か月〔歳〕でしたか. | ― How many months〔How old〕was he〔she〕? |

## 用語・表現ファイル

### 病名　その2　小児に多い病気

#### 1. 感染症

| | |
|---|---|
| 麻疹 | measles |
| 風疹［三日ばしか］ | rubella［German measles］ |
| 流行性耳下腺炎 | mumps |
| 水痘 | chickenpox |
| 突発性発疹 | exanthema subitum（roseola） |
| 溶血性連鎖球菌感染症 | hemolytic streptococcal infection |
| しょう紅熱 | scarlet fever |
| リウマチ熱 | rheumatic fever |
| 百日咳 | whooping cough［pertussis］ |
| 脳炎 | encephalitis |
| 髄膜炎 | meningitis |
| 反復する中耳炎 | recurrent middle-ear infection［otitis media］ |

#### 2. アレルギー性疾患

| | |
|---|---|
| アレルギー性鼻炎 | allergic rhinitis |
| アトピー性皮膚炎 | eczema［atopic dermatitis］ |
| 喘息 | asthma |
| 花粉症 | hay fever |

#### 3. その他

| | |
|---|---|
| 鼠径ヘルニア | inguinal hernia |
| 頭部外傷 | injury of the head |
| 骨折 | bone fracture |
| 熱傷 | burn |
| 熱性痙攣 | febrile convulsion |

☞「主要な病気」(189ページ).

## ➲ 薬歴

☞「薬歴」(194ページ).

今までに薬を飲みましたか.
- [ ] Has he〔she〕taken any drugs or medications in the past?

何か薬を常用していますか.
- [ ] Does he〔she〕take any drugs or medications regularly?

---

### 名句・ことわざ

**All we know is still infinitely less than all that still remains unknown.**

**これまで知り得たことの全ては,いまだ知り得ぬことに比べると極めてわずかにすぎない**

英国の解剖学者・医師ハーヴェイ(William Harvey, 1578-1657, *De Motu Cordis et Sanguinis*)の名言.彼は血液循環説を初めて唱えたことで名高い.

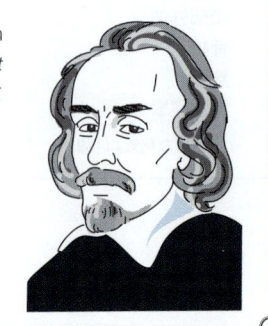

## 家族歴・ペット

ご家族で…の人はいますか.

1. 結核
2. 遺伝性の病気

3. アレルギー性疾患
4. 神経系疾患

ペットを飼っていますか.
―どんなペットですか.
1. 犬.
2. 猫.
3. 鳥.

☐ Has anyone in his〔her〕immediate family had...
1. tuberculosis?
2. a disease which runs in his〔her〕family?
3. allergic disease?
4. neurological disease?

☐ Do you have pets in your house?
— What type of pets?
1. Dogs?
2. Cats?
3. Birds?

## 薬剤投与

☞「薬剤投与」(297 ページ).

薬はシロップ〔錠剤／丸薬〕がよいですか.
―粉薬はジュース〔アイスクリーム／ヨーグルト〕に混ぜると飲ませやすいです.
―乳酸飲料〔スポーツ飲料〕に混ぜると苦くなります.

―スポイトを使うと飲ませやすいです.

☐ Would you like to have syrup〔tablets/pills〕for your child?
— It'll be easy to give the powder to your child if you mix it with juice〔ice cream/yoghurt〕.
— If you mix it with a lactic acid beverage〔sports drink〕, it'll become bitter.
— It'll be easy to give the medication to your child if you use a dropper.

# 予防接種・健診

## ● 予防接種

☞「予防接種」(198, 400 ページ).

| | |
|---|---|
| これまでにどんな予防接種を受けましたか. | ☐ What vaccinations has he〔she〕had? |
| —母子(健康)手帳を見せて下さい. | — Let me see *Boshi-techo*〔the Mother and Child Health Handbook〕. |
| 今日は…の予防注射をしましょう. | ☐ I'm going to give him〔her〕 ____ vaccine today. |
| —しっかり抱っこしていて下さい. | — Please hold him〔her〕firmly. |
| —今日は激しい運動は控えさせて下さい. | — He〔She〕shouldn't exercise hard today. |
| —お風呂に入れてもいいですよ. | — He〔She〕can have a bath. |
| —少し腫れるかもしれませんが,心配ないでしょう. | — He〔She〕may have slight swelling, but don't worry. |
| —心配なときは 03−xxxx−xxxx までお電話下さい. | — Please call us at 03−xxxx−xxxx when you have concerns. |
| 次回の予防接種は 1 か月後です. | ☐ The next vaccination is going to be in about 1 month. |

## ● 健診

| | |
|---|---|
| 前回の健診はいつでしたか. | ☐ When was his〔her〕last health checkup? |
| —何か異常所見はありましたか. | — Have you been told that he〔she〕has a problem? |
| —何の異常ですか. | — What was the problem? |
| —どのような指導,治療を受けましたか. | — What kind of instructions or treatments did he〔she〕get? |

| 専門医の診察を受けたことがありますか. | ☐ Has he〔she〕had an exam by a specialist? |
| --- | --- |
| —いつですか. | — When was it? |
| —何と言われましたか. | — What did the doctor tell you about his〔her〕problem? |

| 4か月〔18か月／3年〕健診は6月7日,火曜日です. | ☐ His〔Her〕4-month 〔18-month/ 3-year〕health checkup is Tuesday, June 7. |
| --- | --- |
| —市の広報でチェックして下さい. | — Please check the schedule in your local city bulletin. |

---

### 名句・ことわざ

**Prevention is better than cure.**

予防にまさる治癒はなし

英国の法律家ブラクトン(Henry of Bracton, 1210?-1268, *De Legibus*). 日本のことわざ「転ばぬ先の杖」に相当する.

## 用語・表現ファイル

### 予防接種

#### 1. 定期接種

| | |
|---|---|
| BCG | BCG [bacille Calmette-Guerin] vaccine |
| 三種混合［ジフテリア・百日咳・破傷風］ | DPT [diphtheria-pertussis-tetanus combined] vaccine |
| 二種混合［ジフテリア・破傷風］ | DT [diphtheria-tetanus combined] vaccine |
| ポリオ | IPV [inactivated polio vaccine] |
| 麻疹・風疹混合 | MR [measles-rubella combined] vaccine |
| 麻疹 | measles vaccine |
| 風疹 | rubella vaccine |
| 日本脳炎 | Japanese encephalitis vaccine |

#### 1. Routine Vaccination

#### 2. 任意接種

| | |
|---|---|
| 流行性耳下腺炎 | mumps vaccine |
| 水痘 | chickenpox vaccine |
| インフルエンザ | influenza vaccine |
| A 型肝炎 | hepatitis A vaccine |
| B 型肝炎 | hepatitis B vaccine |
| 肺炎球菌感染症 | PCV [pneumococcal conjugate vaccine] |
| ロタウイルス | RV [rotavirus vaccine] |
| ヒトパピローマウイルス | HPV [human papillomavirus vaccine] |
| インフルエンザ菌 b 型 | Hib [*Haemophilus influenzae* type b] vaccine |

#### 2. Voluntary Vaccination

☞「予防接種」(198 ページ).

chapter 12

# リハビリテーション

## Rehabilitation

リハビリテーションの案内　402
リハビリテーション専門医の診察　403
理学療法　404
作業療法　406
言語聴覚療法　407

## リハビリテーションの案内

私たちは，あなたが可能な限り自立した生活に戻ることができるよう，必要なリハビリテーションを行います．

- [ ] We provide you with the rehabilitation therapy needed to return to the highest level of independent living as possible.

リハビリテーション専門医があなたに合ったリハビリテーション計画を立てます．

- [ ] The physiatrist, a doctor specially trained in rehabilitation medicine, will make a treatment plan specifically for you.

医師の指示を受けて理学療法士・作業療法士・言語聴覚士がリハビリテーションを行います．

- [ ] Physical therapists, occupational therapists, and speech-language-hearing therapists will perform the rehabilitation therapy under the direction of the physiatrist.

## リハビリテーション専門医の診察

| | |
|---|---|
| 初めまして．私は医師の阿部です． | ☐ Nice to meet you. I'm [My name is] Dr.Abe. |
| スペンサーさんですね． | ☐ Are you Mr.〔Mrs./Ms./Miss〕Spencer? |
| お待たせしてすみません． | ☐ I'm sorry to have kept you waiting. |
| どなたのご紹介ですか．<br>—紹介状をお持ちですか． | ☐ Who sent you to our office?<br>— Do you have a referral letter from him〔her〕? |
| それでは，いくつか質問します． | ☐ Now, can you tell me a little about yourself? |
| あなたは理学療法〔作業療法／言語療法〕を受ける必要があります． | ☐ You need to have some physical therapy〔occupational therapy/speech therapy〕. |
| リハビリテーション計画を立てましょう． | ☐ Let's make [set up] your rehabilitation plan. |
| 手続きはこちらで行います．ご都合はいつがいいですか． | ☐ We'll make the necessary arrangement. When is it convenient for you? |
| ゆったりした楽な服装とスニーカーでお越し下さい． | ☐ Wear loose fitting, comfortable clothes and sneakers. |
| ご質問はありますか． | ☐ Do you have any questions? |

chapter 12 リハビリテーション

## 理学療法

### ➡ 平行棒を使った歩行訓練

| | |
|---|---|
| こんにちは．理学療法士の金子です．ミラーさんですね． | ☐ Hello, I'm Mr. 〔Ms.〕 Kaneko, a physical therapist. Are you Ms. Miller? |
| 調子はいかがですか． | ☐ How are you feeling [doing]?<br>☐ How's your condition now? |
| あなたは脳卒中を起こして右半身が麻痺しているのですね． | ☐ I understand you're paralyzed on the right side of your body as a result of a stroke. |
| 平行棒を使って歩いてみましょう． | ☐ Let's walk on the parallel bars. |
| ご気分が悪いときや痛みがあるときにはおっしゃって下さい． | ☐ Please let me know if you feel sick or have any pain. |
| では，平行棒の間に真っ直ぐ立ちましょう．<br>―左手で，足元より数 cm 手前で手すりを握って下さい．<br>―麻痺した右足を少し踏み出し，その足に体重をかけます．<br>―次に，素早く左足を踏み出して，左足に体重を移動させます． | ☐ Now, let's stand upright between the parallel bars.<br>— With your left hand, grab onto the bar several centimeters in front of your feet.<br>— Place your paralyzed right foot a little forward, and shift your weight over onto that leg.<br>— Next, quickly step your left foot forward, and re-shift your weight onto the left leg. |
| 心配しないで下さい．そばについていますよ．<br>―そうそう，いいですよ！　続けて下さい． | ☐ Don't worry! I'll be here beside you.<br>— That's it! Go on. |
| よくできましたね．平行棒の端まで来ましたよ． | ☐ (You did a) good job! Now, you have reached the end of the parallel bars. |

| | |
|---|---|
| 今回はうまくできなくても練習していけば大丈夫ですよ. | ☐ Even though you can't do very well at this time, you'll improve by practicing this exercise. |
| これからもご一緒にリハビリテーションを頑張りましょう. | ☐ Let's work together on your rehabilitation. |
| お帰りになる前に次回の予約をして下さい. | ☐ Before you leave the hospital, please make a return appointment. |
| ―受付で予約カードをもらって下さい. | ― Please go to the reception counter and get your appointment card. |

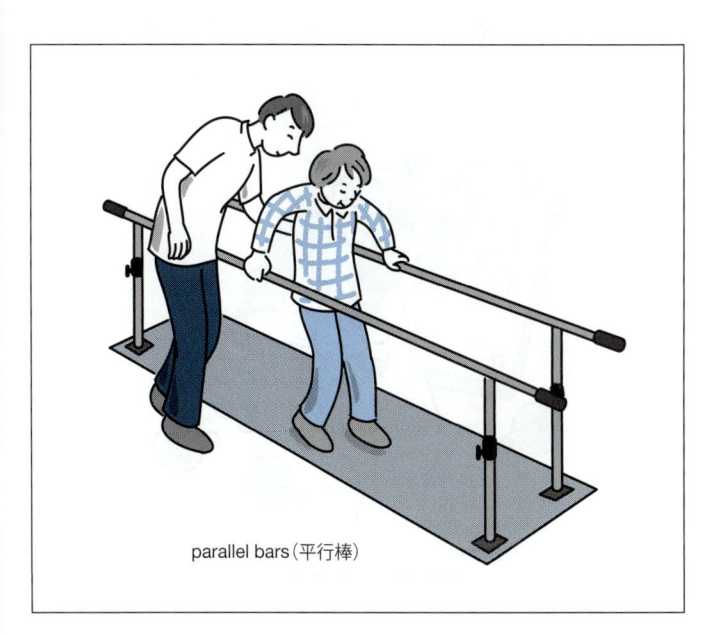

parallel bars(平行棒)

## 作業療法

### ペグボードを使った機能回復訓練

| | |
|---|---|
| おはようございます．作業療法士の清水です．ナラヤンさんですね． | ☐ Good morning, I'm Ms.〔Mr.〕Shimizu, an occupational therapist. Are you Mr. Narayan? |
| お変わりありませんか． | ☐ How have you been doing? |
| これはペグボードです．<br>―穴が開いていますから，こんなふうに棒（ペグ）を穴に入れる練習をしましょう．<br>―さあどうぞ．<br>―大変けっこうです． | ☐ Here's a peg board.<br>― Here're several holes on it. Let's practice inserting pegs into the holes, like this.<br>― Here you go!<br>― Very good! You're doing fine. |
| 今度はできるだけ早く入れてみて下さい． | ☐ This time, place the pegs in the holes as fast as you can. |
| さあ，終わりました．よく頑張りましたね． | ☐ It's all over. Well done! |

pegboard（ペグボード）

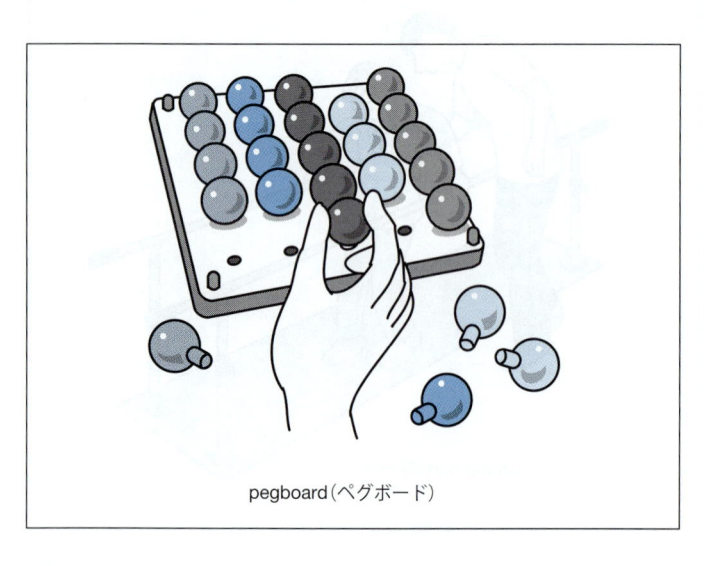

# 言語聴覚療法

## ● 顔面筋肉訓練

| | |
|---|---|
| こんにちは．言語聴覚士の森田です．リーさんですね． | Good afternoon, I'm Ms.〔Mr.〕 Morita, a speech therapist. Are you Mrs. Lee? |

ご気分はいかがですか．　　　　　How are you today?

顔の筋肉を動かす練習をしましょう．
— 私の口を見て，真似して下さい．
— まず唇をすぼめて口笛を吹くときのように前に突き出して下さい．
— それから，口を開いて思いっきり笑います．こんなふうに．

Let's do the exercise to move your facial muscles.
— Look at my mouth, and do likewise.
— First, purse your lips and push them out as if you're whistling.
— Then, let the lips come apart and smile as wide as you can, like this.

次に，英語の母音を発音してみましょう．
— できるだけ口を大きく開いて，大きな声で　母音の「エィ，イー，アィ，オゥ，ウー」を言って下さい．

Next, we're going to pronounce English vowels.
— Open your mouth as wide as you can and say the vowels out loud, "A, E, I, O, U."

もう一度やってみましょう．　　　Let's try again.

この練習は毎日繰り返すことが大切です．　　It's important to repeat these exercises every day.

鏡の前で練習するとよいでしょう．　　It can be helpful to practice them in front of a mirror.

## 用語・表現ファイル

## 呼吸法

### 1. 口すぼめ呼吸

| | |
|---|---|
| 口を閉じて,いつも通りに鼻から息を吸って下さい. | With your mouth shut, please breathe through your nose normally. |
| 口笛を吹くときのように唇をすぼめて下さい. | Purse your lips as if you're whistling. |
| すぼめた口からゆっくり息を吐いて下さい. | Breathe out slowly through your pursed lips. |
| 息を吐くとき,無理に空気をしぼり出そうとしないで下さい. | Be careful not to push yourself too hard to force the air out. |
| 吸うときの2倍くらいの時間をかけてゆっくり吐きます. | Breathe out twice as slowly as you breathed in. |
| 慣れてきたら,息を吐く時間を少しずつ長くして,呼吸の回数を減らすようにしてみましょう. | After some practice try to gradually increase the time to breathe out [make breathing out longer] and slow [reduce] your breathing rate. |

### 2. 腹式呼吸

| | |
|---|---|
| まず仰向けに寝て下さい. | First, please lie on your back. |
| リラックスして,お腹に手を当てて下さい. | Relax, and place your hand(s) on your abdomen. |
| 鼻からゆっくり息を吸って下さい.息を吸うとき,お腹が膨らむことを意識するようにして下さい. | Breathe in slowly through your nose. Try to feel that your abdomen gets larger as you breathe in. |

### 用語・表現ファイル（つづき）

| | |
|---|---|
| 唇をすぼめてゆっくり息を吐いて下さい．息をはくときは，お腹が引っ込むことを意識するようにして下さい． | Breathe out slowly through your pursed lips. Try to feel that your abdomen falls inward as you breathe out. |

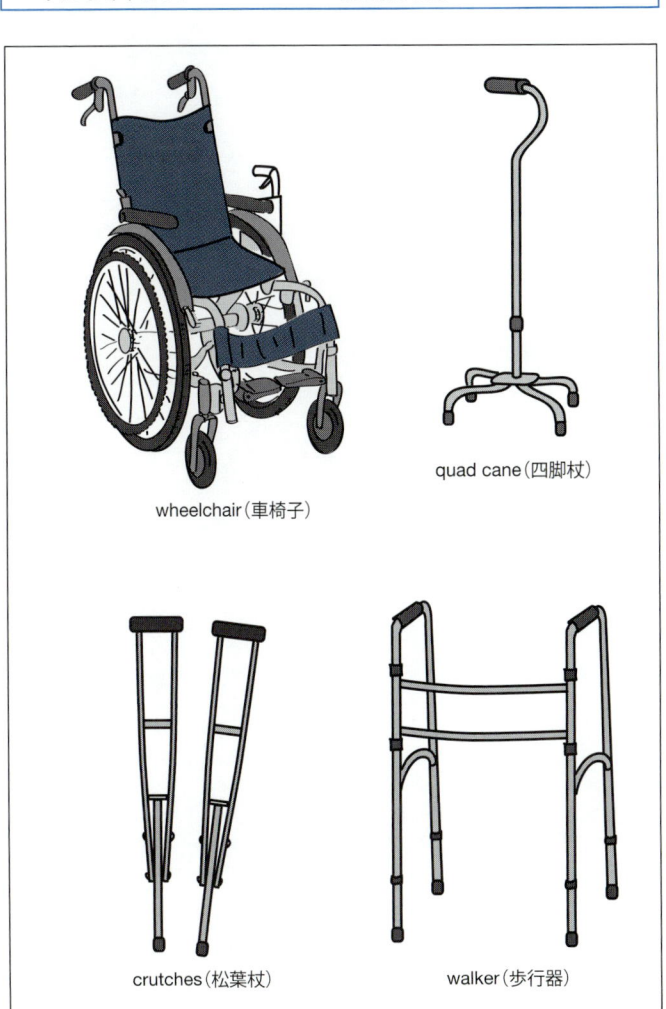

wheelchair（車椅子）

quad cane（四脚杖）

crutches（松葉杖）

walker（歩行器）

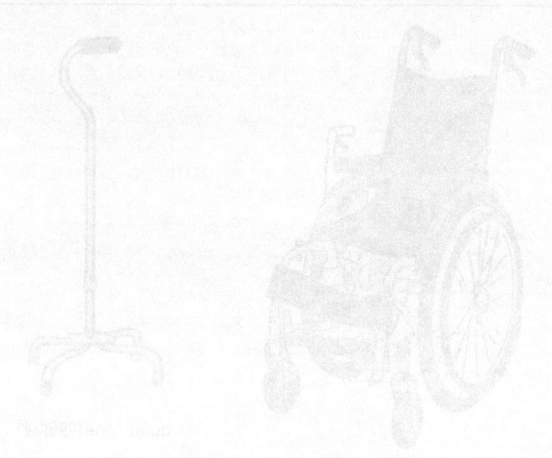

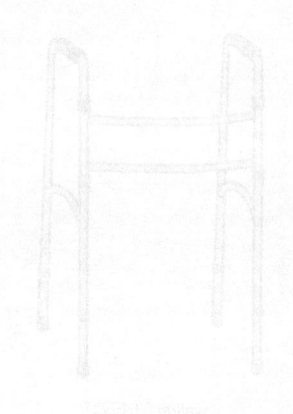

chapter 13

# 医療福祉相談

## Medical Social Work

**相談室の案内** 412
**相談当日** 414
**相談内容** 415
　受診 415
　入院生活 416
　退院後の生活 417
　経済問題 421
　その他の心配事 425

## 相談室の案内

医療福祉相談室では，社会面，心理面，経済面などさまざまな生活問題についてあなたやあなたのご家族を支援いたします．★

☐ At the Social Work Office we help you and your family by providing support in a wide variety of areas of your life including social, psychological, and financial adjustment and more.

ご質問や心配事があるときや援助を必要とするときには，お気軽にお越し下さい．

☐ If you have any questions, concerns, or if you need assistance, please feel free to visit the Office.

—お待ちしております．

— We'll be happy to help.

ご相談のある方は直接相談室にお越しいただくか，電話をおかけ下さい．看護師や医師にその旨をお伝えいただいても結構です．

☐ You may contact us directly by stopping in the Office or by making a phone call, or by informing your nurse or physician of your interest in our services.

—ベッドサイドでご相談をお受けすることもできます．

— Medical social workers are also available at your bedside.

ご相談は無料です．

☐ Our services are free of charge.

ご相談内容の秘密は厳守いたします．

☐ All information is strictly confidential.

相談室は本館の1階にあります．

☐ The Office is located on the first floor of the main building.

---

★ 医療ソーシャルワーカーの業務は多岐にわたり，地域や病院により業務内容が異なるため，1つの病院においてすべてを網羅することはできない．しかも異なる文化背景や言語をもつ外国人の患者さんには特有の相談があるので，その点にも留意したい．

| 医療相談室の受付時間は　平日の午前9時から午後4時です. | ☐ The Office is open: Monday through Friday from 9:00 am to 4:00 pm. |

### 名句・ことわざ

We should all know that diversity makes for a rich tapestry, and we must understand that all the threads of the tapestry are equal in value no matter their color; equal in importance no matter their texture.

**多様性とは味わい深いタペストリーのようなもの．織りなす糸はすべて，色が違ってもその価値は同じ，生地は違ってもその重要性は同じであることを，私たちは自覚すべきである**

米国の評論家・詩人アンジェロウ Maya Angelou（1928-, *Wouldn't Take Nothing for My Journey Now*）の名言．最近わが国でも，ダイバーシティー［多様性］という語がよく使われるようになってきた．人種・国籍・性・年齢を問わず，さまざまな違いを尊重して受け入れようという取り組みである．

## 相談当日

こんにちは．私は医療ソーシャルワーカーの石井です．

☐ Hello, I'm [my name is] Ms. [Mr.] Ishii, a medical social worker.

どうなさいましたか．
―不安や心配事がありますか．

―何でも遠慮なくお話し下さい．

☐ How can I help you?
— Are you concerned or worried about something?
— Please feel free to talk to us about any issues that you may have.

それでは，この用紙にご記入下さい．活字体でお願いします．
―姓のほうのお名前はどう発音するのですか．

☐ Then, please fill out this form. Write in block letters, please.
— How do you pronounce your family [last] name?

## 相談内容

気にかかっていることは何ですか.  □ What are your concerns?

ご相談は何についてですか.  □ What would you like to talk about?

1. 受診.
2. 入院生活.
3. 退院後の生活.
4. 経済問題.
5. その他の心配事.

1. Consultation?
2. Life in the hospital?
3. Life after discharge?
4. Financial problems?
5. Other concerns?

もっと詳しくお話し下さい.  □ Please tell me more about it.

### ➲ 受診

受診のことで何かお困りのことがありますか. 例えば, …

1. 診察申込書の記入の仕方がわからない.
2. （あなたの症状に対して）どの医師に診てもらうべきかわからない.
3. 医師, 看護師, ほかの病院スタッフとのコミュニケーションで困っている.
4. その他.

□ Do you have any concerns about your consultation?
For example, ...
1. you don't know how to fill out [in] the application form for the examination?
2. you don't know which type of doctor you should see (for your symptom)?
3. you're in trouble with communicating with your doctor, nurses, or other hospital staff?
4. any other problems?

通訳が必要ですか.
―通訳が必要ならば, こちらで手配いたします.
―通訳サービスは有料となっております.
―通訳サービスを受けるには最低3,000円の料金をお支払いいただきます.

□ Do you need an interpreter?
― If you need an interpreter, we'll make the arrangements for you.
― We offer interpreting services for a fee.
― You'll be asked to pay a three thousand yen minimum charge for interpreting services.

―通訳サービスは無料となっております.

― Interpreting services are offered free of charge.

## ⮕ 入院生活

入院のことで何かご質問がありますか.

☐ Do you have any questions about your admission?

入院手続きのことで何かお困りのことがありますか. 例えば, …
―入院手続きの書類をどう書いてよいかわからない.

☐ Do you have any concerns about your admission procedures?
― You don't know how to complete the admission paper work?

お知りになりたいのは…についての情報ですか.
1. 面会時間
―面会時間は, 平日は午後3時から8時, 日曜・祭日は午前10時から午後8時までです.

2. 差額病室［差額ベッド］
―差額病室の費用は保険適用になりません.

―別に差額病室代として1万円かかります.

―多床室［大部屋］には追加料金はかかりません.
3. 入院中の食事
―病院の食事でお困りですか.

―菜食主義者ですか.
―宗教上, 食事についてのご要望や制約はありますか.
  a. 宗教上の理由で食べられないものはありますか.

☐ Do you need information about...
1. visiting hours?
— Visiting hours are from 3:00 pm to 8:00 pm on weekdays and from 10:00 am to 8:00 pm on Sundays and holidays.
2. special charge rooms [extra-charge beds/pay beds]?
— Additional fees for special charge rooms are not covered by health insurance.
— We'll charge you an additional ten thousand yen for a special charge room.
— There's no additional fee for multiple occupancy rooms.
3. hospital meals?
— Are you having trouble with hospital meals?
— Are you a vegetarian?
— Do you have any religious needs or dietary restrictions?
  a. Are there any kinds of food that you can't eat for religious reasons?

| | |
|---|---|
| b. 宗教上の理由で肉〔豚肉〕を食べないのですか. | b. Do you avoid meat〔pork〕for religious reasons? |
| —食事についてもっと詳しくお知りになりたければ，病院の栄養士がご相談にのります. | — If you would like more information about your meals, our hospital dietitian will be able to help you. |
| 入院中お子さんのことがご心配ですか. | ☐ Are you concerned about your child〔children〕while you're in the hospital? |
| その他，何かご要望はありますか. | ☐ Do you have any other needs? |

## ● 退院後の生活

| | |
|---|---|
| 退院の手続きのことでご質問がありますか. | ☐ Do you have any questions about discharge procedures? |
| お知りになりたいのは…についての情報ですか.<br>1. 退院後の転出先<br>2. 退院後の在宅介護<br>3. 社会復帰<br>4. その他 | ☐ Do you need information about...<br>1. where to go after discharge?<br>2. home care〔care in your home〕after discharge?<br>3. return to normal life?<br>4. something else? |

### 退院後の転出先

| | |
|---|---|
| お知りになりたいのは…への転出についての情報ですか.<br>1. ほかの病院<br>  a. リハビリテーション病院<br>  b. 療養型医療施設<br>  c. 精神科病院<br>  d. 緩和ケア病院［ホスピス］ | ☐ Do you need information about transfer to...<br>1. another hospital?<br>  a. a rehabilitation [recuperative care] hospital?<br>  b. a long-term medical care facility?<br>  c. a psychiatric [mental] hospital?<br>  d. a palliative care hospital [hospice]? |

- e. 大学病院
- f. その他
2. ほかの施設
    - a. 介護老人福祉施設［特別養護老人ホーム］
    - b. 介護老人保健施設
    - c. 有料老人ホーム
    - d. 認知症共同生活介護施設［認知症グループホーム］
    - e. 身体障害者更生施設
    - f. その他

- e. a university hospital?
- f. any other hospital?
2. another facility?
    - a. a special nursing home for elderly people [for seniors]?
    - b. a long-term (health) care facility for elderly people [for seniors]?
    - c. a private residential home for elderly people [for seniors]?
    - d. a group home for dementia patients?
    - e. a rehabilitation facility for people with a physical disability?
    - f. any other facility?

### 退院後の在宅介護

どんなケアが必要ですか．
1. 身体面でのケア：入浴，食事，着替え，排泄など．
2. 家事：料理，掃除，買い物など．
3. 医療ケア：薬の管理，痰の吸引，傷の手当など．
4. 心のケア：仲間や友人，カウンセリング，自助グループなど．

在宅ケアサービスを必要としますか．

☐ What kind of care is needed?
1. Personal care, such as bathing, eating, dressing, or toileting?
2. Household care, such as cooking, cleaning, or shopping?
3. Healthcare, such as medication management, suctioning, or wound treatment?
4. Emotional care, such as companionship, counseling, or self help [peer support] group?

☐ Do you need home care services?

―どんなサービスが必要ですか.

1. 訪問介護［ホームヘルプサービス］.
2. 訪問入浴.
3. 通所介護［デイサービス］.
4. 通所リハビリテーション.
5. 介護タクシー.
6. 配食サービス.
7. 短期入所生活介護［ショートステイ］.

これは在宅ケアサービス事業所のリストです．ご自由にお持ちください．

必要ならば，ケアプランを作ってくれるケアマネージャーを紹介いたします．

市〔区〕の相談窓口，社会福祉協議会，最寄りの地域包括支援センターでも相談にのってくれます.

在宅ケアのための住宅整備や日常生活用具の情報が必要ですか.

―どんな情報が必要ですか.

1. 移動［歩行用］の手すり，つかまるための手すり，車椅子用のスロープ.

— What kind of services are needed?
1. Home care (and housekeeping) service?
2. Bathing service?
3. Day care service?
4. Outpatient [Ambulatory] rehab [rehabilitation]?
5. Care taxi [cab]?
6. Meal service?
7. Short-stay [Short-term] care facility?

☐ Here's a list of home care agencies. Feel free to take it.

☐ If it's necessary, I'm going to refer you to a care manager (for an appointment). She'll [He'll] make a care plan for you.

☐ If it's necessary, we'll make the arrangements for a care manager. She'll [He'll] make a care plan for you.

☐ You could go and ask for help at the consultation counter of your city [ward], the social welfare council, or the nearest regional comprehensive support center.

☐ Do you need information about housing arrangements and equipment for home care?

— What kind of information is needed?
1. Handrails, grab bars, or a ramp for a wheelchair?

| | |
|---|---|
| 2. ケアベッド,車椅子,杖,松葉づえ,歩行器. | 2. A care bed, a wheelchair, a cane, crutches, or a walker? |
| 3. その他. | 3. Other? |

### 社会復帰

| | |
|---|---|
| 普通の生活に戻るご予定ですか. | ☐ Are you planning to return to your normal life? |
| 職場への復帰［社会復帰］をご希望ですか. | ☐ Would you like to return to work [go back to your job]? |
| 復学をご希望ですか. | ☐ Would you like to return [go back] to school? |
| ―仕事に復帰〔復学〕するには担当医の許可が必要です. | ― You need your doctor's approval before you can return to work〔school〕. |
| 社会復帰プログラムに参加することができます. | ☐ You can take part in the return-to-work program. |

### その他

| | |
|---|---|
| その他の情報が必要ですか. 例えば…など. | ☐ Do you need any other information, such as... |
| 1. カウンセリング | 1. information about counseling? |
| 2. 患者会,家族会,自助グループなどの支援グループ | 2. information about patients' associations, family associations, or self-help [peer support] groups? |
| 3. 葬儀会社 | 3. information about funeral homes? |
| 帰国をご希望されますか. | ☐ Would you like [Do you want] to go back to your country? |
| ―ご帰国の予定ですか. | ― Are you planning to go back to your country? |

## ➔ 経済問題

### 医療費

医療費の支払いのことで不安をおもちですか.

- ☐ Are you concerned about the payment of your medical expenses?

―お知りになりたいのは何についての情報ですか.
1. 健康保険.
2. 医療費助成.
3. 介護保険.
4. 労働災害補償保険[労災].
5. その他.

― What kind of information do you need?
1. Health insurance?
2. Public medical support?
3. Long-term care insurance?
4. Workers' accident compensation insurance?
5. Other?

### ▶ 健康保険

日本の公的医療保険に入っていますか.

☐ Do you have Japanese public health insurance?

―医療費は3割自己負担です.

― You'll have to pay 30 percent of your (medical) expenses.

―医療費は全額自己負担です.

― You'll have to pay all your medical expenses.

―75歳以上の高齢者の医療費負担は1割で,一定額以上の収入のある人は3割です.

― Elderly people aged 75 years and older will pay 10 percent, and those whose income exceeds a certain amount will pay 30 percent of the medical expenses.

この薬には保険が使えません.

☐ This medication is not covered by insurance.
☐ Insurance does not cover the cost of this medication.

正常な妊娠や健康診断に保険は使えません.

☐ Normal pregnancy and health checkups are not covered by insurance.

| | |
|---|---|
| 民間の保険に入っていますか． | ☐ Do you have private insurance? |
| 申し訳ありませんが，当院では外国の保険は扱えません． | ☐ I'm sorry, but we can't accept foreign insurance at our hospital. |

### ▶ 医療費助成

公的保険に加入している人は医療費助成を受けることができます．例えば，…など．

1. 高額療養費
2. 乳幼児［こども］医療費
3. ひとり親家庭等の医療費
4. 心身障害者〔児〕の医療費
5. 特定疾患［難病］の医療費
6. 結核患者の医療費

☐ People who have public insurance are eligible for medical support [medical subsidy], such as...

1. high-cost medical care support.
2. medical care support for infants and children.
3. medical care support for single parents.
4. medical support for people [children] with physical and intellectual disabilities.
5. medical support for patients with intractable diseases.
6. medical support for tuberculosis patients.

―医療費が一定額を超えた場合，申請により超えた金額を高額療養費として受け取ることができます．

— Medical expenses above a certain level will be reimbursed as high-cost medical care benefits if the proper paperwork is submitted.

―このタイプの医療費助成の対象者や助成額は住む地域によって異なります．

— Eligible persons and the amount subsidized for this type of medical care support depend on where they live.

―特定疾患［難病］には医療費助成があります．

— There is some financial assistance for patients with intractable diseases.

―結核患者の医療費は免除あるいは減額されます．最寄りの保健所で公費負担の申請をして下さい．

— Medical expenses for tuberculosis patients will be waived or reduced. Please go to the nearest public health center and apply for public assistance for your medical expenses.

医療費の払い戻しをするかどうか，会社に問い合わせるとよいでしょう．

☐ You should make an inquiry to your company as to whether they may reimburse you for your medical expenses.

### ▶ 介護保険

介護保険は長期にわたる支援や介護を必要とする高齢者のための保険です．
― 65歳以上の高齢者が支援や介護を受けられます．

☐ Long-term care insurance is for elderly people who need long-term support and care.
— Persons 65 years and older can receive the support and care services.

― 40〜64歳までの人も病気の種類によってはサービスを受けることができます．

— Persons 40 to 64 years old can receive the services only if care is necessary due to certain types of illnesses.

介護申請は市［区］の窓口か当該機関で行って下さい．

☐ Please apply for approval on need for long-term support and care at the counter in the city [ward] office or other agencies concerned.

### ▶ 労働災害補償保険

仕事中の怪我や病気には，労働災害補償保険［労災］が医療費を支払ってくれます．

☐ When you suffer a job-related injury or illness, the workers' accident compensation insurance will cover the medical expenses.

—労災の給付を受けるには当該機関で申請する必要があります．

— You need to apply for these benefits at the agencies concerned.

### 生活費

生活費のことで不安をおもちですか．

―お知りになりたいのは何についての情報ですか．
1. さまざまな手当［給付金］，例えば…など．
    a. 障害手当
    b. 傷病手当
    c. 出産手当
    d. 育児休業給付金
    e. 児童手当
    f. 児童扶養手当（ひとり親家庭などの）
2. 生活保護費
3. 雇用保険
4. 日本の公的年金
5. その他

☐ Are you concerned about the cost of living?

— What kind of information do you need?
1. Various kinds of allowance [benefits] such as...
    a. disability allowance?
    b. injury and disease allowance?
    c. maternity allowance?
    d. child care leave allowance?
    e. child allowance?
    f. family allowance for single parents?
2. Public assistance payments [Welfare payments]?
3. Unemployment insurance?
4. Japanese public pension?
5. Other?

#### ▶ 手当・生活保護

生活保護は病気や障害などによって生活が苦しくなったときに，必要な援助を行うものです．

☐ Public assistance is to help people who have difficulty making a living because of diseases or physical disability.

手当［給付金］や生活保護を受けるにはいくつかの要件があります．

☐ There are several requirements in order to receive benefits or public assistance.

手当［給付金］や生活保護を受けるには市〔区〕役所の窓口で申請する必要があります．

☐ You need to apply for benefits or public assistance at the counter of the city〔ward〕office.

### ▶ 雇用保険

雇用保険は失業して就職活動中の人に給付されます．

☐ Unemployment insurance benefits are paid to people who have become unemployed and are looking for new jobs.

―病気，怪我，出産などで働くことができない人には給付されません．

— The benefits are not paid to people who cannot work because of an illness, injury, childbirth, and so on.

雇用保険の適用を受けるには，働いていた事業所から離職証明書をもらって，直ちにハローワーク［公共職業安定所］に申請して下さい．

☐ To receive unemployment insurance benefits, you need to obtain the separation notice from the agency where you worked, and apply promptly at Hello Work [the public employment offce].

## ● その他の心配事

他に疑問や心配をおもちですか．

☐ Do you have any other questions or concerns?

―どんな疑問や不安ですか．例えば，…

— What are they? For example....

1. 医師や看護師から病気や治療の説明を受けたがよく理解できない．

2. 治療についてのセカンドオピニオンを受けたい．

3. 処方された薬や食事についてもっと詳しく知りたい．

4. 緩和ケアについて知りたい．

5. 家族や職場の人間関係がうまくいかない．

1. you can't understand your doctor's or nurses' explanation about your disease or treatments.

2. you'd like to have a second opinion about your treatment.

3. you'd like to have more detailed information on your medications and diet.

4. you'd like to know about palliative care.

5. you have difficulty keeping up good (personal) relationships at work or with your family.

6. 夫〔妻〕が亡くなってどうしてよいかわからない．
7. 病気や怪我による生活の変化に対処できない．
8. 仕事や子育てがあって介護の責任が果たせない．
9. 病院の医療ケアやサービスに不満がある．

6. you don't know how to deal with the loss of your husband〔wife〕.
7. you can't cope with life changes due to illness or injury.
8. you have some difficulty fulfilling caregiver responsibilities because of your job or childcare.
9. you're not happy about the medical care and services you receive in the hospital.

---

名句・ことわざ

**Health is better than wealth.**
健康は富にまさる

"Health is a jewel [great riches]."（健康は宝石［富］である）ということわざもある．

# インフォームド・コンセントのサンプル

## Consent to Surgical, Diagnostic or Therapeutic Procedures

I hereby authorize and give my consent to Dr._____, and such physicians
(担当医師の氏名)
and assistants he/she may select, to perform： _____
(手術名・検査名・治療内容)

1. I have received information about my condition. I have been told:
    1. The nature and purpose of the proposed surgery or procedure.
    2. The benefits and the related risks or complications, serious injury, or even death from both known and unknown causes.
    3. The alternative methods of treatment, if applicable.

    My questions have been answered. I know that each person reacts in a different way to surgery or procedures and I acknowledge that no guarantee has been made as to result or cure.

2. I understand that, during the surgery or procedure, additional services might be needed. I give my consent to the above named people to do these services.

3. I give my consent to receive anesthesia and/or medications I may need. I have been informed of the nature and risks of the anesthetic procedure.

4. I give my consent to the hospital authorities to dispose of any tissues or parts removed in accordance with accustomed practice.


**Patient**(患者)
Print Name_____Signature_____Date_____
　　　(活字体)　　　　　　　　　(署名)　　　　　　　　(日付)

**Witness**(同席者)
Print Name_____Signature_____Date_____
　　　(活字体)　　　　　　　　　(署名)　　　　　　　　(日付)

**Interpreter**(通訳)
Print Name_____Signature_____Date_____
　　　(活字体)　　　　　　　　　(署名)　　　　　　　　(日付)

# 問い合わせ手紙文のサンプル

06/8/13
Kumi Yamada, MD
Department of Internal Medicine
Central Hospital
5-3 Hongo, Bunkyo-ku, Tokyo 113-0001
Japan
Fax:03-xxx-xxxx
E-mail:ky@central-hospital com.

Dr. Susan Ford
Department of Surgery
Memorial Hospital
………

Dear Dr. Ford:

Re : Alicia White (F)
　　Date of Birth: 25/7/57

　I am writing this letter in reference to the above patient of mine in Central Hospital, Tokyo, Japan. Mrs. White came to my office for problems associated with several months' history of progressively worsening breathlessness and dry cough. Her chest X-ray showed bilateral reticulonodular opacities of central distribution, and her chest CT revealed bilateral interstitial septal thickening and centrilobular small nodules, consistent with lymphangitis carcinomatosa.

　As she mentioned that she had had a history of cancer in the right breast and undergone mastectomy 5 years before at your hospital, I would be grateful if you could provide me with the relevant information about her medical history.

　I would appreciate hearing from you soon.

　Thank you for your time and attention.

　　　　　　　　　　　　　　　　　　　　Sincerely,

　　　　　　　　　　　　　　　　　　　　*Kumi Yamada*

## 紹介状サンプル(1)

05/11/13
Ichiro Tanaka, MD
Cardiology Department
Central Hospital
5-3 Hongo, Bunkyo-ku, Tokyo 113-0001
Japan
Fax:03-xxx-xxxx
E-mail:it@central-hospital com.

Dear Dr. Miller: [*]

Re : Roger Smith (M)
   Date of Birth : 20/9/65

Mr. Smith has been a patient of mine since May 25, 2012. He is returning to the United States, so I would be grateful if you could see him fairly soon.

**Chief Complaint :** Chest pain.

**History :** Mr. Smith had noticed chest pain which radiated to the left shoulder for the past two weeks before he was admitted to our hospital. The pain usually had occurred with exercise and its maximum duration had been 10 minutes. He had several coronary artery disease risk factors such as hypercholesterolemia, hypertension and cigarette smoking.

   On examination, he had normal heart sounds, and other physical examination was normal. His chest X-ray, Troponin I and CPK tests were negative, and his resting ECG was within normal limits. The echocardiogram showed a normal heart motion and a normal cavity size of the left ventricle. He underwent treadmill testing which was stopped at low workload because of chest pain and ST segment depression in antero-lateral leads. His coronary angiography showed a severe stenosis of the proximal left anterior descending coronary artery and of the first diagonal branch, and he underwent coronary angioplasty for both stenosis (residual stenosis< 20%).

**Diagnosis :** Angina pectoris

**Present Medications :** His medications continue to be nifedipine 40 mg per day, atorvastatin 5 mg per day, panaldine 200 mg per day and aspirin 81 mg per day.

**Other Comments :** He has been remaining asymptomatic and he is planning to go back to his hometown.

I am referring Mr. Smith to you for further consultation. If there is any further information that I can provide you with, don't hesitate to contact me.

                          Sincerely,

                          *Ichiro Tanaka*

\* 紹介先の医師名がわからないときには，To whom it may concern:

# 紹介状サンプル(2)

05/9/13
Koichi Hayashi, MD
Department of Pulmonary Medicine
Central Hospital
5-3 Hongo, Bunkyo-ku, Tokyo 113-0001
Japan
Fax:03-xxx-xxxx
E-mail:kh@central-hospital com.

To whom it may concern:

Re : Peter Cain (M)
    Date of Birth : 16/4/90

  I am writing this letter in reference to the above 23-year-old student who visited our outpatient clinic for problems associated with his left back pain. His blood chemistry findings indicated mild inflammation. Chest radiography revealed a massive left pleural effusion. Cytological and bacteriological studies of the pleural effusion were all negative, and polymerase chain reaction to tuberculosis was also negative. The pleural fluid was exudates with high lymphocyte counts and elevated adenosine deaminase activity (ADA; 64.6 IU/l), and interferon-gamma release assay was positive, both of which indicated tuberculous pleuritis. Since his diagnosis was not confirmed by histopathology or culture, we recommended that he undergo a further examination such as re-thoracocentesis or pleural biopsy. Unfortunately, however, he had no Japanese health insurance, so he refused further examinations.

  He was started on isoniazid 300 mg, rifampicin 600 mg, ethanbutol 750 mg, and pyrazinamide 1,500 mg per day. He has taken them since July 19. His clinical symptoms improved after antituberculous chemotherapy, but his pleural effusion has not yet completely improved.

  As he is planning to go back to his home country, I would certainly appreciate your treatment and follow-up.

  If there is any further information that I can provide you with, don't hesitate to contact me.

Sincerely,

*Koichi Hayashi*

# 患者満足度アンケート(例)

## Patient Satisfaction Questionnaire

We would like to know how you feel about the services we provide. All responses will be anonymous and kept confidential. We hope you will help us improve our services.
当院が提供するサービスについてお伺いいたします．回答は無記名とし個人が特定されることはありません．当院のサービス改善に役立つようご協力をお願いいたします．

1. **How old, what gender and what nationality are you?**
   年齢，性別，国籍を記入して下さい．

   Age: _____ years old.
   年齢　　　　歳

   Gender:　Male ☐　Female ☐
   性別　　　男性　　　女性

   Nationality:　American ☐　British ☐　Australian ☐
   国籍　　　　米国　　　　英国　　　　オーストラリア

   　　　　　　New Zealander ☐　Filipino ☐　Chinese ☐　Korean ☐
   　　　　　　ニュージーランド　フィリピン　中国　　　韓国

   　　　　　　Other _____
   　　　　　　その他

2. **Did you receive any interpreter services during your visit [stay]?**
   通院中［入院中］通訳をつけましたか．

   Yes ☐　No ☐
   はい　　いいえ

   — If yes, who interpreted for you?
   　通訳をしてくれたのはどなたですか．

   　Your family ☐　Your friend(s) ☐　A bilingual hospital staff ☐
   　家族　　　　　友人　　　　　　　当院のスタッフ

   　A professional interpreter ☐　A telephone interpreter ☐
   　通訳　　　　　　　　　　　　電話通訳

   — What is your native language [mother tongue]?
   　あなたの母語は何語ですか．

   　English ☐　Spanish ☐　Portuguese ☐　Chinese ☐　Korean ☐
   　英語　　　スペイン語　ポルトガル語　　中国語　　　韓国語・朝鮮語

   　Other _____
   　その他

3. Have you received the services as _____ ?
   サービスを受けたのは…としてですか．

   an inpatient ☐   an outpatient ☐
   入院患者         通院患者

4. **Did the doctor explain details about your illness, related procedures and medications clearly in the way you could understand?**
   医師の病状，処置，薬についての説明はわかりやすかったですか．

   Very well. ☐      OK. ☐        Fairly. ☐   Poorly. ☐
   大変わかりやすかった  まあまあだった   ふつう      わかりにくかった

5. **Did the nurse(s) explain details about procedures and medications clearly in the way you could understand?**
   看護師の処置や薬についての説明はわかりやすかったですか．

   Very well. ☐      OK. ☐        Fairly. ☐   Poorly. ☐
   大変わかりやすかった  まあまあだった   ふつう      わかりにくかった

6. **Did you have enough opportunities to ask questions to your doctor or nurses?**
   医師や看護師に質問する機会は十分にありましたか．

   Always. ☐    Often. ☐      Sometimes. ☐   Rarely. ☐
   いつもあった  頻繁にあった   時々あった      めったになかった

   Never. ☐
   なかった

7. **Were the other hospital staff friendly and helpful?**
   病院の他のスタッフは親切で協力的でしたか．

   Always. ☐       Most of the time. ☐    Some of the time. ☐
   いつもよかった   おおむねよかった         一部はよかった

   Seldom. ☐
   あまりよくなかった

8. **How satisfied were you with the medical care you received?**
   当病院で受けた医療ケアに満足しましたか．

   Very satisfied. ☐   Satisfied. ☐      Neither satisfied nor dissatisfied. ☐
   大変満足した         おおむね満足した    ふつう

   Dissatisfied. ☐     Very dissatisfied. ☐
   やや不満だった       大変不満だった

9. Would you recommend this hospital to your family and friends?
   ご家族や友人に当病院を推薦しますか.

   Yes, definitely. ☐   Maybe. ☐   No. ☐
   絶対に勧める       どちらともいえない  勧めない

10. Please tell us anything else you think we should know about your hospital visit [stay].
    通院中［入院中］のことで私どもに知ってもらいたいことがあればお教え下さい.

    _____
    _____
    _____

11. Please let us know of any suggestions you have to help us improve our services.
    その他，当病院の改善に対するご提案がございましたらご記入下さい.

    _____
    _____
    _____

Thank you for your cooperation.
ご協力ありがとうございました.

# 参考文献

American Cancer Society: Breast awareness and self-exam. Available from http://www.cancer.org/cancer/breastcancer/

Baile, W.F. et al.: SPIKES-A six-step protocol for delivering bad news: application to the patient with cancer. *Oncologist* 5(4): 302-311, 2000.

Bartlett, J.: *Familiar Quotations*, 16th ed. Little Brown and Company, 1992.

Canadian Lung Association: COPD; breathing techniques. Available from http://www.lung.ca/diseases-maladies/copd-mpoc/breathing-respiration/index_e.php

Goldmann, D.R. and Horowitz, D.A. (eds): *American College of Physicians; Home Medical Adviser*. DK Publishing Inc., 2002.

Simpson, J.: *The Consice Oxford dictionary of Proverbs*. Oxford University Press, 1985.

Springhouse Publishing Co. Staff (eds): *English and Spanish Medical Words and Phrases*, 2nd ed. Springhouse, 1999.

The U. S. National Library of Medicine: MedlinePlus. Available from http://www.nlm.nih.gov/medlineplus/

Venes, D. et al. (eds): *Taber's Cyclopedic Medical Dictionary*, 19th ed. F.A. Davis Co., 2001.

池田彌三郎・ドナルド・キーン監修:『日英故事ことわざ辞典』. 朝日イブニングニュース社, 1986.

岩崎春雄・忍足欣四郎・小島義郎編:『英語の常識百科』. 研究社出版, 1988.

大塚高信・高瀬省三編:『英語諺辞典』, 縮刷版. 三省堂, 1986.

金澤一郎, 永井良三編:『今日の診断指針』, 第6版. 医学書院, 2010.

カルペニート, リンダ J.・朝倉稔生:『医師とナースのための問診とフィジカルアセスメントの英語—— *Bedside English for Doctors and Nurses*』. 医学書院, 1998.

仁木久恵ほか:『臨床看護英語 *Let's Listen, Speak and Learn*』. 医学書院, 2012.

日本呼吸管理学会呼吸リハビリテーションガイドライドライン作成委員会ほか編:『呼吸リハビリテーションマニュアル—運動療法』. 照林社, 2003.

日野原重明監訳:『診察術マニュアル——問診―診察―記録』. 医学書院, 1982.

日野原重明・仁木久恵訳:『平静の心—オスラー博士講演集 *Aequanimitas*』. 医学書院, 2003.

山口徹ほか編:『今日の治療指針2013年版』. 医学書院, 2013.

# 索引

## 欧文

A 型肝炎　198, 400
ATM　343
B 型肝炎　101, 114, 125, 190, 198, 400
BCG　198, 400
C 型肝炎　101, 190
CT　282, 292
CT 室　344
E メールアドレス　3
HIV 感染症　114, 125, 189
ID バンド　342
LSD 幻覚剤　206
MRI　282, 292
MRI 室　344
NST　369
PTSD　191
X 線検査　280, 292

## あ

あいさつ　340
　――，再診の　17
　――，初診の　16
　――，診察室での　16
　――，入院患者さんへの　340
　――，入院当日の　342
アキレス腱縫合術　325
顎　70
顎の痛み　71
あざ　160
アトピー性皮膚炎　191, 201, 395
アバネーシィ　15
アメリカ人　3
アリストテレス　51
アルコール　205
アルコール依存　177
アルコール依存症　191
アルコール消毒　275, 312
アレルギー，既往歴　195
アレルギー検査　292
アレルギー性鼻炎　395
アレルギー専門医　261
アレルギーと薬　302
アンジェロウ　413
安静の指示　265, 352

## い

胃潰瘍　39, 190
医学生　91
息切れ　79
イギリス人　3
育毛剤　166
医師　89
意識，小児の　382
意識障害　148
意識状態の診察　229
イスラム教　10
痛み　27
　――，顎の　71
　――，咽頭の　66
　――，筋・骨格の　139
　――，男性生殖器の　110
　――，乳房・女性生殖器の　118, 120
　――，鼻の　65
　――，歯の　70

437

痛み（つづき）
　——，耳の　61
　——，目の　56
痛みの表現　31
一般医　89
一般開業医　262
一般外科　52
一般外科医　261
一般事務（職員）　90
一般情報　2
一般内科　52
遺伝　188, 200, 201
遺伝子診療部　53
移動の指示　352
居眠り　81
いびき　81
医療ソーシャルワーカー
　　　　　　　4, 89, 253, 414
医療通訳　4, 91
医療費　421
医療費助成　422
医療福祉相談室　345, 412
入れ歯　75, 220, 282
慰労　242
胃瘻　252
咽喉頭　66
咽喉の診察　220
飲酒　177, 205
インターベンション治療医　261
インチ　216
院長　90
咽頭の痛み　66
インド人　3
陰嚢　110
インフォームド・コンセント
　——，検査と　270
　——，サンプル　427
　——，手術と　324
インフルエンザ　198, 400

## う

うがい薬　307
受付　14
受付事務（職員）　90
うつ病　191
運動　207
　——，小児の　390
運動機能の診察　231
運動障害　153
運動制限　142
運動の指示　265
運動負荷検査　293

## え

エイズ　114, 125, 189
栄養, 小児の　389
栄養士　89, 266, 417
栄養相談室　345
腋窩　223
エコー　283
エホバの証人　10
嚥下障害　92
嚥下造影検査　293
遠視　55, 191
延命治療　252, 253

## お

黄疸　100
嘔吐　93
黄熱　198
オーストラリア人　3
お薬手帳　300
おしゃぶり　391
オスラー　241, 371
お腹　36

おなら 285
オムツかぶれ 384
おりもの 122
オルガスム 113
悪露 378
音叉 219, 232
温度 24, 215, 216
温熱療法 257

## か

ガーナ人 3
海外渡航歴 199
海外旅行保険 11
会計受付 343
会計事務（職員） 90
会計窓口 359
介護員 90
介護保険 423
外傷 50, 160
外転神経の診察 ☞ 眼 54
回診 350
回復室 344, 377
潰瘍 65, 162
外来棟 343
カイロプラクティック 194
カウンセラー 253
カウンセリング 418
かかりつけの医師 187
過換気症候群 190
核医学検査室 344
喀痰検査 293
確認 242
隔離病棟 345
学歴 7
　——, 精神・心理 184
華氏 216
下肢静脈造影検査 293
下肢の診察 227

過食症 102
ガス 37
家族 5, 380
家族構成 200
家族の仕事 9
家族の病気 200
家族歴 200
　——, 筋・骨格 144
　——, 呼吸器 81
　——, 消化器 101
　——, 小児の 397
　——, 神経 158
　——, 心・血管 87
　——, 腎・泌尿器 108
　——, 精神・心理 184
　——, 代謝・内分泌 132
　——, 乳房・女性生殖器 125
　——, 眼 58
下腿部 40
科長（…科の） 90
学校教育 7
滑車神経の診察 ☞ 眼 54
合併症 324
かつら 166
カテーテル 108
カトリック 10
カナダ人 3
カニューラ 353
化膿 256
カフ 213
カフェテリア 343, 348
下腹部 40
カプセル 303
花粉症 66, 191, 201, 395
かゆみ 56, 62, 160
空咳 76
ガリウムシンチグラフィ 296
カルシウム 301
川崎病 190

がん 189
眼圧検査 292
肝炎 190
眼科 52
眼科医 261
感覚機能の診察 232
感覚障害 156
肝機能異常 101
看護学生 91
看護師 89
看護師長 90
看護主任 90
看護助手 90
看護部長 90
鉗子分娩 365, 377
関節 139, 145
関節炎 145, 201
関節リウマチ 146
感染症, 小児の 388, 395
感染対策専門医 261
乾燥 160
浣腸薬 294
眼底検査 292
冠動脈疾患集中治療部 344
冠動脈造影検査 293
冠動脈バイパス術 325
顔面筋肉訓練 407
顔面神経の診察 230
丸薬 298, 303, 373
緩和ケア科 53
緩和ケア専門医 262
緩和ケア病棟 345

## き

既往歴 187
——, 筋・骨格 144
——, 呼吸器 81
——, 消化器 101
——, 小児の 392
——, 神経 158
——, 心・血管 87
——, 腎・泌尿器 108
——, 精神・心理 184
——, 代謝・内分泌 132
——, 男性生殖器 114
——, 乳房・女性生殖器 125
——, 歯・口腔 75
——, 鼻 65
——, 耳 62
——, 眼 58
記憶の障害 150
気管支炎 189
気管支鏡検査 293
利き手 231
訊きにくい質問 116
キケロ 20, 188
機嫌, 小児の 382
義肢装具士 89
傷口 256
基礎体温 121
基礎体温測定 294
貴重品 339, 347
喫煙 205, 350
喫茶室 343
機能回復訓練 406
ギプス 257
逆行性腎盂造影検査 294
逆行性尿道造影検査 294
逆行性膀胱造影検査 294
きゅう (灸) 194
吸引分娩 365, 377
嗅覚 65, 152
嗅覚検査 292
救急入口 344
救急医療専門医 262
救急救命士 90
救急車の読み方 215

救急部 53
嗅神経の診察 ☞ 耳鼻咽喉・頸部 60
吸入器 307
吸入麻酔 327
吸入薬 307
救命救急室 343
胸腔鏡検査 293
胸腔穿刺 293
狂犬病 198
狭心症 87
胸水検査 293
胸痛 32
胸背部の診察 222
恐怖 171
胸部 X 線〔CT／MRI〕 293
局所麻酔 327
拒食症 102
巨大児 365
切り傷 51
キログラム 216
禁煙 350
緊急用カード 316
緊急連絡先 3, 338
筋・骨格 139
——, 痛み 139
——, 家族歴 144
——, 既往歴 144
——, 小児の 387
——, 生活歴 144
近視 55, 191
筋電図検査 296
筋肉 139, 145
筋肉内注射 312

## く

駆血帯 275
くしゃみ 63
薬 255, 298
口 70, 72
口すぼめ呼吸 408
唇 72
クラーク 348
クラミジア感染症 114, 125
クリーム 310
クリップ 282
グループホーム 418
車椅子 352
クレジットカードの読み方 214

## け

ケアマネージャー 419
計画分娩 373
経管栄養 252
敬称 15
経食道心臓超音波検査 293
計測値の読み方 215
形成外科 52
形成外科医 261
経腟超音波検査 295
経腟分娩 365
経直腸超音波検査 294
頸椎牽引 257
系統的レビュー 54
頸動脈超音波検査 293
経尿道的膀胱腫瘍切除術 325
警備員 90
警備室 344
頸部 68
痙攣 148, 191
怪我 50
——, 既往歴 192
外科 52
外科医 89, 261
外科外来 343
外科的処置の説明 256

441

外科病棟　345
血圧　213
血液　134
血液型，既往歴　194
血液検査　275, 292
血液内科　52
血液内科医　261
血液培養検査　292
結核　146, 190, 201
月経　118, 367
月経期間　119
月経周期　119, 367
結婚　5
血栓性静脈炎　190
血痰　78
ゲップ　93, 281, 285
血便　96
結膜　218
下痢　96, 204
腱　145
減塩食　372
幻覚　182
検眼士　90
玄関ホール　344
言語，小児の　390
健康保険　11, 421
言語聴覚士　89, 402, 407
言語聴覚療法　257, 407
言語（聴覚）療法室　345
検査一般　270
検査着　280
検査結果の説明　245
検査室　239
検査値の読み方　215
検査の説明　238
研修医　89
健診，既往歴　198
健診，小児の　378, 398
健診異常　186

健診センター　53, 345
倦怠感　42
検尿　276
腱反射　232
現病歴　24
——，筋・骨格　139
——，血液　134
——，呼吸器　76
——，耳鼻咽喉・頸部　60
——，主要症状　24
——，消化器　92
——，小児の　382
——，神経　147
——，心・血管　84
——，腎・泌尿器　103
——，精神・心理　168
——，代謝・内分泌　127
——，男性生殖器　110
——，乳房・女性生殖器　117
——，歯・口腔　70
——，皮膚　159
——，眼　54
減量　180

## こ

誤飲　388
コインランドリー　343, 348
口角　72
口渇　129
睾丸　110
口腔　70, 72
口腔外科　53
口腔外科医　89, 262
高血圧　189, 201
膠原病　145
高コレステロール血症　189
口臭　74
甲状腺腫　201

甲状腺シンチグラフィ 293
甲状腺超音波検査 293
高中性脂肪血症 189
交通事故 50
口内炎 75
高尿酸血症 189
高熱 24
更年期症状 122
後発医薬品 298
広汎子宮全摘術 325
硬膜外麻酔 327
肛門 225, 309
声がれ 67
コールボタン 347
コカイン 206
呼吸器 76
——, 家族歴 81
——, 既往歴 81
——, 小児の 385
——, 生活習慣 81
呼吸器科医 261
呼吸器外科 52
呼吸器内科 52
呼吸機能検査 286, 293
呼吸機能検査室 344
国籍 2
固形食 331
腰 39
個室 345
鼓室形成術 325
個人特性, 小児の 391
骨格, 小児の 387
骨格の診察 227
骨シンチグラフィ 295
骨髄生検 295
骨髄穿刺 295
骨折 395
骨粗鬆症 145, 146
骨盤の診察 226

骨密度測定 295
鼓動 84
子供 6, 380
粉薬 298, 303
鼓膜 62
こむらがえり 149
雇用保険 425
コレラ 198
こわばり 142
婚姻歴 5
コンタクトレンズ 55, 217
根治 324
コンピュータ 8

## さ

細菌検査 292
細隙灯顕微鏡検査 292
採血 275
採血室 344
最終学歴 7
最終月経 119, 367
菜食主義者 203, 416
再診のあいさつ 17
再発 250
在宅介護 417, 418
細胞診 292
再来受付 343
差額病室［ベッド］ 416
さかご 365
作業療法 257, 406
作業療法士 89, 402, 406
作業療法室 345
酒 101, 205
嗄声 67
サプリメント 301
坐薬 254, 298, 309
ざらざら感 160
産科 52

産科医　261
産科病棟　345
産業医　262
散剤　298
三叉神経の診察　230
三種混合　400
酸素マスク　353
産徴［おしるし］　375
残尿感　160

## し

痔　190
自慰行為　113
シェイクスピア　332, 371
ジェネリック医薬品　298
シェリー　358
歯科　53
歯科医　75, 89, 262
歯科衛生士　90
歯科技工士　90
歯科矯正医　262
色覚異常　59
色覚検査　292
磁気共鳴血管造影検査　295
磁気共鳴胆管膵管造影検査　294
子宮鏡検査　295
子宮頸がん検診　125, 199
子宮頸部擦過細胞診　295
子宮口　375
子宮内膜組織診　295
子宮の診察　226
子宮卵管造影検査　295
事故　50
　——, 既往歴　192
　——, 小児の　388
思考の障害　150
時刻の読み方　214
仕事, 家族の　9

仕事の環境　8
しこり　48, 68
　——, 乳房の　117
自殺　201
死産　365
指示, 日常生活への　265
脂質異常症　35, 87, 189
四肢の腫脹　86
四肢の疼痛　86
四肢の冷感　86
歯周病　74
視神経の診察　☞ 眼　54
事前指示書　253
自然分娩　373
自宅ケア, 手術と　333
舌　72
舌の炎症　72
歯痛　70
耳痛　61
失語　151
失行　152
失神　148
失認　151
湿疹　☞ 発疹　159, 195
湿布薬　254, 298, 311
自動販売機　343, 348
視能訓練士　89
死の伝え方　360
支払い　11
市販薬　300
耳鼻咽喉科　52
耳鼻咽喉科医　261
耳鼻咽喉・頸部　60
耳鼻咽喉の診察　219
自費診療　11
ジフテリア　198, 400
事務室　343
事務長　90
耳鳴　61

視野　54, 152
社会性，小児の　391
社会福祉協議会　419
社会復帰　417, 420
視野検査　292
射精　113
宗教　10, 416, 417
住所　3
集中治療部　344
十二指腸潰瘍　39
終夜睡眠ポリグラフィ　293
手術　258, 323
　——，既往歴　193
手術室　344
手術の説明　258, 325
主訴　18
　——，小児の　382
腫脹　48
　——，四肢の　86
出血傾向　136, 190
出生前・出生時情報　392
出生地　2
授乳　352, 389
　——，既往歴　197
　——，薬剤と　314
主任看護師　90
趣味　207
主要症状　24
腫瘍専門医　261
腫瘍内科　52
腫瘤　48
循環器科医　261
循環器内科　52
昇圧剤　252
紹介，専門医への　260
紹介状　16
紹介状サンプル　429, 431
消化器　92
　——，家族歴　101

　——，既往歴　101
　——，小児の　386
消化器科医　261
消化器外科　52
消化器内科　52
消化器の診察　224
消化不良　93
しょう紅熱　189, 395
錠剤　254, 298, 303, 373
上肢の診察　227
消灯　349
床頭台　347
消毒　256, 348
小児科　52
小児科医　261
小児科病棟　345
小児外科　52
小児外科医　261
小脳機能の診察　232
小脳系症状　155
上部消化管造影検査　294
上部消化管内視鏡検査　285, 294
静脈性腎盂造影検査　294
静脈造影検査　293
静脈内注射　312
静脈麻酔　327
静脈瘤　190
職業　7
食事の指示　266
食習慣　202
食堂　343
食物繊維　301
食欲　99
　——，小児の　383
職歴　7
　——，精神・心理　184
助産師　89, 370
初診のあいさつ　16
女性生殖器　117

初乳　378
処方箋　255, 298
処方薬　300
自律神経障害　157
視力　54, 152
視力検査　55, 289, 292
視力検査技師　90
視力の測り方の違い　291
耳漏　61
シロップ　303, 397
腎炎　190
新館　343
新患受付　343
鍼灸　196
心筋血流シンチグラフィ　293
心筋梗塞　88, 190, 201
神経　147
　——, 家族歴　158
　——, 既往歴　158
神経科医　261
神経症　191, 201
神経内科　52
神経の診察　229
心・血管　84
　——, 家族歴　87
　——, 既往歴　87
　——, 小児の　386
腎結石　190
人工関節　282
人工呼吸器　252
深刻な説明　247
診察　212, 217
　——, 身体の　211
診察券　339
診察券の読み方　214
診察室　343
診察室でのあいさつ　16
診察の終了　234
診察予約　263

腎シンチグラフィー　294
新生児室　345
新生児集中治療部　344
心臓　84
腎臓　103, 108
心臓カテーテル検査　293
心臓血管外科　52
心臓血管外科医　261
心臓超音波検査　293
腎臓内科　52
腎臓内科医　261
腎臓病　201
心臓マッサージ　252
靱帯　145
身体計測　212
診断内容の説明　246
身長　212
陣痛室　345, 375
陣痛促進剤　377
心的外傷後ストレス障害　191
心電図（検査）　276, 293
心電図室　344
腎・泌尿器　103
　——, 家族歴　108
　——, 既往歴　108
　——, 生活習慣　108
心理　168
診療科　52
心療内科　52
診療部長　90
診療部門　52
診療放射線技師　89

## す

髄液検査　296
錐体外路系症状　154
錐体路系症状　153
水痘　164, 189, 198, 395, 400

髄膜炎　395
髄膜刺激症状の診察　233
睡眠　202
睡眠時無呼吸　81
睡眠時無呼吸症候群　190
睡眠障害　168
睡眠専門医　261
睡眠の指示　265
スウィフト　133
杉田玄白　428
頭痛　27
ステッキ　145
ストーマ療法士　89
ストレス　161, 169
スポーツ医　262
擦り傷　160

## せ

精液　111
精液検査　294
性格変化　182
生活習慣　202
──, 呼吸器　81
──, 小児の　390
──, 腎・泌尿器　108
生活費　424
生活歴, 筋・骨格　144
性感染症　108
性器　108, 110, 117
性機能　112
性器ヘルペス　114, 125
整形外科　52
整形外科医　261
整形外科病棟　345
性行為感染症　114, 125, 189
性交後試験　295
性交渉　101
性習慣　112

正常分娩　365
生殖器, 小児の　387
生殖器の診察　226
精神科　52
精神科医　261
精神・心理　168
──, 学歴　184
──, 家族歴　184
──, 既往歴　184
──, 職歴　184
精神遅滞　191
精神的な問題　191
精神保健福祉士　89
性生活　114, 123
清掃員　90
成長発達　390
生年月日　2
精密検査　186, 199, 238
生命維持装置　252
性欲　112
生理用ナプキン　119
西暦年号の読み方　214
セカンドオピニオン　252, 260
咳　76
脊髄腔造影検査　295
脊柱の診察　228
脊椎麻酔　327
舌咽神経の診察　230
舌下錠　298, 306
舌下神経の診察　231
セックス　112
摂氏　216
摂食障害　102, 180
説明
──, 検査の　238
──, 深刻な　247
──, 診断の　245
──, 治療の　254
背中　39

尖圭コンジローマ 114, 125
前頸部腫瘤 130
染色体検査 295
全身倦怠感 42
全身麻酔 327
喘息 81, 190, 201, 395
センチメートル 216
前庭蝸牛神経の診察 ☞ 耳鼻咽喉・頸部 60
先発医薬品 298
喘鳴 80
洗面所 344
専門医 260, 261
専門医への紹介 260
前立腺 108
前立腺肥大 190

## そ

造影剤 282
騒音 61
総合案内 343
総合診療科 52
躁状態 176
双生児 365
ソーシャルワーカー ☞ 医療ソーシャルワーカー
鼠径の診察 225
鼠径ヘルニア 395
組織診 292
蘇生術 252
ソフトレンズ 55

## た

退院 359
ダイエット 99, 180, 204
体温 14, 24, 213
体温計 213

太極拳 194
帯下 122
代謝・内分泌 127
――, 家族歴 132
――, 既往歴 132
代謝・内分泌内科 52
体重 212
――, 小児の 383
体重変化 100, 127
退職 8
大腿部 40
大腸内視鏡検査 285, 294
胎動 367
大動脈造影検査 293
大脳高次機能の診察 229
胎盤 376
体毛 164
多飲 129
唾液 74, 92
尋ねにくい質問 116
立会い出産 373
立ちくらみ 157
脱毛 165
脱毛剤 166
脱毛症 166
脱力感 42
多尿 129
タバコ 67, 205
打撲傷 51
だるさ 42
痰 76
男性生殖器 110
――, 痛み 110
――, 既往歴 114
胆石 39, 190
担当医 89, 253
痰培養検査 292
タンポン 119

## ち

チアノーゼ 382
地域包括支援センター 419
地下 343, 348
乳首の陥没 117
腟拡大鏡検査 295
腟の診察 226
チャペル 345
中央病棟 343
中耳炎 395
駐車場 344
注射の説明 254
注射薬 312
中心静脈栄養 252
虫垂炎 39
虫垂切除術 325
注腸造影検査 294
超音波検査 283, 292
超音波検査室 344
超音波内視鏡検査 294
聴覚検査技師 89
調剤 255
調剤薬局 298
腸チフス 198
聴能訓練士 89
聴力 60, 153
聴力検査 61, 290, 292
直腸 309
直腸診 225
治療の説明 254

## つ

痛風 145, 189
通訳 4, 91, 338, 415
付き添い 339
突っ張り 142

つば 92, 217
ツベルクリンテスト 293
爪 166

## て

帝王切開 365, 377
低血圧 189
ティンパノメトリー 292
デジタル減算血管造影検査 295
鉄欠乏性貧血 190
テニスン 319
テレビ 350
てんかん 191, 201
点眼薬 219, 298, 308
電気ショック 252
電気療法 257
点耳薬 308
点滴 256, 312
転倒 50
点鼻薬 308
臀部 40
電話，携帯の 350
電話，公衆の 344
電話番号 3
電話番号の読み方 214

## と

問い合わせ手紙文のサンプル 428
同意書 270
動眼神経の診察 ☞ 眼 54
動悸 84
同居人 5
頭頸の診察 217
動作，小児の 390
当日検査の説明 239
透析センター［室］ 345
疼痛，四肢の 86

糖尿病　189, 201
糖尿病 ID カード　316
頭髪　164
頭部 X 線　295
頭部外傷　395
動脈血ガス分析　293
動脈硬化　189
動脈瘤　190
投薬の説明　254
独身　5
図書室　345
突発性発疹　395
トリコモナス感染症　114, 125
トレッドミル負荷心電図検査　277

## な

ナースステーション　345, 348
内科　52
内科医　89, 261
内科外来　343
内科病棟　345
内視鏡検査　285, 292
内視鏡室　344
内視鏡的逆行性胆管膵管造影検査　294
ナイチンゲール　341
内服薬　248, 303
内分泌　127
内分泌科医　261
慰め　242
名前　2, 15
涙　56
喃語　390
軟膏　248, 298, 310

## に

におい　65

肉体労働　8
二種混合［ジフテリア，破傷風］　400
日常生活への指示　265
日本語能力　4
日本脳炎　198, 400
入院　258, 337
　──，既往歴　192
入院受付　343
入院患者さんへのあいさつ　340
入院棟　343
入院の説明　258
乳がん　126
乳腺外科医　261
乳腺・内分泌外科　52
乳頭　223
乳房　117
乳房 X 線検査　294
乳房温存術　325
乳房・女性生殖器，家族歴　125
乳房・女性生殖器，既往歴　125
乳房診察　125, 223
乳房超音波検査　125, 294
乳房の自己触診　125, 288
乳房変化　117
尿意　105, 106
尿器　352
尿検査　276, 292
尿失禁　105
尿線　106
尿道　107, 108
尿道括約筋筋電図　294
尿道口　107, 111
尿道造影検査　294
尿道膀胱鏡検査　294
尿の性状　103
尿培養検査　292
尿流測定　294
尿量　104

尿路結石 39, 190
人間ドック ☞ 健診センター
――, 既往歴 198
妊娠 363, 367
――, 既往歴 197
――, 薬剤と 314
妊娠高血圧症候群 392
妊娠試験 295
妊娠週数・月数の数え方 368
妊娠中絶 364
妊娠中毒症 ☞ 妊娠高血圧症候群
妊娠歴 364
認知症 147
認知障害 150

## ね

熱 14, 24, 213
熱傷 395
熱性痙攣 395
年齢 2, 380

## の

脳 CT〔MRI〕 295
脳炎 395
脳血管造影検査 295
脳血流 SPECT 296
脳梗塞 191
脳死 252
脳出血 191
脳神経外科 52
脳神経外科医 261
脳神経障害 152
脳神経の診察 229
脳卒中 201
脳動脈瘤クリッピング 325
脳波検査 296

のど 66, 219
飲み忘れ・飲みすぎ 314
ノンストレステスト 369

## は

歯 70
パートナー 5
ハーヴェイ 396
ハードレンズ 55
肺炎 81, 190
肺炎球菌 198
肺炎球菌感染症 400
肺がん 82
配偶者 5
肺結核 82
肺血流シンチグラフィ 293
バイタルサイン 213
売店 343
梅毒 114, 125, 189
排尿 104, 106, 129
排尿回数 104
排尿困難 106
排尿時膀胱尿道造影検査 294
排尿痛 106
背部痛 39
培養検査 292
肺葉切除術 325
吐き気 93
歯ぎしり 75
歯茎 70, 71, 72
白内障 59, 191
白内障手術 325
励まし 242
破傷風 198, 400
破水 375
白血病 201
抜糸 256, 332
発熱 24

パップスメア検査 125, 199
鼻 63
　──, 小児の 384
鼻アレルギー 65
鼻血 64
鼻の痛み 65
鼻の診察 220
鼻水 63
歯の痛み 70
母親学級 373
パピローマウイルス感染症 125
はり（鍼） 194
バリウム 281
パルスオキシメーター 213
腫れ 48, 68
　──, 筋・骨格 143
　──, 乳房の 117
判断の障害 150

## ひ

鼻咽喉内視鏡検査 292
皮下出血 136
皮下注射 312
ひきつけ 382
鼻汁 63
鼻出血 64
ビタミン剤 301
左利き 231
日付の読み方 214
ヒトパピローマウィルス 400
泌尿器 103
　──, 小児の 387
泌尿器科 52
泌尿器科医 261
微熱 24
皮膚 159
　──, 小児の 384
皮膚科 53

皮膚科医 261
鼻閉 63
ヒポクラテス 209
肥満 189
秘密厳守 112, 412
百日咳 189, 198, 395, 400
ヒューナーテスト 295
病院案内 343
病院生活 349
病室 345, 347, 416
病室番号の読み方 215
病棟 343, 344
病棟案内 347
病棟事務（職員） 90
病理医 262
病理検査 292
病理診断科 53
病歴 21
　──, 小児の 384
病歴をとるためのヒント 22
疲労感 42
貧血 134, 190
ヒンズー教 10

## ふ

不安 171
フィート 216
フィリピン人 3
風疹 164, 189, 198, 395, 400
不快感, のどの 66
副院長 90
腹腔鏡下胆嚢摘出術 325
腹腔鏡検査 295
腹腔穿刺 294
副作用, 薬剤の 255, 318
腹式呼吸 408
副神経の診察 231
腹水検査 294

腹痛 36
副鼻腔 X 線〔CT/MRI〕 292
副鼻腔炎 66
腹部 X 線〔CT/MRI〕 294
腹部超音波検査 293, 294
服薬上の注意 313
服用歴 300
浮腫 46
婦人科 52
婦人科医 261
婦人科病棟 345
不正出血 121
不整脈 88, 190
2 人部屋 345
普通食 331
二日酔い 178
仏教 10
ブドウ糖錠剤 316
ブドウ糖負荷試験 295
ブラウン 311
ブラクトン 399
ブランド医薬品 298
プロテスタント 10
分泌物 111
分娩 363, 375
分娩室 345, 376
分娩歴 364

## へ

ヘイウッド 332
閉経 121
平衡機能検査 292
平行棒 404
ペースメーカー 282
ペグボード 406
へこみ, 乳房の 117
ペスト 198
へそ 36

へその緒 365
別居 5
ペット 208, 397
ペニス 111, 125
ヘルペス 189
ヘロイン 206
便器 352
便検査 292
便通 204
便通異常 96
便秘 96, 204

## ほ

包茎 387
縫合 250
膀胱 103, 108
膀胱造影検査 294
膀胱内圧測定 294
放射線科 53
放射線技師 89
放射線診断医 261
放射線治療医 261
放射線部 344
放射線療法医 261
包帯 257
訪問看護部 345
保管上の注意, 薬剤の 317
補完代替医療 194
補完代替医療品 301
牧師 91
ほくろ 164
保険 11
保健師 89
保険証 11, 339
保険申請書 11
母語 4
歩行器 145
歩行訓練 404

母子（健康）手帳 373, 380, 398
母子同室 339, 373
保証人 338
ホスピス・緩和ケア専門医 262
補聴器 61
勃起 113
発疹 159, 195
母乳 378, 389
哺乳瓶 389
骨 139
ボランティア 91
ポリオ 198, 400
ホルター心電図（検査） 278, 293
ホルモン 127
本館 343
ポンド 216

## ま

マウスピース 307
麻疹 164, 189, 198, 395, 400
麻疹・風疹混合 400
麻酔科 53
麻酔科医 261
麻酔の説明 327
マスク 14, 353
待合室 344
マッサージ 194, 257
松葉杖 145
まばたき 219
まぶた 58, 218
麻薬 206
マラリア 189
マリファナ 206
慢性閉塞性肺疾患 83, 190
マンモグラフィ検査 125, 287

## み

味覚 73, 152
味覚検査 292
右利き 231
未熟児 365
水薬 254, 298
みぞおち 36
三日ばしか 189, 395
ミッチェル 342
ミネラル 301
耳 60
——, 既往歴 62
——, 小児の 384
耳掻き 62
耳栓 62
耳だれ 62
耳鳴り 61
耳の痛み 61
耳の診察 219
脈 213

## む

無関心 158
無気力 157
むくみ 46
虫歯 71
無痛分娩 373
胸の痛み 32
胸焼け 93

## め

目（眼） 54
——, 家族歴 58
——, 既往歴 58
——, 小児の 385

迷走神経の診察 230
眼鏡 55, 282
目薬 298, 308
目の痛み 56
目のかゆみ 56
目の診察 217
目の中の異物 57
めまい 43
目やに 56
面会 349
面会室 345, 349
面談室 345
綿棒 239

## も

妄想 181
盲目 59
もたれ 93
問診の最後に 209

## や

夜間・休日出入口 344
薬剤 298
薬剤師 89, 255
薬剤投与，小児の 397
薬剤の副作用 255, 318
薬剤の保管上の注意 317
薬剤部長 90
薬草 301
薬物依存症 191
薬歴 194
　——，小児の 396
やけど（火傷） 51, 160
薬局 255, 298, 343
夜尿 387, 391

## ゆ

ユウェナリス 185
ユークリッド 91
郵便受け 343
輸液 252
輸血 101, 252, 256, 324
輸血歴 194
ユダヤ教 10
指しゃぶり 391

## よ

溶血性連鎖球菌感染症 189, 395
羊水穿刺 295
腰椎穿刺 296
腰痛 39
陽電子放出断層撮影 296
用法，薬剤の 255, 303
用務員 90
用量，薬剤の 303
ヨガ 194
抑うつ状態 173
夜泣き 391
予防接種，既往歴 198
予防接種，小児の 398, 400
読み書き 4
予約 263, 264, 405
予約検査の説明 240
予約取り消し 271

## ら

ラウンジ 345
ラジオ 350
ラマーズ法 373
乱視 55, 191

## り

リウマチ科医　261
リウマチ内科　52
リウマチ熱　189, 395
理学療法　257, 404
理学療法士　89, 402, 404
理学療法室　345
離婚　5
離乳食　389
リハビリテーション　257, 401, 402
リハビリテーション科　53
リハビリテーション科医　261
リハビリテーションセンター　345
リハビリテーションの説明　257
リビングウィル　253
流行性耳下腺炎　189, 198, 395, 400
流産　364
流動食　331
理容室　343
両親　6
両親学級　373
療法士　89
緑内障　59, 191
淋菌感染症　114, 125, 189
臨床検査技師　89
臨床検査室　344
臨床工学技士　90
臨床心理士　89
臨床治験室　345
リンパ節腫大　48
リンパ節生検　295

## れ

霊安室　345
冷感, 四肢の　86
冷蔵庫　350
裂傷　51
レントゲン　280
レントゲン室　239, 344

## ろ

老人病専門医　262
労働災害補償保険　423
老年内科　52
ローション　310
ロタウィルス　400
ロッカー　344
ロビー　344

## わ

悪い知らせの伝え方　249

## 頻度の表現

### 1. よく使う表現

| | |
|---|---|
| 毎時間 | every hour |
| 毎日 | every day |
| 6時間ごと | every six hours |
| 4時間に1回 | once every four hours |
| 1日おき | every other day |
| 3日に1回 | every three days |
| 1日〔週〕1回〔2／3回〕 | once〔twice / three times〕a day〔week〕 |
| | |
| 朝に | in the morning |
| 食前に | before meals |
| 食後に | after meals |
| 食間に | between meals |
| 就寝時に | at bedtime |
| 必要に応じて | when you need it |

### 2. 頻度を表わす副詞

"How often...?" と尋ねた場合，患者の表現には個人差があり，主観的要素が含まれるが，おおよその目安として頻度の高い順にあげると，

always → usually → often (frequently) → sometimes →
いつも　　たいてい　　　頻繁に　　　　　　　　時々

occasionally → rarely [seldom] → never
たまに　　　　　まれに　　　　　　一度もない